Anesthesiology: A Practical Approach

Anesthesiology: A Practical Approach

Edited by Dennis Hanks

hayle medical
New York

Hayle Medical,
750 Third Avenue, 9th Floor,
New York, NY 10017, USA

Visit us on the World Wide Web at:
www.haylemedical.com

ISBN: 978-1-63241-781-7

The publisher's policy is to use permanent paper from mills that operate a sustainable forestry policy. Furthermore, the publisher ensures that the text paper and cover boards used have met acceptable environmental accreditation standards.

Printed in China.

Cataloging-in-Publication Data

Anesthesiology : a practical approach / edited by Dennis Hanks.
p. cm.
Includes bibliographical references and index.
ISBN 978-1-63241-781-7
1. Anesthesiology. 2. Anesthesia. 3. Surgery. I. Hanks, Dennis.
RD81 .A54 2019
617.96--dc23

Table of Contents

Preface

This book has been a concerted effort by a group of academicians, researchers and scientists, who have contributed their research works for the realization of the book. This book has materialized in the wake of emerging advancements and innovations in this field. Therefore, the need of the hour was to compile all the required researches and disseminate the knowledge to a broad spectrum of people comprising of students, researchers and specialists of the field.

The medical study of anesthetics and the clinical application of these are under the domain of anesthesiology. A physician who is trained in this field is known as an anesthesiologist. Medications are either injected or inhaled to induce a loss of sensation in patients before performing procedures that can cause excruciating pain. Various invasive and non-invasive organ support techniques are required to control the vital functions of patients while they are under the effect of anesthesia. Active airway management, ultrasonography, echocardiography imaging and hemodynamic monitoring are crucial responsibilities of anesthesiologists. They are also responsible for the non-surgical management of pain through prescription of pain medicine and provision of care to patients in intensive care units through critical care medicine. This book aims to shed light on some of the unexplored aspects of anesthesiology and the recent researches in this field. While understanding the long-term perspectives of the topics, it makes an effort in highlighting their impact as a modern tool for the growth of the discipline. With state-of-the-art inputs by acclaimed experts of this field, this book targets students and professionals.

At the end of the preface, I would like to thank the authors for their brilliant chapters and the publisher for guiding us all-through the making of the book till its final stage. Also, I would like to thank my family for providing the support and encouragement throughout my academic career and research projects.

Editor

1

Ethanol locks for the prevention of catheter-related bloodstream infection: a meta-analysis of randomized control trials

Peng Zhang, Jun-Hao Lei, Xin-Jun Su* and Xing-Huan Wang*

Abstract

Background: Current evidence regarding the efficacy of ethanol locks in preventing catheter-related bloodstream infection (CRBI) is inconclusive.

Methods: Electronic databases, including PubMed, Web of Science, Embase, and the Cochrane Library (until April 2018),were systematically searched for relevant studies. Two reviewers independently screened the retrieved records and identified RCTs that met the inclusion criteria. Relevant data were extracted for pooled analyses using Review Manager 5.3 software. Subgroup analysis was performed according to the study quality, duration of the ethanol lock, disease type and CRBI definition. Eggs' method was applied to detect publication bias. Sensitivity analysis was conducted to check the stability of the meta-analysis results.

Results: Ten RCTs involving 2760 patients were included in the analysis. The overall pooled result indicated that ethanol locks significantly reduced the incidence of CRBI (RR 0.66, 95% CI 0.51–0.86). Subgroup analysis suggested that an ethanol lock significantly decreased the incidence of CRBI in patients with hematological diseases (RR 0.50, 95% CI 0.31–0.80). An ethanol lock significantly reduced the incidence of CRBI in a2-hour ethanol lock group (RR 0. 49, 95% CI 0.33–0.73). The meta-analysis showed that an ethanol lock significantly reduced the incidence of CRBI according to analysis of high-(RR 0.66, 95% CI 0.47–0.94) or low-(RR 0.66, 95% CI 0.46–0.95) quality studies. Meta-analysis of studies with a strict CRBI definition showed that an ethanol lock can significantly prevent CRBI (RR 0.61, 95% CI 0.42–0.89). The results of sensitivity analysis suggested that the pooled result was stable. Meta-analysis of adverse events showed that an ethanol lock did not increase the incidence of thrombosis (RR 1.05, 95% CI 0.51–2. 18) or mortality (RR 0.99, 95% CI 0.90–1.08) but did result in increased nausea (RR 1.54, 95% CI 1.01–2.35), dizziness (RR 4.21, 95% CI 2.40–7.39),elevated blushing rates (RR 3.27, 95% CI 2.05–5.22) and altered taste rates (RR 2.61, 95% CI 1.93–3.54).

Conclusions: An ethanol lock may play a role in the prevention of CRBI, especially in immunocompromised patients with hematological diseases.

Keywords: Catheter-related bloodstream infection, Ethanol lock, Meta-analysis

* Correspondence: 1919519046@qq.com; wangxinghuan@whu.edu.cn
Department of Urology, Zhongnan Hospital, Wuhan University, 169 Donghu load, Wuchang district, Wuhan 430071, Hubei, People's Republic of China

Background

Tunneled central venous catheters(CVCs) are widely used for long-term venous access to deliver blood and its products, chemotherapy and parenteral nutrition [1]. However, despite improved international guidelines on CVC placement and catheter care, the use of CVCs carries a high risk of developing catheter-related bloodstream infection (CRBI) [2]. Furthermore, CRBIs are related to increased healthcare costs, morbidity, hospitalization and death [3].

There are many ways to reduce CRBIs, including antimicrobial lock solutions, catheter care procedures, and agents that reduce nasal colonization of *Staphylococcus aureus*, and one meta-analysis showed that antimicrobial lock solutions significantly reduce the risk of CRBI [4]. Overall, ethanol locks are considered a promising lock solutions because they are inexpensive, universally available, and effective against a broad spectrum of bacteria and fungi [5]. Nevertheless, study results to date on ethanol locks are controversial.

For example, Bertrand Souweine et al. observed that a 2-min ethanol lock does not decrease the frequency of infection of dialysis catheters(DCs) in intensive care unit (ICU) patients [6]. A randomized pilot study showed that a 30% ethanol/4% sodium citrate appears to prevent CRBI and may improve catheter survival compared to heparin [7], and a randomized controlled multi-center trial showed that ethanol locks can prevent CRBI in pediatric oncology patients [8]. However, ethanol lock therapy has not been observed to affect patients after major heart surgery (MHS) [9].

Here, we present the results of a meta-analysis to investigate the association between ethanol locks and CRBI.

Methods

This study was performed according to the preferred reporting items of the systematic review and meta-analysis (PRISMA) guidelines.

Systematic search strategy

We conducted an electronic search of the PubMed (1966 to April2018), Embase (1974 to April2018), Science Citation Index (1974 to April 2018) and Cochrane (April 2018) databases for relevant studies on the efficacy of ethanol locks in preventing CRBI.

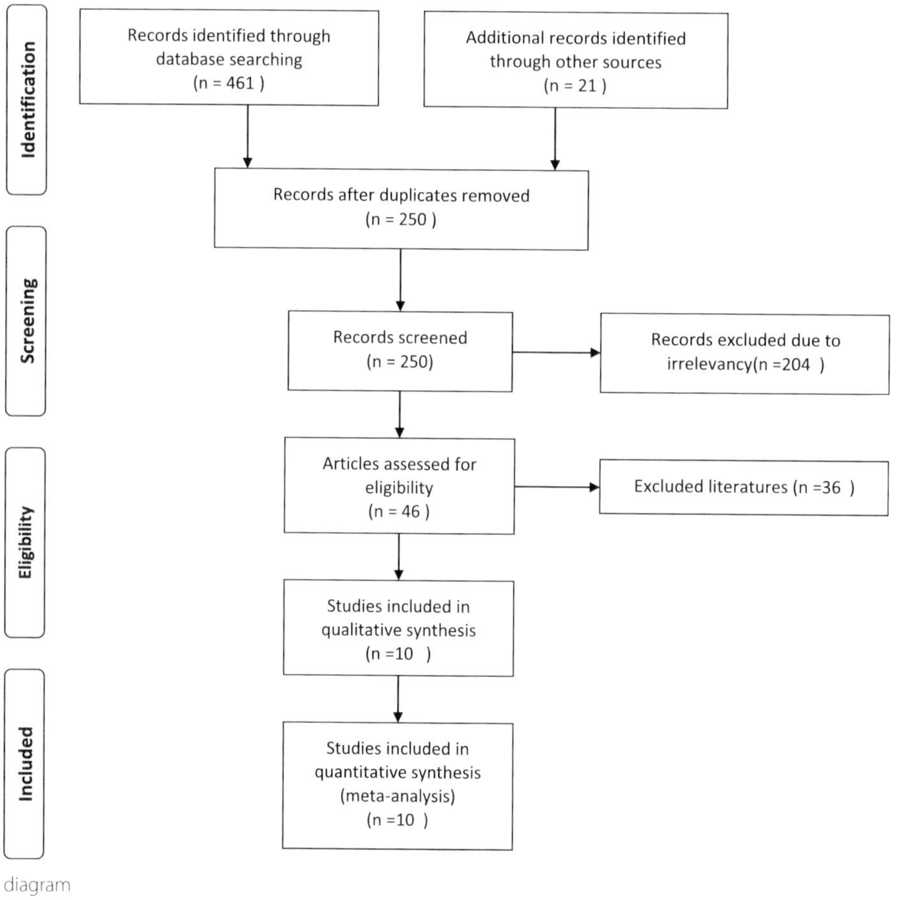

Fig. 1 PRISMA flow diagram

Table 1 Characteristics of included studies

NO.	Country	Sample size(T/C)	Gender(T/C, %)	Age(T/C)	Inclusion criteria	Exclusion criteria	Intervention	Control	Diagnosis of CRBSI	Catheter types	Follow up
Bradley R.S. 2017 [12]	USA	18/20	M(33/30)	49/52	Adult patients providing consent, non-medicare insur ance, or medicare in surance with a sup plementary insurance, anticipated duration on home parenteral nutrition(HPN) > 3 m not previously on HPN at Mayo Clinic or elsewhere, patients with single lumen, sili cone Hickman ® cath eters, and no known alcohol addiction	Failure to provide consent, medicare insurance without supplemental private insurance, patients with a catheter type other than a single lumen Hickman ®, patients who were anticipated to be on HPN for less than three months, pregnant patients, patients who have previously proven addiction and/or dependence to alcohol	3 ml 70% ethanol lock until next PN infusion	Heparin lock plus saline infusion	(1)Bacteremia or fungemia in a patient who had an intravascular device and > 1 positive blood culture result obtained from the peripheral vein; (2)Clinical manifestations of infection (e.g., fever, chills, and/or hypotension), and no apparent source for blood stream infection other than the central venous catheter.	Single lumen, silicone Hickman ® catheters	NA
Lavern M.V. 2016 [7]	Canada	20/19	M(60/47)	63/62.3	Eligible participants were 18 years of age or older with end-stage renal disease and planned vascular access with a catheter or current hemodialysis patients requiring exchange of an existing catheter	(1) they were critically ill in the ICU setting, (2) had acute kidney injury and were unlikely to require prolonged vascular access, (3) had a maturing or planned arteriovenous fistula/graft creation within 2 months, or (4) planned antibiotic treatment courses lasting longer than 4 weeks from the date of the new catheter insertion.	2.5 ml 30% ethanol/4% sodium citrate for a 6-month period	Heparin 1000 units/mL	Two or more positive blood cultures of the same organism (species, antibiogram) from any source (peripheral or intravascular device cultures) from a patient with clinical and microbiologic data suggesting no other source for the bacteremia except the intravascular device.	Inserted dual-lumen tunneled, cuffed catheters made of carbothane, an alcohol-resistant polymer with silicone extensions (Tal Palin drome, Tyco Health care Kendall/Covi dien, Mansfield, MA, USA)	If an outcome occurred, an additional 30 days for safety was added
Bertrand 2015 [6]	France	730/730	M(60.8/61.1)	65/66	Patients required insertion of DCs with an expected duration of use longer than 48 h in ICU	Ethanol intolerance and pregnancy	60% wt/wt EL locks for 2 min	0.9% saline lock	In patients with one or more blood cultures positive for coagulase-negative staphylococci, identity of pulse-field gel elec trophoresis patterns in the catheter tip and blood cultures was re quired for a diagnosis of CRBSI	A nontunneled, nonantimicrobial-impregnated double-lumen dialysis cathe ters (DC)	Until death or 48 h after ICU discharge
Reineke A 2015 [8]	Netherlands	153/154	M(58/56)	9.8/7.8	Paediatric oncology patients (1–18 years) with a newly inserted, tunnelled central venous catheters (CVC)	≤1 year at diagnosis, a primary immunological disorder, an ethanol allergy or a CVC inserted in a vessel	70% ethanol locks for 2 h	100 IU/ml heparin locks	At least one of the following criteria: (1) recognised pathogen cultured from ≥1 blood cultures, not	Tunnelled CVC(port-a-cath (PAC) or Broviac)	Time to CABSI or death due to CABSI, during a maximum

Table 1 Characteristics of included studies *(Continued)*

NO.	Country	Sample size(T/C)	Gender(T/C, %)	Age(T/C)	Inclusion criteria	Exclusion criteria	Intervention	Control	Diagnosis of CRBSI	Catheter types	Follow up
						with previously confirmed thrombosis			related to an infection at another site (2) Clinical manifestations of infection and a common skin microorganism (such as coagulase-negative staphylococci (CoNS), diphtheroids, Bacillus spp., or micrococci) cultured from ≥2 blood cultures drawn on separate occasions		follow-up period of six months
L.J. Worth 2014 [16]	Australia	42/43	M(28/24)	47.0/48.1	Patients with haematological malignancy or planned BMT were eligible for enrolment at time of insertion of a dual lumen, non-antibiotic-impregnated, tunnelled, cuffed, intravascular catheter (Hickman catheter) into subclavian or internal jugular veins, where the intended period of catheterization was 30 days.	NA	70% ethanol locks for 2 h	Heparinized saline	A positive blood culture with a recognized pathogen or common commensal, with confirmation of infection by isolation of the same organism following culture of catheter tip, or a differential time to positivity for centrally and peripherally drawn blood cultures of 2 h	A dual lumen, non-antibiotic-impregnated, tunnelled, cuffed, intravascular catheter (Hickman catheter)	Until a device-related bloodstream infection occurred, or planned study end-date
Sishir 2014 [15]	India	35/35	NA	NA	Hemodialysis population	NA	70% ethanol lock for 20 min	Heparin lock (1000 U/ml)	NA	Double lumen polyurethane hemodialysis cathete	NA
Mara 2014 [14]	Spain	113/87	M(55/54)	67.3/65.2	Recent MHS admission with Central Vascular Catheters (CVC) inserted >48 h; Age >18 years; No evidence or suspicion of CRBSI at enrolment: No signs of infection neither general nor at catheter site entrance	Allergy or intolerance to ethanol or chronic liver disease;Pregnancy	70% ethanollock for 2 h	Conventional catheter-care	Microbiologically proven CRBSI considered when the same microorganism was recovered from blood and a catheter tip within less than 8 days.	Conventionalcatheter	Enrolled patients were prospectively followed for the occurrence of CR-BSI until catheter withdrawal, hospital discharge or death
Jennifer K 2012 [13]	Australia	25/24	M(52/46)	52/64	Adults > 18 years, the presence of a tunnelled intravenous catheter and the ability to give informed consent	Pregnancy or breast feeding, religious or personal objection to the use of ethanol, intolerance of ethanol, and a history of an exit site, tunnel or blood stream	70% ethanol for 48 h	Thrice weekly standard heparin locks(Heparin sodium 5000 U/Ml)	(1)Positive blood cultures for the presence of bacteria with or without Clinical manifestations of infection	A tunnelled central venous catheter	NA

Table 1 Characteristics of included studies *(Continued)*

NO.	Country	Sample size(T/C)	Gender(T/C, %)	Age(T/C)	Inclusion criteria	Exclusion criteria	Intervention	Control	Diagnosis of CRBSI	Catheter types	Follow up
						infection associated with the current catheter.					
Lennert Solbbe 2010 [11]	Netherlands	226/222	M(57.5/56.3)	51.7/49.8	Eligible study-participants were all consecutive adult (age>17 years) hematology patients with a tunnelled silicone CVC, inserted in the preceding 72 h before study-entry	Patients with an alcohol-intolerance or concomitant treat ment with metronidazole	70% ethanol lock for 15 min per day	0.9% NaCl	A positive central or peripheral blood culture; For (coagulase-negative staphylococci) or other skin-colonizers, 2 blood cultures had to be posi tive when no peripheral cultures were available [19]	A tunnelled silicone CVC	NA
Sanders 2008 [10]	New Zealand	32/28	M(53/57)	52.4/47.2	An age >18 years or older and admission as an inpatient to receive intensive chemotherapy likely to produce neutropenia (<0.5 × 109 L) for the treatment of haematological disease, including haematopoietic stem cel transplantation.	Abnormal liver function tests or a history of alcohol abuse	70% ethanol for 2 h	Control	The culture of a recognized pathogen from one or more blood cultures, unrelated to infection at another site [18].	Identical dual lumen Hickman central venous catheters	The study period ended with either diagnosis of CABSI, removal or failure of catheter, discharge from hospital, death or end of study period after an arbitrary 30 days.

	Random sequence generation (selection bias)	Allocation concealment (selection bias)	Blinding of participants and personnel (performance bias)	Blinding of outcome assessment (detection bias)	Incomplete outcome data (attrition bias)	Selective reporting (reporting bias)	Other bias
Bertrand 2015	+	+	+	?	+	?	?
Bradley R.S. 2017	+	+	+	?	+	?	?
Jennifer K 2012	+	+	−	?	+	+	+
L.J. Worth 2014	?	?	?	?	−	+	?
Lavern M.V. 2016	+	+	−	?	+	+	?
Lennert Solbbe 2010	+	+	+	+	+	+	?
Mara 2014	?	?	?	?	−	+	?
Reineke A 2015	+	+	+	?	−	+	+
Sanders 2008	+	+	+	?	+	+	?
Sishir 2014	?	?	?	?	?	?	?

Fig. 2 Risk of bias assessment for the included RCTs

The two keywords used to search the above electronic databases were 'ethanol lock' and 'infection.' All reference sections of eligible studies were hand-reviewed for potential inclusion, and no limits on language were imposed.

Eligibility criteria

We included studies if they met the following criteria: (1) study participants were patients with indwelling central venous catheters,(2) the intervention group received ethanol locks and the control group heparin/NaCl locks, and (3) the studies were randomized controlled trials (RCTs).

Study selection and data extraction

Two reviewers independently screened and assessed titles and abstracts to confirm whether the inclusion criteria were met. Data, including study characteristics (title, publication time, and sample size), detailed information in the PICOS approach (participant, intervention, comparison, outcomes, and study design), and other characteristics, were extracted by two authors using standard data extraction forms. Where necessary, the authors of the original studies were contacted for missing information.

Methodological quality assessment

The Cochrane Collaboration tool for assessing the risk of bias was used to evaluate the methodological quality of each included RCT. There were seven items for assessing bias including random sequence generation (selection bias), allocation concealment (selection bias), blinding of participants and personnel (performance bias), blinding of outcome assessment (detection bias), incomplete outcome data (attrition bias), selective reporting (reporting bias) and other biases. Each item was categorized as a low risk of bias, an "unclear" (either lack of information or uncertainty about the potential for bias) risk of bias, or a high risk of bias under the guidelines in the Cochrane Handbook.

Data synthesis and analysis

The meta-analysis was performed using Review Manager 5.3 software based on PRISMA guidelines. Heterogeneity was assessed by examining the clinical characteristics of the included studies and by formal statistical $\chi^2$and I^2tests. For main outcomes (incidence of CRBI), Mantel-Haenszel estimates with a random-effects analytical model (due to the considered between-trial heterogeneity) were used to calculate relative risks (RRs) and their 95% confidence intervals (CIs). The funnel plot methods of Egger's test were used to assess publication bias. We performed subgroup analysis according to study quality, duration of the ethanol lock, disease type and CRBI definition. Sensitivity analysis was conducted to determine the stability of the meta-analysis results using Stata 12.0 software.

Results

Characteristics of the included studies

The initial results of databasesearchingproduced461 records and 10 studies [6–8, 10–16] that met the inclusion criteria and were ultimately included after screening and reviewing by the authors. The selection flowchart is shown in Fig. 1. Reasons for the exclusion of 36 studies in the literature screening process are presented in Additional file 1.

The characteristics of the 10 included trials are listed in Table 1. A total of 2760 patients were

Study or Subgroup	Ethanol lock Events	Ethanol lock Total	Control Events	Control Total	Weight	Risk Ratio M-H, Fixed, 95% CI
1.2.1 Hematopathy						
L.J. Worth 2014	9	42	16	43	13.6%	0.58 [0.29, 1.16]
Lennert Solbbe 2010	10	226	16	222	13.8%	0.61 [0.28, 1.32]
Sanders 2008	3	34	11	30	10.0%	0.24 [0.07, 0.78]
Subtotal (95% CI)		**302**		**295**	**37.4%**	**0.50 [0.31, 0.80]**
Total events	22		43			
Heterogeneity: Chi² = 1.91, df = 2 (P = 0.38); I² = 0%						
Test for overall effect: Z = 2.89 (P = 0.004)						
1.2.2 Hemodialysis patients						
Bertrand 2015	14	730	13	730	11.1%	1.08 [0.51, 2.28]
Jennifer K 2012	1	25	3	24	2.6%	0.32 [0.04, 2.87]
Lavern M.V. 2016	0	20	1	19	1.3%	0.32 [0.01, 7.35]
Sishir 2014	18	35	21	35	18.0%	0.86 [0.56, 1.31]
Subtotal (95% CI)		**810**		**808**	**33.1%**	**0.87 [0.59, 1.27]**
Total events	33		38			
Heterogeneity: Chi² = 1.51, df = 3 (P = 0.68); I² = 0%						
Test for overall effect: Z = 0.73 (P = 0.47)						
1.2.3 Paediatric oncology patients						
Reineke A 2015	16	153	29	154	24.8%	0.56 [0.31, 0.98]
Subtotal (95% CI)		**153**		**154**	**24.8%**	**0.56 [0.31, 0.98]**
Total events	16		29			
Heterogeneity: Not applicable						
Test for overall effect: Z = 2.03 (P = 0.04)						
1.2.4 Others						
Bradley R.S. 2017	4	18	1	20	0.8%	4.44 [0.55, 36.18]
Mara 2014	2	113	4	87	3.9%	0.38 [0.07, 2.05]
Subtotal (95% CI)		**131**		**107**	**4.7%**	**1.09 [0.36, 3.28]**
Total events	6		5			
Heterogeneity: Chi² = 3.21, df = 1 (P = 0.07); I² = 69%						
Test for overall effect: Z = 0.15 (P = 0.88)						
Total (95% CI)		**1396**		**1364**	**100.0%**	**0.66 [0.51, 0.86]**
Total events	77		115			
Heterogeneity: Chi² = 10.66, df = 9 (P = 0.30); I² = 16%						
Test for overall effect: Z = 3.15 (P = 0.002)						
Test for subgroup differences: Chi² = 4.37, df = 3 (P = 0.22), I² = 31.3%						

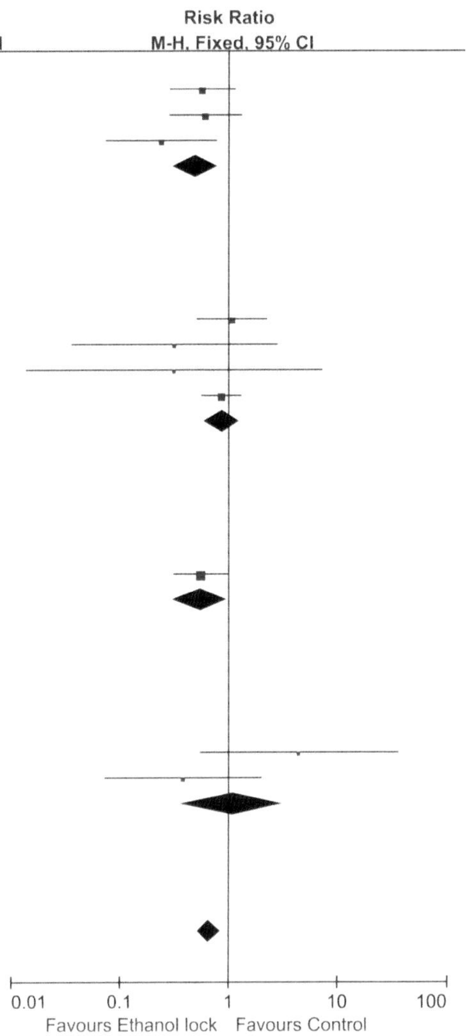

Fig. 3 Forest plot for subgroup analysis of the incidence of CRBI according to patients with different diseases (RR, relative risk; CI, confidence interval)

included in the meta-analysis, among whom1396received an intervention with ethanol locks. Three studies [10, 11, 16] included only patients with hematological diseases, and 4 included hemodialysis patient [6, 7, 13, 15]. Pediatric oncology patients were included only in one study [8], and the remaining two studies involved home parenteral nutrition patients [12] or those after major heart surgery [9].

Risk of bias

There were seven studies [6–8, 10–13] that were considered to have a low risk of bias for "Random sequence generation" and "Allocation concealment." "Blinding of participants and personnel" was judged to have a low risk of bias in five studies [6, 8, 10–12] and a high risk in two studies [7, 13]. There was only one study that was deemed to have a low risk of bias for the item "Blinding of outcome assessment" [11]. For "Incomplete outcome data", six studies had a low risk of bias [6, 7, 10–13] and three a high risk [8, 14, 16]. There were seven studies [7, 8, 10, 11, 13, 14, 16] that could be judged as having a low risk of bias in the item "selective reporting." The risk of bias assessment results are shown in Fig. 2.

CRBI

Definitions of CRBI among the included studies are shown in the Table 1, and a positive blood culture was necessary to diagnose CRBI [17, 18]. All included studies reported the incidence of CRBI. The total pooled results showed that there was a significant difference between ethanol locks and conventional catheter-care (RR 0.66, 95% CI 0.51 to 0.86), without

Table 2 the pathogens involved in the infections

NO.	Ethanol lock(n)	Control(n)
Bradley R.S. 2017 [12]	Candida species(2); Staphylococcus species(1); Escherichia coli plus Klebsiella species plus Pseudomonas(1).	Unidentified gram positive cocci
Lavern M.V. 2016 [7]	NA	Klebsiella Pneumonia
Bertrand 2015 [6]	Staphylococcus epidermidis(20) Staphylococcus aureus(2) Enterococcus species (0) Other coagulase negative Staphylococci(31) Other Gram-positive (5) Escherichia coli (2) Proteus species (0) Pseudomonas aeruginosa (10) Enterobacterspecies (2) Other Gram-negative (2) Fungi (5) Polymicrobial(20)	Staphylococcus epidermidis(9) Staphylococcus aureus(0) Enterococcus species (1) Other coagulase negative Staphylococci(27) Other Gram-positive (6) Escherichia coli (1) Proteus species (2) Pseudomonas aeruginosa (9) Enterobacterspecies (0) Other Gram-negative (3) Fungi (3) Polymicrobial(17)
Reineke A 2015 [8]	Staphylococcus epidermidis(2) Other coagulase-negative Staphylococc(4) Staphylococcus aureus(0) Streptococcus parasanguis(1) Other alpha-haemolytic streptococci (1) Enterococcus faecalis(0) Bacillus sp.(0) Streptomyces sp.(0) Escherichia coli(1) Citrobacter freundii(1) Brevundimonas vesicularis(1) Gram-negative rod (1) Polymicrobial(3) Candida sp.(1)	Staphylococcus epidermidis(1) Other coagulase-negative Staphylococc(8) Staphylococcus aureus(2) Streptococcus parasanguis(0) Other alpha-haemolytic streptococci (0) Enterococcus faecalis(1) Bacillus sp.(2) Streptomyces sp.(1) Escherichia coli(3) Citrobacter freundii(0) Brevundimonas vesicularis(0) Gram-negative rod (0) Polymicrobial(0) Candida sp.(2)
L.J. Worth 2014 [16]	Coagulase-negative Staphylococcus spp. (3), Staphylococcus aureus (1), Listeria monocytogenes (1), Klebsiella pneumoniae (2), Escherichia coli (1), Pseudomonas aeruginosa (1), E. coli (2)and C. glabrata (1).	Coagulase-negative Staphylococcus spp. (7), Staphylococcus aureus (1), Enterococcus faecium (1), Klebsiella pneumoniae (2), Escherichia coli (1), Pseudomonas aeruginosa (1), Enterobacter cloacae(1), E. coli and E. faecium (1), and Candida parapsilosis (1).
Sishir 2014 [15]	NA	NA
Mara 2014 [14]	Gram positive cocci(0) Enterobacteriaceae(2) Gram negative non-fermenting rods(0) Fungi(0)	Gram positive cocci(1) Enterobacteriaceae(2) Gram negative non-fermenting rods(1) Fungi(0)
Jennifer K 2012 [13]	Staphylococcus aureus(1)	Staphylococcus aureus(1) Enterobacter cloacae(1) Staphylococcus hominis (1)
Lennert Solbbe 2010 [11]	n = episodes Coagulase-negative staphylococci.(49) Other skin colonizers(2) Staphylococcus aureus(2) Other gram-positive cocci(12) Gram-negatives(4) Polymicrobial(20) Yeasts(2)	n = episodes Coagulase-negative staphylococci.(57) Other skin colonizers(2) Staphylococcus aureus(3) Other gram-positive cocci(10) Gram-negatives(5) Polymicrobial(13) Yeasts(1)
Sanders 2008 [10]	n = episodes A-haemolytic Streptococcus(1) Streptococcus group B (agalactiae)(0), S. epidermidis(0), Staphylococcus aureus(0), Stomatococcus rothia mucilaginosa(1), Escherichia coli(1), Pseudomonas aeruginosa(0), Klebsiella pneumoniae(0), non-speciated Gram-negative bacilli(0).	n = episodes A-haemolytic Streptococcus(1) Streptococcus group B (agalactiae)(1), S. epidermidis(3), Staphylococcus aureus(1), Stomatococcus rothia mucilaginosa(0), Escherichia coli(4), Pseudomonas aeruginosa(1), Klebsiella pneumoniae(1), non-speciated Gram-negative bacilli(1).

significant heterogeneity (I^2 = 16%, Fig. 3). The pathogens involved in the reported infections are shown in Table 2.

Subgroup analysis showed that an ethanol lock can reduce the incidence of CRBI in patients with hematological diseases (RR 0.50, 95% CI 0.31 to 0.80, I^2 = 0%, Fig. 3). There was no significant difference between ethanol lock and conventional catheter care groups (RR 0.87, 95% CI 0.59 to 1.27) among hemodialysis patients, without significant heterogeneity (I^2 = 0%, Fig. 3). In addition, an ethanol lock was more effective than traditional controls at preventing CRBI in pediatric oncology patients (RR 0.56, 95% CI 0.31 to 0.98, Fig. 3). Meta-analysis of high-quality studies (random sequence generation, allocation concealment and blinding of participants and personnel in the study can be evaluated as low risk) showed that an ethanol lock significantly reduced CRBI in patients with central venous catheters (RR 0.66, 95% CI 0.47to 0.94),and meta-analysis of low-quality studies also suggested a significant difference in the incidence of CRBI between ethanol lock and control groups (RR 0.66, 95% CI 0.46to 0.95) (Fig. 4). Subgroup analysis indicated that there was a significant difference between 2-h ethanol lock and conventional catheter care groups (RR 0.49 95% CI 0.33 to 0.73), without significant heterogeneity (I^2 = 0%, Fig. 5). There was no significant difference between less than 20-min ethanol lock and conventional catheter care groups (RR 0.84, 95% CI 0.59 to 1.19), again without significant heterogeneity (I^2 = 0%, Fig. 5), or48-hour ethanol lock and conventional catheter care groups (RR 1.29, 95% CI 0.37 to 4.47).Meta-analysis of studies with a strict CRBI definition revealed that an ethanol lock can significantly prevent CRBI (RR 0.61, 95% CI 0.42–0.89),though pooled analysis of studies with a less strict CRBI definition suggested no significant change in the incidence of CRBI between ethanol lock and control lock groups (RR 0.65, 95% CI 0.39–1.07) (Fig. 6).

Sensitivity analysis results showed that the results were relatively consistent (Fig. 7), and no obvious publication bias was detected, as based on Eggers' funnel plots (Fig. 8).

Adverse events

The results of meta-analysis involving adverse events are depicted in Fig. 7. An ethanol lock did not significantly increase the incidence of a thrombus (RR 1.05, 95% CI 0.51 to 2.18) or mortality (RR 0.99, 95% CI 0.90 to 1.08) but did increase nausea (RR 1.54, 95% CI 1.01 to 2.35), dizziness (RR 4.21, 95% CI 2.40 to 7.39), and blushing (RR 3.27, 95% CI 2.05 to 5.22) and altered taste (RR 2.61, 95% CI 1.93 to 3.54) (Fig. 9).

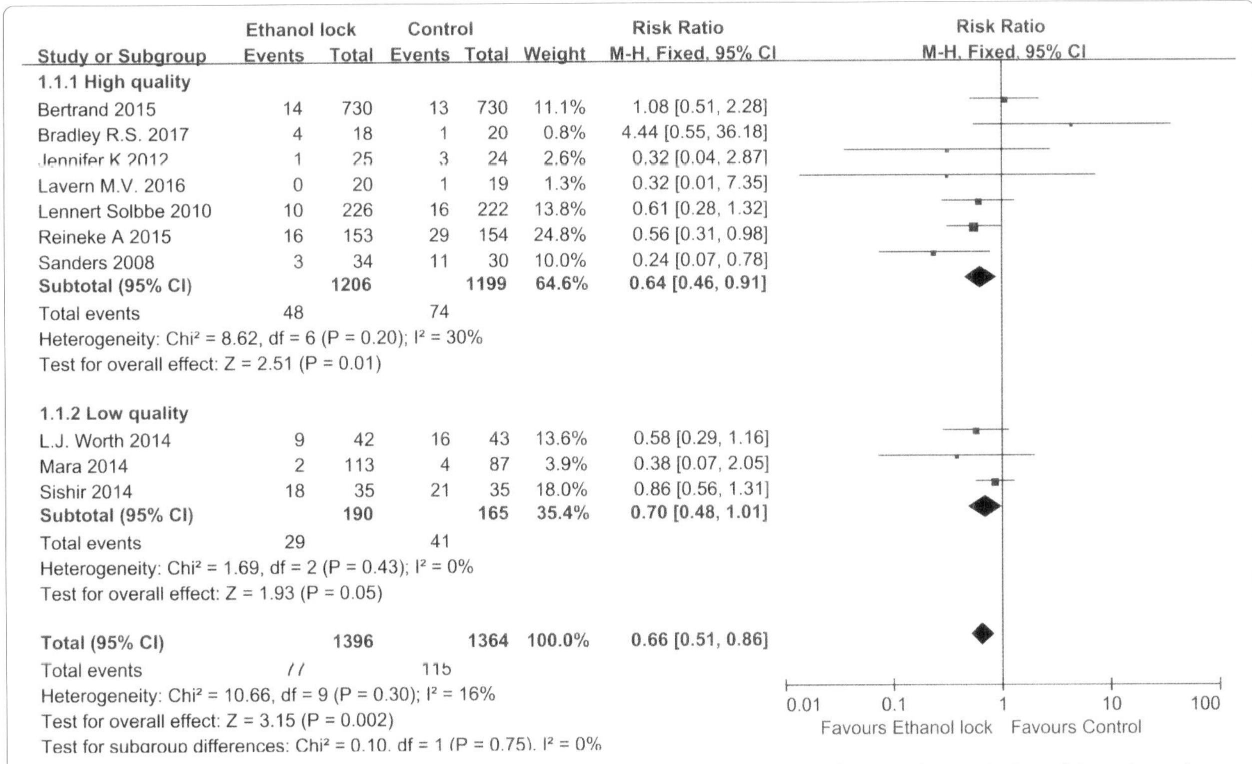

Fig. 4 Forest plot for subgroup analysis of the incidence of CRBI according to different study quality (RR, relative risk; CI, confidence interval)

Study or Subgroup	Ethanol lock Events	Ethanol lock Total	Control Events	Control Total	Weight	Risk Ratio M-H, Fixed, 95% CI
1.9.1 <20min						
Bertrand 2015	14	730	13	730	11.1%	1.08 [0.51, 2.28]
Lennert Solbbe 2010	10	226	16	222	13.8%	0.61 [0.28, 1.32]
Sishir 2014	18	35	21	35	18.0%	0.86 [0.56, 1.31]
Subtotal (95% CI)		**991**		**987**	**43.0%**	**0.84 [0.59, 1.19]**
Total events	42		50			
Heterogeneity: Chi² = 1.07, df = 2 (P = 0.58); I² = 0%						
Test for overall effect: Z = 0.99 (P = 0.32)						
1.9.2 2 hours						
L.J. Worth 2014	9	42	16	43	13.6%	0.58 [0.29, 1.16]
Mara 2014	2	113	4	87	3.9%	0.38 [0.07, 2.05]
Reineke A 2015	16	153	29	154	24.8%	0.56 [0.31, 0.98]
Sanders 2008	3	34	11	30	10.0%	0.24 [0.07, 0.78]
Subtotal (95% CI)		**342**		**314**	**52.2%**	**0.49 [0.33, 0.73]**
Total events	30		60			
Heterogeneity: Chi² = 1.88, df = 3 (P = 0.60); I² = 0%						
Test for overall effect: Z = 3.53 (P = 0.0004)						
1.9.3 48 hours						
Bradley R.S. 2017	4	18	1	20	0.8%	4.44 [0.55, 36.18]
Jennifer K 2012	1	25	3	24	2.6%	0.32 [0.04, 2.87]
Subtotal (95% CI)		**43**		**44**	**3.4%**	**1.29 [0.37, 4.47]**
Total events	5		4			
Heterogeneity: Chi² = 2.89, df = 1 (P = 0.09); I² = 65%						
Test for overall effect: Z = 0.41 (P = 0.68)						
1.9.4 6 months						
Lavern M.V. 2016	0	20	1	19	1.3%	0.32 [0.01, 7.35]
Subtotal (95% CI)		**20**		**19**	**1.3%**	**0.32 [0.01, 7.35]**
Total events	0		1			
Heterogeneity: Not applicable						
Test for overall effect: Z = 0.72 (P = 0.47)						
Total (95% CI)		**1396**		**1364**	**100.0%**	**0.66 [0.51, 0.86]**
Total events	77		115			
Heterogeneity: Chi² = 10.66, df = 9 (P = 0.30); I² = 16%						
Test for overall effect: Z = 3.15 (P = 0.002)						
Test for subgroup differences: Chi² = 5.24, df = 3 (P = 0.15), I² = 42.8%						

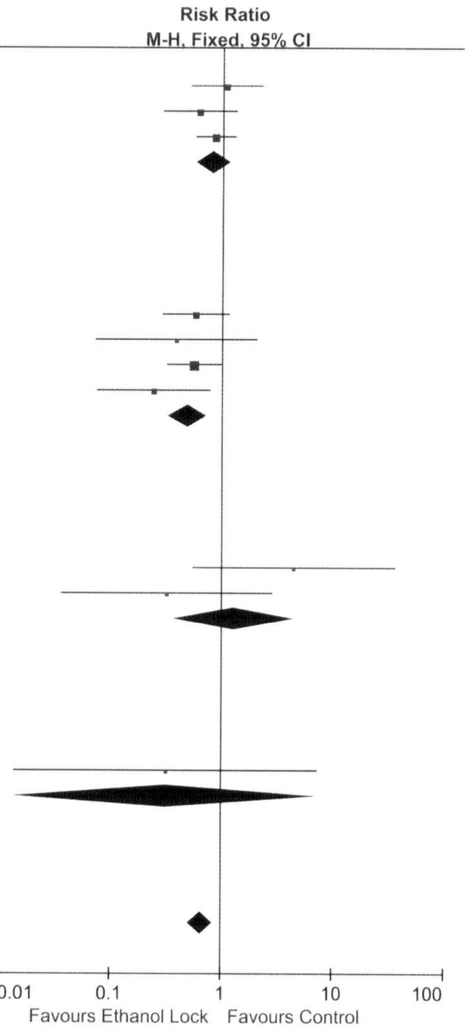

Fig. 5 Forest plot for subgroup analysis of the incidence of CRBI according to different ethanol lock duration (RR, relative risk; CI, confidence interval)

Discussion

Our meta-analysis first identified the efficacy of ethanol locks in preventing CRBIs. We found that ethanol locks significantly reduced the incidence of CRBI (RR 0.66, 95% CI 0.51–0.86). Subgroup analysis suggested that an ethanol lock significantly decreased CRBI incidence in patients with hematological diseases (RR 0.50, 95% CI 0.31–0.80), and a meta-analysis that only included high-quality studies showed that an ethanol lock significantly reduced CRBI incidence (RR 0.64, 95% CI 0.46–0.91). A 2-h ethanol lock diminished the frequency of CRBI, but a shorter (less than 20 min) ethanol lock did not decrease infection risk. Additionally, a meta-analysis of studies with strict CRBI definitions showed that an ethanol lock can significantly prevent a CRBI. Although an ethanol lock did not significantly increase thrombus and mortality rates, it did increase certain adverse reactions, such as nausea, dizziness, blushing and altered taste, in patients.

Tunneled CVCs are used for long-term venous access to deliver blood and blood products, chemotherapy and parenteral nutrition. The prevalence of CRBI is high in patients with indwelling CVCs, which also leads to a severe result [19], and internal colonization in long-term tunneled CVCs more frequently contributes to bacteremia [20, 21]. Many methods have been employed to prevent catheter-related sepsis, including the use of cutaneous antisepsis at the time of insertion, catheter tunneling, intraluminal antibiotic locks, antiseptic hubs and anti-microbial coating of catheters [22, 23]. However, these methods may fail to decrease the risk of infection and may instead increase the risk of hypersensitivity and development of anti-microbial resistance. Ethanol-based catheter locks may provide a

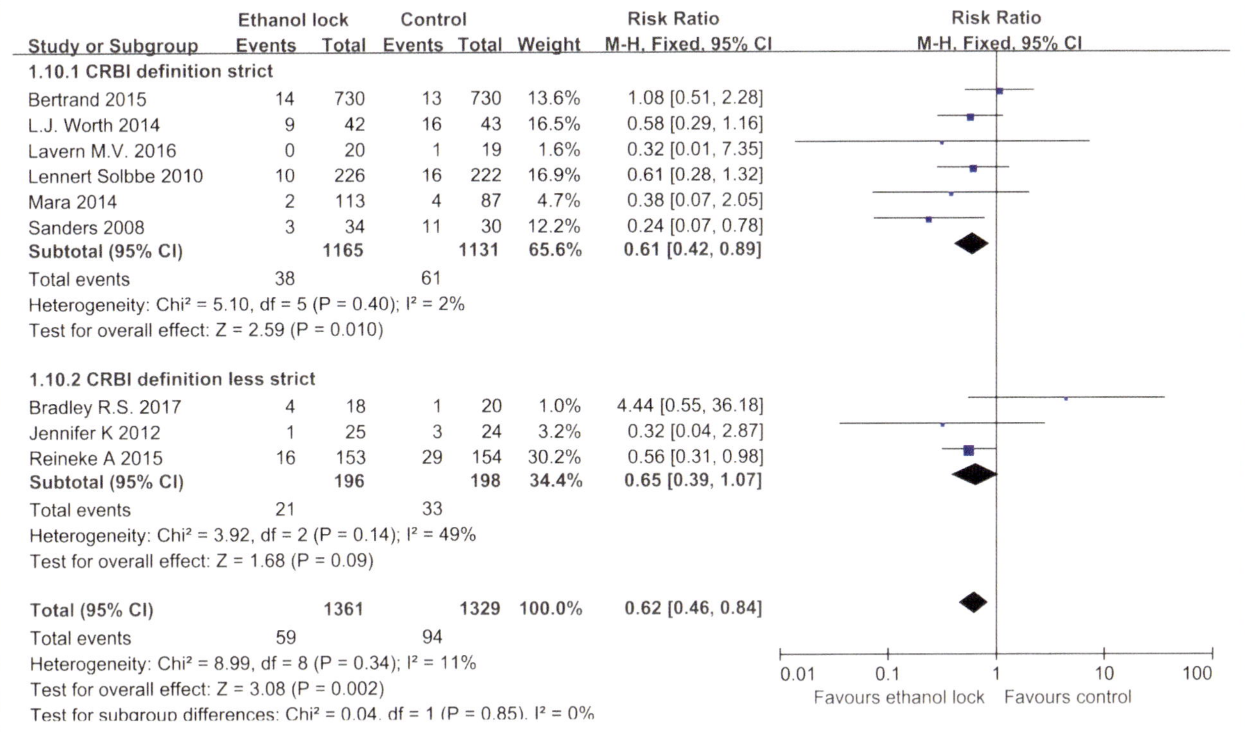

Fig. 6 Forest plot for subgroup analysis of the incidence of CRBI according to CRBI definition (RR, relative risk; CI, confidence interval)

better alternative because ethanol is a widely used antiseptic with no known acquired resistance [24]. A meta-analysis of observational studies found that ethanol locks are effective alternatives to heparin locks for preventing CRBI in pediatric patients with intestinal failure [25], with the ethanol lock dwell time ranging from more than 2 h per day to 4 h 3 days per week.

To the best of our knowledge, this report describes the first meta-analysis of RCTs to investigate the efficacy of ethanol locks in the prevention of CRBI. Ten RCTs were included in our meta-analysis, and the high quality of the included studies enhances current evidence. Moreover, we performed subgroup analysis based on differences in study quality, duration of the ethanol lock and disease type.

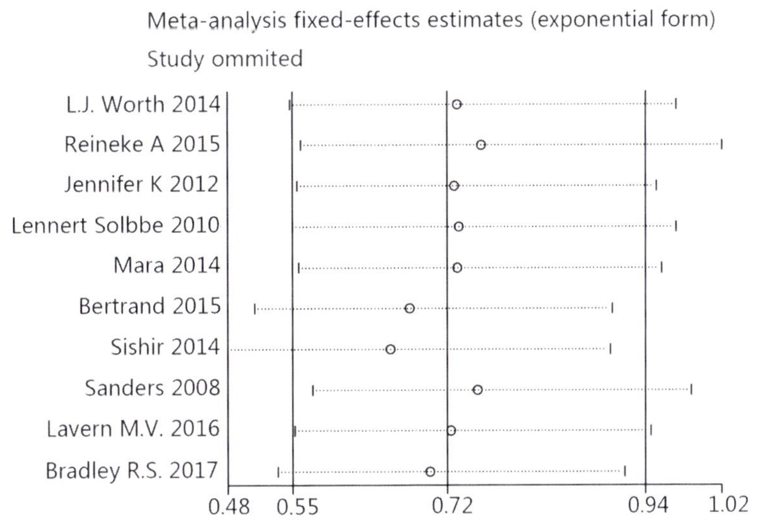

Fig. 7 Sensitivity analysis of CRBI results

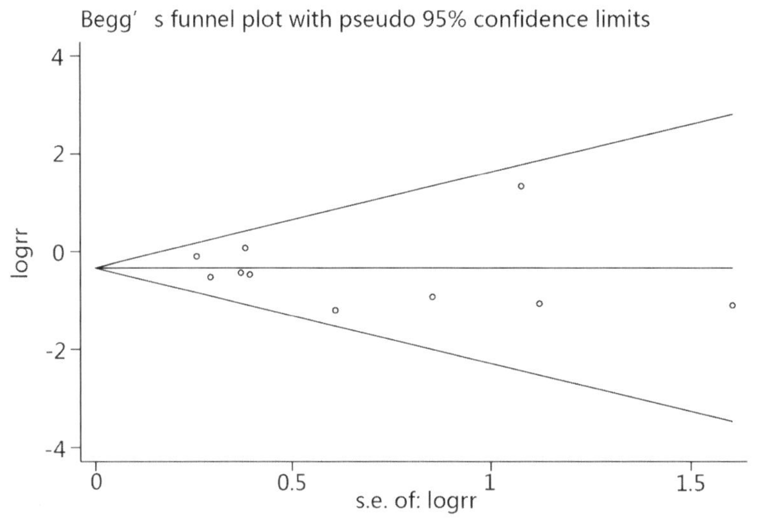

Fig. 8 Begg's funnel plot

Three studies reported the incidence of CRBI in patients with hematological diseases whose immune system was suppressed, and pooled analysis of these three studies suggested that an ethanol lock significantly reduces CRBI in immunosuppressed patients. Despite no significant difference according to the subgroup analysis in CRBI in hemodialysis patients, immune status or homeostasis may have an effect on the incidence of CRBI with an ethanol lock, which can result in bias among studies. In addition, to exclude bias by differences in study quality, subgroup analysis of relative high-quality or low-quality studies was performed, and the results suggested that an ethanol lock can significantly reduce CRBI risk. However, our definition of high-quality study was different from the Cochran high-quality trial definition; the latter requires all seven domains of the risk of bias assessment tool to be at "low risk of bias". Consequently, our subgroup analysis results regarding study quality are not very accurate. More high-quality studies that meet the Cochran definition are needed.

Three studies reported that the CVCs were locked with ethanol for 2 min, 15 min, and 20 min. The incidences of CRBI in these studies were determined by pooled analysis, though the short time frame for the ethanol lock did not effectively prevent CRBIs. In addition, the follow-up times were only 48 h, or shorter in the study by Bertrand et al., who used a 2-min ethanol lock. In combination with the low incidence of CRBI in that study, this situation might have contributed to the low efficiency in calculating a difference. In the remaining two studies, ethanol locks exhibited a tendency to prevent CRBIs, though without statistical significance. Interestingly, our findings showed that a 2-h ethanol lock (2-h duration of the lock) significantly decreased the frequency of CRBI. The preferable baseline similarity in the included four studies with a 2-h ethanol lock also enhanced the reliability of our meta-analysis results. Raadet al. found that prolonged exposure to lock solutions containing 25% ethanol in ethylenediaminetetraacetic acid (EDTA) can effectively enhance antibacterial activity in the silicone disk biofilm colonization model [26]. We did not find that a 48-h or 6-month lock can effectively prevent CRBI in our meta-analysis, and this may be due to their smaller size.

The strict definition of CRBI is such that clinical symptoms are not included and only blood culture results are used. Interestingly, meta-analysis of the studies with a strict CRBI definition showed that an ethanol lock can significantly prevent CRBI; however, this was not the result of pooled analysis of studies with a less strict CRBI definition. This finding may be the reason why a less strict CRBI definition reduced the sample weight. Because there was one study that included pediatric patients, the subgroup analysis on age was achieved by sensitivity analysis. Sensitivity analysis showed the results of pooled analysis were relatively stable. Statistical significance was lost when the trial by Reineke et al. was removed, which was due to the large sample size (307) of the study, resulting in its larger weight in the pooled result. It is noteworthy that an ethanol lock did not reduce the incidence of mortality, but there was a notable lack of mortality data in most of the trials. No obvious publication bias was detected, enhancing the value of the meta-analysis results. In addition, based on data of the pathogens involved in the infections, we determined that *Staphylococcus* has an important role as a cause of CRBI.

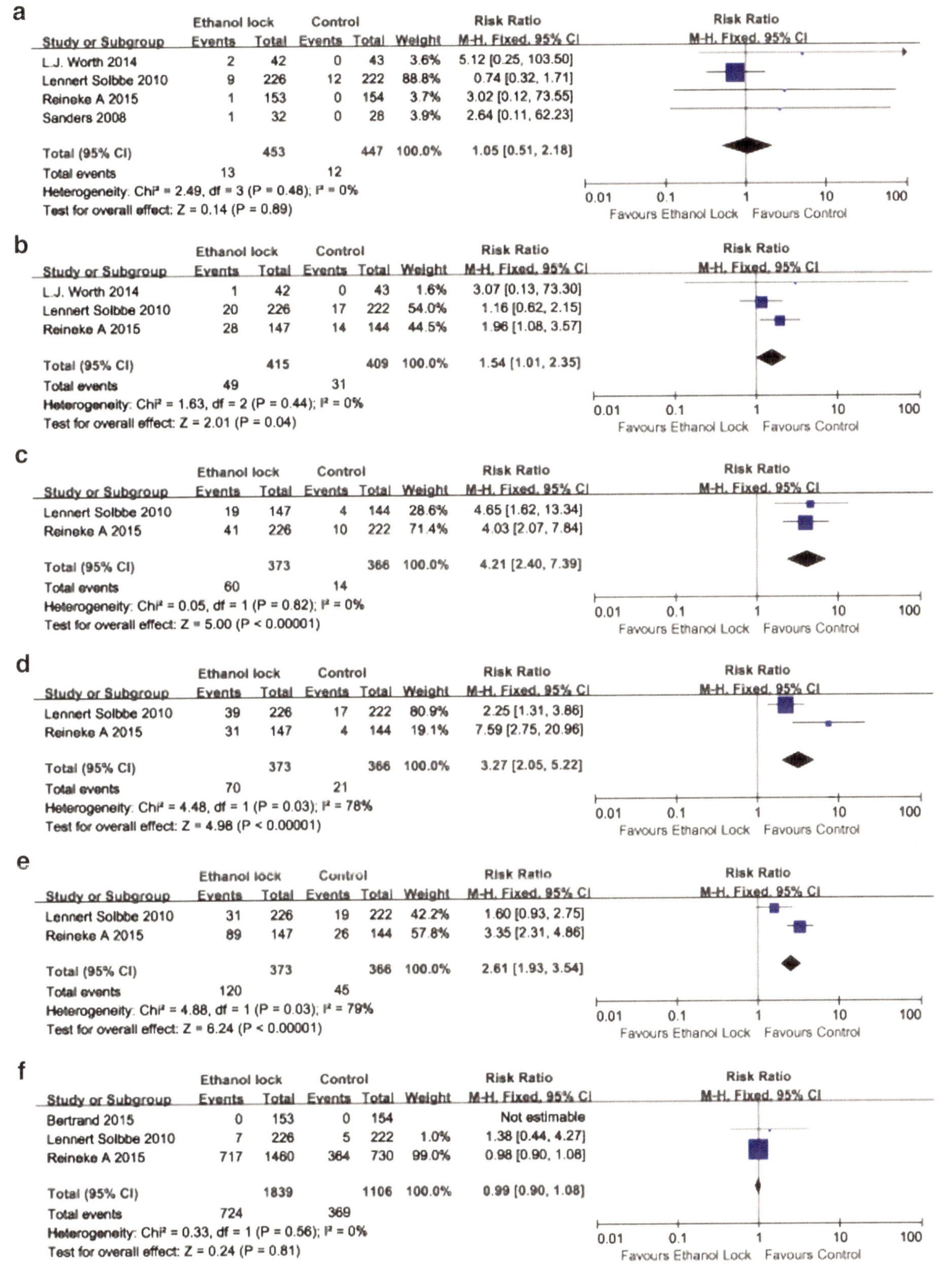

Fig. 9 Forest plot for adverse events including thrombus (**a**), nausea (**b**), dizziness (**c**), blushing (**d**), altered taste (**e**) and mortality (**f**)

There were also several limitations to our meta-analysis. First, we included only the abstract of studies for which we could not find the full text. Second, although a significant difference was detected in CRBI between ethanol lock and control lock groups according to subgroup analysis, the analyzable number of studies was low, which can result in bias risk. Third, very small differences in catheter type, such as dialysis catheter, and inserting catheters for parenteral nutrition may also lead to bias risk. Fourth, we did not find a significant difference in the incidence of CRBI between ethanol locks and control locks in hemodialysis patients, which was according to meta-analysis results of four studies, and the incidence of CRBI can be influenced by disturbed homeostasis. Sixth, the inclusion of the pediatric population of one study with a large sample might represent a small bias (adult and pediatric populations are different). Finally, patients with an ethanol lock may have certain adverse reactions, such as nausea, dizziness, blushing and altered taste, which might becaused by the ethanol lock solution entering into the bloodstream during catheter use.

Conclusions

Ethanol locks may play a role in preventing CRBI, though the strength of evidence is limited by the number of studies in the analysis.

Abbreviations

CI: Confidence interval; CRBI: Catheter-related bloodstream infection; CVC: Central venous catheters; DCs: Dialysis catheters; MHS: Major Heart Surgery; PRISMA: Preferred reporting items of the systematic review and meta-analyses; RCTs: Randomized controlled trials; RR: Relative risk

Authors' contributions

PZ and JH-L participated in the project development, literature search, statistical analysis, and manuscript writing; XJ-S and XH-W did the project development. All authors read and approved the final manuscript.

Competing interests

The authors declare that they have no competing interests.

References

1. Eggimann P. Prevention of intravascular catheter infection. Curr Opin Infect Dis. 2007;20(4):360–9.
2. Worth LJ, McLaws ML. Is it possible to achieve a target of zero central line associated bloodstream infections? Curr Opin Infect Dis. 2012;25(6):650–7.
3. Vassallo M, Dunais B, Roger PM. Antimicrobial lock therapy in central-line associated bloodstream infections: a systematic review. Infection. 2015;43(4): 389–98.
4. Labriola L, Crott R, Jadoul M. Preventing haemodialysis catheter-related bacteraemia with an antimicrobial lock solution: a meta-analysis of prospective randomized trials. Nephrol Dial Transplant. 2008;23(5):1666–72.
5. Tan M, Lau J, Guglielmo BJ. Ethanol locks in the prevention and treatment of catheter-elated bloodstream infections. Ann Pharmacother. 2014;48(5): 607–15.
6. Souweine B, Lautrette A, Gruson D, Canet E, Klouche K, Argaud L, Bohe J, Garrouste-Orgeas M, Mariat C, Vincent F, et al. Ethanol lock and risk of hemodialysis catheter infection in critically ill patients. A randomized controlled trial. Am J Respir Crit Care Med. 2015;191(9):1024–32.
7. Vercaigne LM, Allan DR, Armstrong SW, Zacharias JM, Miller LM. An ethanol/ sodium citrate locking solution compared to heparin to prevent hemodialysis catheter-related infections: a randomized pilot study. J Vasc Access. 2016;17(1):55–62.
8. Schoot RA, van Ommen CH, Stijnen T, Tissing WJ, Michiels E, Abbink FC, Raphael MF, Heij HA, Lieverst JA, Spanjaard L, et al. Prevention of central venous catheter-associated bloodstream infections in paediatric oncology patients using 70% ethanol locks: a randomised controlled multi-Centre trial. Eur J Cancer. 2015;51(14):2031–8.
9. Hannan MM, O'Sullivan KE, Higgins AM, Murphy AM, McCarthy J, Ryan E, Hurley JP. The Combined Impact of Surgical Team Education and Chlorhexidine 2% Alcohol on the Reduction of Surgical Site Infection following Cardiac Surgery. Surgical Infections. 2015;16(6):799–805.
10. Sanders J, Pithie A, Ganly P, Surgenor L, Wilson R, Merriman E, Loudon G, Judkins R, Chambers S. A prospective double-blind randomized trial comparing intraluminal ethanol with heparinized saline for the prevention of catheter-associated bloodstream infection in immunosuppressed haematology patients. J Antimicrob Chemother. 2008;62(4):809–15.
11. Slobbe L, Doorduijn JK, Lugtenburg PJ, Barzouhi AE, Boersma E, van Leeuwen WB, Rijnders BJA. Prevention of catheter-related bacteremia with a daily ethanol lock in patients with tunnelled catheters: a randomized, placebo-controlled trial. PLoS One. 2010;5(5)
12. Salonen BR, Bonnes SL, Vallumsetla N, Varayil JE, Mundi MS, Hurt RT. A prospective double blind randomized controlled study on the use of ethanol locks in HPN patients. Clin Nutr. 2017;37(4):1181–85.
13. Broom JK, Krishnasamy R, Hawley CM, Playford EG, Johnson DW. A randomised controlled trial of heparin versus EthAnol lock THerapY for the prevention of catheter associated infecTion in Haemodialysis patients–the HEALTHY-CATH trial. BMC Nephrol. 2012;13:146.
14. Perez-Granda MJ, Barrio JM, Munoz P, Hortal J, Rincon C, Rabadan PM, Pernia MS, Bouza E. Ethanol lock therapy (E-lock) in the prevention of catheter-related bloodstream infections (CR-BSI) after major heart surgery (MHS): a randomized clinical trial. PLoS One. 2014;9(3):e91838.
15. Sishir G, Bhupeshkumar K, Umapati H, Kalpesh G, Mohan R. To study the efficacy of intraluminal 70% ethanol vs heparin lock prior to hemodialysis in prevention of infections in non-tunneled hemodialysis catheters: a randomised study. Nephrology. 2014;19:181–2.
16. Worth LJ, Slavin MA, Heath S, Szer J, Grigg AP. Ethanol versus heparin locks for the prevention of central venous catheter-associated bloodstream infections: a randomized trial in adult haematology patients with Hickman devices. J Hosp Infect. 2014;88(1):48–51.
17. O'Grady NP, Alexander M, Dellinger EP, Gerberding JL, Heard SO, Maki DG, Masur H, RD MC, Mermel LA, Pearson ML, et al. Guidelines for the prevention of intravascular catheter-related infections. The hospital infection control practices advisory committee, Center for Disease Control and Prevention, U.S. Pediatrics. 2002;110(5):e51.
18. Mermel LA, Allon M, Bouza E, Craven DE, Flynn P, O'Grady NP, Raad II, Rijnders BJ, Sherertz RJ, Warren DK. Clinical practice guidelines for the diagnosis and management of intravascular catheter-related infection: 2009

update by the Infectious Diseases Society of America. Clin Infect Dis. 2009; 49:1):1–45.
19. Hajjej Z, Nasri M, Sellami W, Gharsallah H, Labben I, Ferjani M. Incidence, risk factors and microbiology of central vascular catheter-related bloodstream infection in an intensive care unit. J Infect Chemother. 2014;20(3–4):163–8.
20. Buchman AL, Spapperi J, Leopold P. A new central venous catheter cap: decreased microbial growth and risk for catheter-related bloodstream infection. J Vasc Access. 2009;10(1):11–21.
21. Decicco M, Chiaradia V, Veronesi A, Santini G, Panarello G, Fracasso A, Testa V, Tesio F. Source and route of microbial colonization of parenteral-nutrition catheters. Lancet. 1989;2(8674):1258–61.
22. Sawyer M, Weeks K, Goeschel CA, Thompson DA, Berenholtz SM, Marsteller JA, Lubomski LH, Cosgrove SE, Winters BD, Murphy DJ, et al. Using evidence, rigorous measurement, and collaboration to eliminate central catheter-associated bloodstream infections. Crit Care Med. 2010;38(8):S292–8.
23. Crnich CJ, Maki DG. The promise of novel technology for the prevention of intravascular device-related bloodstream infection. II. Long-term devices. Clin Infect Dis. 2002;34(10):1362–8.
24. Metcalf SCL, Chambers ST, Pithie AD. Use of ethanol locks to prevent recurrent central line sepsis. J Infect. 2004;49(1):20–2.
25. Oliveira C, Nasr A, Brindle M, Wales PW. Ethanol locks to prevent catheter-related bloodstream infections in parenteral nutrition: a meta-analysis. Pediatrics. 2012;129(2):318–29.
26. Raad I, Hanna H, Dvorak T, Chaiban G, Hachem R. Optimal antimicrobial catheter lock solution, using different combinations of minocycline, EDTA, and 25-percent ethanol, rapidly eradicates organisms embedded in biofilm. Antimicrob Agents Chemother. 2007;51(1):78–83.

2

Comparison of upper airway patency in patients with mild obstructive sleep apnea during dexmedetomidine or propofol sedation: a prospective, randomized, controlled trial

Hyun-Jung Shin[1], Eun-Young Kim[2], Jung-Won Hwang[1], Sang-Hwan Do[1] and Hyo-Seok Na[1*]

Abstract

Background: In addition to propofol, dexmedetomidine is a suitable alternative for intraoperative sedation in procedures requiring regional anesthesia. To date, however, little is known about the influences of each drug on upper airway patency. Accordingly, the authors investigated differences between dexmedetomidine and propofol sedation in the occurrence of upper airway obstruction and requirements for airway intervention in patients with mild obstructive sleep apnea.

Methods: Patients with an apnea/hypopnea index of 5–14/h according to Watch-PAT 200 analysis were enrolled in this study. Spinal anesthesia was routinely performed for surgery. Intraoperative sedation was initiated using either dexmedetomidine or propofol infusion at a level of modified observer's assessment of alertness/sedation scale 3. The primary outcome was the proportion of patients exhibiting signs of upper airway obstruction. A sign of upper airway obstruction was defined as no detection of end-tidal carbon dioxide for at least 10 s despite respiratory efforts.

Results: A total of 50 patients were included in the final analysis (dexmedetomidine [$n = 26$]; propofol [$n = 24$]). During the intraoperative sedation period, there was a significantly lower proportion of patients exhibiting signs of upper airway obstruction in the dexmedetomidine group than in the propofol group (11.5% vs. 41.7%, $P = 0.035$). An artificial airway was inserted in 1 patients (3.8%) and 5 patient (20.8%) in the dexmedetomidine and propofol groups, respectively ($P = 0.093$).

Conclusion: Dexmedetomidine sedation was associated with a lower incidence of upper airway obstruction than propofol sedation in patients with mild obstructive sleep apnea.

Keywords: Dexmedetomidine, Obstructive sleep apnea, Propofol, Sedation

* Correspondence: hsknana@gmail.com
[1]Department of Anesthesiology and Pain Medicine, Seoul National University Bundang Hospital, 82, Gumi 173, Bundang, Seongnam, Gyeonggi 13620, South Korea
Full list of author information is available at the end of the article

Background

Various agents have been used to sedate patients in operating rooms, intensive care units, procedure rooms, and diagnostic rooms. When sedation is induced, close attention is required for potential adverse events such as upper airway obstruction, hypoventilation, or apnea, as well as for any cardiovascular complications [1, 2]. Obstructive sleep apnea (OSA) is a challenging condition during intraoperative sedation. OSA patients have been associated with higher rates of postoperative complications, including significant postoperative hypoxemia [3, 4].

Dexmedetomidine acts as a selective α_2 adrenergic receptor agonist, with both sedative and analgesic effects [5]; thus, it has been favored in procedural sedation or monitored anesthesia care [6–8]. Moreover, dexmedetomidine has been known to induce sleep characteristics similar to physiological sleep [9, 10], and to be less associated with sleep apnea/hypopnea and respiratory depression [10]. In contrast, despite the advantages of propofol, such as rapid onset, short duration, and clear recovery, it has been known to cause respiratory depression, which can be exacerbated when coadministered with opioid [11, 12].

In children with OSA, dexmedetomidine sedation has less effect on airway patency and protective reflexes [13]. In adults, however, less evidence is available. To date, there has been no direct investigative comparison of which drug is better suited in OSA patients for intraoperative sedation during regional anesthesia.

We hypothesized that dexmedetomidine sedation could achieve a more patent airway; accordingly, we evaluated the occurrence of upper airway obstruction or the requirement for airway intervention in patients with mild OSA during intraoperative dexmedetomidine or propofol sedation.

Methods

Ethics approval for this study (B-1411/275–003) was granted by the institutional review board (Seoul National University Bundang Hospital, Seoul, South Korea) on January 4, 2015. This protocol was registered at ClinicalTrial.gov (NCT02993718) on December 2016. Adult patients, who were scheduled to undergo elective surgery under spinal anesthesia, were initially screened for inclusion in this study. The exclusion criteria were as follows: American Society of Anesthesiologists physical status III-V; body mass index $\geq$35 kg/m^2; refusal of intraoperative sedation; lateral decubitus or prone positioning during surgery; congenital or acquired anatomical problem of upper respiratory tract; drug intoxication; chronic alcoholics, or psychotic disorder. Written informed consent was obtained from all patients.

Patients wore the Watch-PAT 200 (Itamar Medical Ltd., Caesarea, Israel) on their wrist and index finger the night before surgery. The Watch-PAT 200, is a wrist-worn device equipped with a non-invasive finger-mounted probe, and is as useful as polysomnography for analyzing sleep patterns and diagnosing OSA [14]. Patients with an apnea/hypopnea index of 5–14 events/h according to the Watch-PAT 200 recording were finally enrolled in this study, and were assigned to either the dexmedetomidine group or the propofol group by one anesthesiologist who did not attend anesthetic care. Randomization was performed by computer-generated group allocation.

On arrival to the operating room, vital signs, including non-invasive arterial pressure, electrocardiogram, and pulse oximetry, were monitored. Spinal anesthesia was performed in a routine manner. After confirming the appropriate sensory and motor block, sedative drugs were administered to the patients. Each patient was positioned supine with a pillow 3 cm high. In the dexmedetomidine group, 0.5 μg/kg of dexmedetomidine was administered over a 10-min period, which was followed by continuous infusion in the range of 0.2–0.8 μg/kg/h. In the propofol group, propofol was infused via a target-controlled infusion device within the range 0.5–2.0 μg/ml. The sedation level was maintained according to the modified observer's assessment of alertness/sedation (OAA/S) scale 3 (response to calling loudly or repeatedly) in all patients [15], which was assessed every 10 min. During the sedation period, oxygen was supplied to patients via face mask and, concurrently, end-tidal carbon dioxide ($ETCO_2$) was monitored using the IntelliVue MP60 monitor (Philips, Boeblingen, Germany).

Signs of upper airway obstruction were defined as no detection of $ETCO_2$ despite inspiratory chest wall movement. If signs of upper airway obstruction were detected, the 3 cm pillow was replaced with a 6 cm pillow to elevate the patient's head and extended the patient's head using a cervical roll to improve airflow through the upper airway. If the signs of upper airway obstruction persisted despite this maneuver, an artificial airway was inserted. An independent investigator monitored events of airway obstruction.

Propofol was discontinued at the end of surgery; however, dexmedetomidine was discontinued earlier, approximately 30 min before the end of surgery. After cessation of each drug, the modified OAA/S scale was evaluated every 5 min until the scale reached 5. Patients were transferred to the post-anesthetic care unit (PACU). A modified Aldrete's scoring system was applied for discharge from the PACU. Most patients could not move their lower extremities voluntarily due to spinal anesthesia; thus, 9 of 10 points were the criteria for discharge from the PACU. In addition, when the modified OAA/S scale reached to 5, and when there was no acute operation-related complication related with operation, spinal anesthesia, and sedation, patients could be discharged from the PACU.

The primary outcome was the proportion of patients who exhibited signs of upper airway obstruction during the intraoperative sedation period. The secondary outcomes included recovery time from discontinuing each sedative drug to reach the modified OAA/S scale 5, the duration of PACU stay, and hemodynamic changes during sedation and the recovery period.

To calculate sample size, it was assumed that the incidences of upper airway obstruction requiring any airway manipulation were approximately 16% in the dexmedetomidine group and 54% in the propofol group, which were representative of pilot data from our center. Assuming an attrition rate of 10%, a total of 52 patients were determined to be an adequate sample size to aim for 80% power and 5% type-1 error.

Data are presented as mean ± SD or number (proportion) as appropriate. The Shapiro-Wilk test was performed to verify the normality of the data. Continuous variables were analyzed using the Student's *t*-test or Mann-Whitney U test, and categorical data were analyzed using the χ^2 test or Fisher's exact test, as appropriate. Changes in mean arterial pressure and heart rate were analyzed using repeated-measures ANOVA. SPSS version 21.0 (IBM Corporation, Armonk, NY, USA) was used for statistical analyses; differences with $P < 0.05$ were considered to be statistically significant.

Results

From January 2015 to June 2017, a total of 52 patients were enrolled in the present study. Two patients dropped out due to conversion of the anesthesia method from spinal to general (Fig. 1). Characteristics of the patients and preoperative Watch-PAT 200 data were summarized in Table 1. The profiles of operation, anesthesia, and recovery, and intraoperative vasopressor requirement were comparable between the two groups (Table 2).

During the intraoperative sedation period, 3 patients (11.5%; 95% Confidence interval, 2.4–33.7%) and 10 patients (41.7%; 95% Confidence interval, 20.0–76.6%) exhibited signs of upper airway obstruction in the dexmedetomidine and propofol group, respectively ($P = 0.035$). An artificial airway was inserted in 1 patient (3.8%; 95% Confidence interval, 0.1–21.4%) and 5 patients (20.8%; 95% Confidence interval, 6.8–48.6%) in the dexmedetomidine and propofol groups, respectively ($P = 0.093$).

Figure 2 showed the modified OAA/S scale during sedation and the PACU stay. In the dexmedetomidine group, the modified OAA/S scale was higher during the first 20 min; however, it was maintained at similar levels between the two groups during the remainder of the operation period. The modified OAA/S scale recovered slower in the dexmedetomidine group than in the propofol group in the PACU. The recovery time was significantly longer in the dexmedetomidine group than in the propofol group (44.4 ± 16.9 min in the dexmedetomidine group vs. 8.4 ± 7.1 min in the propofol group, $P < 0.001$). However, the duration of the PACU stay was similar in the two groups (37.5 ± 13.1 min in the dexmedetomidine group vs. 35.8 ± 11.3 min in the propofol group, $P = 0.627$).

Changes in mean arterial pressure and heart rate were comparable between the two groups during sedation

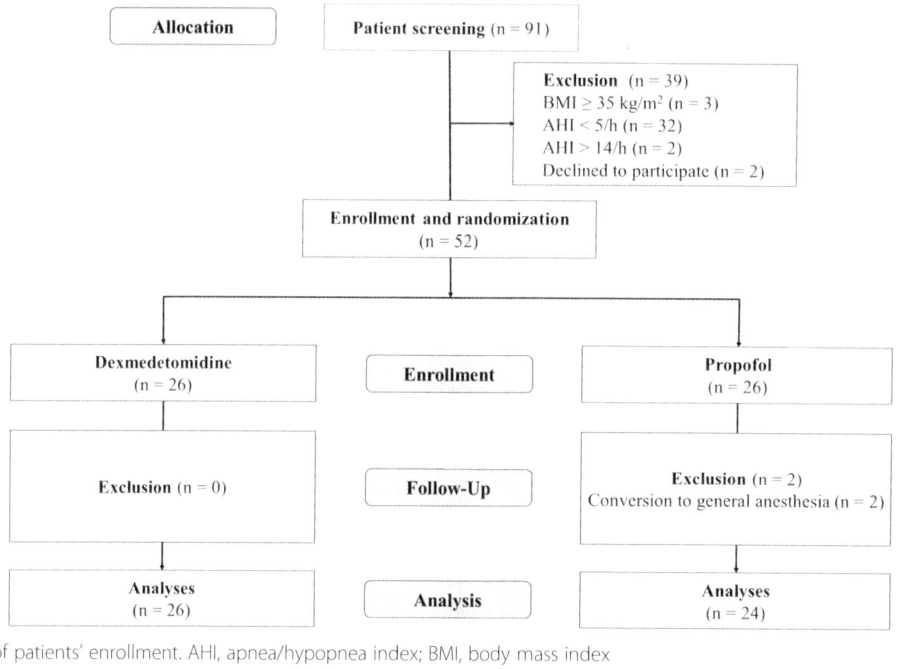

Fig. 1 Flow chart of patients' enrollment. AHI, apnea/hypopnea index; BMI, body mass index

Table 1 The characteristics of patients and preoperative WatchPAT200 analyses

	Dexmedetomidine ($n = 26$)	Propofol ($n = 24$)
Age (years)	56.2 ± 10.0	53.6 ± 11.4
Gender (Male/female)	18/8 (69.2/30.8)	15/9 (62.5/37.5)
Height (cm)	164.3 ± 8.9	163.3 ± 9.6
Weight (kg)	72.2 ± 11.7	68.9 ± 10.4
BMI (kg/m^2)	26.7 ± 3.7	25.8 ± 3.3
ASA (I/II)	9/17 (34.6/65.4)	12/12 (50.0/50.5)
WatchPAT200 analyses		
Mean SpO_2 (%)	95.6 ± 4.3	94.8 ± 3.9
Minimum SpO_2 (%)	87.2 ± 6.7	88.9 ± 8.1
AHI (events/h)	8.5 ± 3.9	7.8 ± 4.4
Sleep architecture (%)		
REM sleep	24.8 ± 8.1	22.2 ± 7.3
Light sleep	52.3 ± 4.6	49.6 ± 9.5
Deep sleep	22.9 ± 9.7	28.2 ± 11.6

BMI body mass index, *ASA* American Society of Anesthesiologists physical status, *AHI* apnea/hypopnea index, *REM* rapid-eye movement

(Fig. 3). However, intraoperative and postoperative mean arterial pressures demonstrated different patterns. The intraoperative mean arterial pressure was higher in the dexmedetomidine group, while the postoperative mean arterial pressure was higher in the propofol group.

Discussion

Patients enrolled in the present study had a mild degree of OSA; consequently, they were vulnerable to the occurrence of upper airway obstruction during sedation. We found that there were fewer occurrences of upper airway obstruction during sedation in the dexmedetomidine group than in the propofol group. The incidence of artificial airway insertion was numerically lower in patients who were administered dexmedetomidine, although the difference was not statistically significant.

Table 2 The characteristics of operation and anesthesia

	Dexmedetomidine ($n = 26$)	Propofol ($n = 24$)	P value
Operation time (min)	147.5 ± 38.9	148.2 ± 43.2	0.952
Anesthesia time (min)	191.0 ± 50.2	201.0 ± 54.2	0.501
Recovery time (min)	44.4 ± 16.9	8.4 ± 7.1	< 0.001
PACU time (min)	37.5 ± 13.1	35.8 ± 11.3	0.627
Phenylephrine (μg)	19.2 ± 8.0	16.3 ± 8.2	0.212
Ephedrine (mg)	1.5 ± 2.4	1.5 ± 3.5	1.000
Atropine (mg)	0.04 ± 0.14	0.02 ± 0.10	0.567

PACU post-anesthesia care unit

It has been reported that patients experience at least mid-level anxiety after spinal anesthesia [16]. Thus, sedation during surgery under regional anesthesia is required to reduce patient anxiety and/or stress. However, sedation remains a challenging task for anesthesiologists because there is a possibility of respiratory complications, including upper airway obstruction, respiratory depression, hypercapnia, and hypoxia [17, 18].

In addition to propofol and benzodiazepine, which have both been universally selected for intraoperative sedation, dexmedetomidine can be administered for intraoperative sedation in regional anesthesia [15]. While dexmedetomidine is known to cause less respiratory depression [10], there are limited studies reporting the safety of dexmedetomidine sedation for adult patients with respect to OSA. It was previously reported that dexmedetomidine sedation resulted in less upper airway obstruction in pediatric patients during radiological evaluation compared with propofol sedation, regardless of the presence of OSA [19, 20]. Moreover, it has also been found that there was no dose-dependent change in airway dimensions during dexmedetomidine sedation [21]. In adults, however, there is little evidence that dexmedetomidine is more advantageous for the maintenance of airway patency under sedation. Results of the present study contribute to a better understanding that dexmedetomidine has significantly less effects on upper airway obstruction compared with propofol in adults with mild OSA.

On the other hand, Watt et al. reported that there was no benefit of dexmedetomidine over propofol in deep sedation regarding upper airway obstruction [22]. Patients sedated with propofol also maintained spontaneous respiration; therefore, dexmedetomidine sedation may not be the only attributing factor to decreased occurrence of upper airway obstruction in the dexmedetomidine group.

The exact mechanism of how dexmedetomidine maintains airway patency warrants further investigation. Previously, it was reported that the anteroposterior diameter of the pharynx at the level of the soft palate decreased after propofol administration [23], and pharyngeal dysfunction was also observed [24]. However, Mahmoud et al. also reported that airway dimensions tended to increase slightly in children with OSA by dexmedetomidine, while propofol had a contrary effect [25]. Although their findings failed to reach statistical significance, we are informed that increased airway dimension induced by dexmedetomidine can result in a reduced incidence of upper airway collapse in patients with OSA. Their results are noteworthy, because it has already been established that patients with OSA have a greater risk for upper airway collapse from anesthesia [26].

Although intraoperative sedation level was maintained at modified OAA/S scale 3 in both groups, it took more

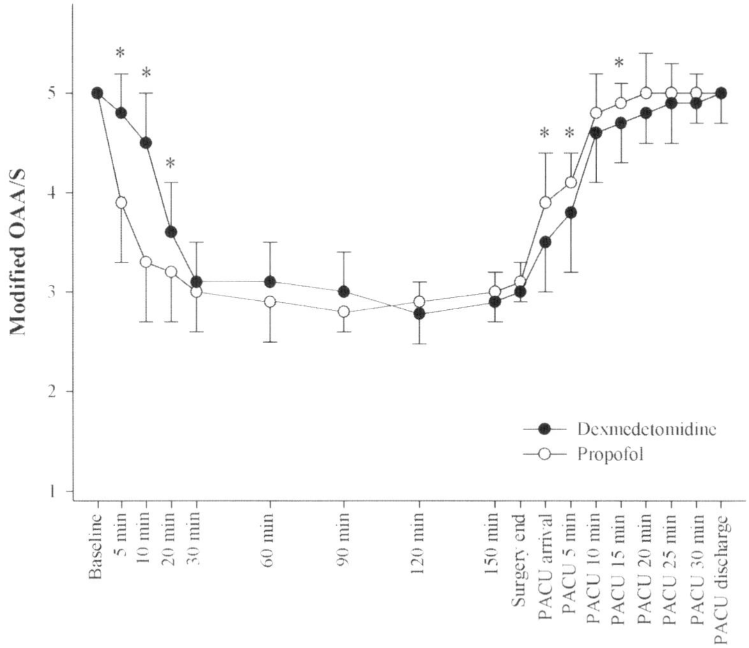

Fig. 2 The change of modified Observer's Assessment of Alertness/Sedation (OAA/S) scale. A stable mid-modified OAA/S scales were presented at 30 min intervals. PACU, post-anesthetic care unit

time for the dexmedetomidine group to recover to a modified OAA/S scale 5, as reported by others [27, 28]. However, we stopped the infusion of dexmedetomidine approximately 30 min before finishing the operation, and this practice helped overcome the extended recovery by dexmedetomidine and did not prolong the PACU stay.

Dexmedetomidine acts as a selective α2 adrenergic receptor agonist and is known to cause hypotension and bradycardia due to decreased centrally mediated sympathetic tone [29]. We did not find any significant differences in the mean arterial pressure and heart rate. However, we found that the mean intraoperative arterial pressure was maintained at a rather higher level in patients sedated with dexmedetomidine. Sympathetic tone was already decreased by spinal anesthesia; therefore, it appears that hypotension was not aggravated by dexmedetomidine. On the other hand, propofol has a direct cardiovascular depressive effect [30]; therefore, patients in the propofol group appeared to exhibit lower mean arterial pressure during the intraoperative sedation period. Due to the short half-life of propofol, the mean arterial pressure increased in the PACU after discontinuing infusion in the

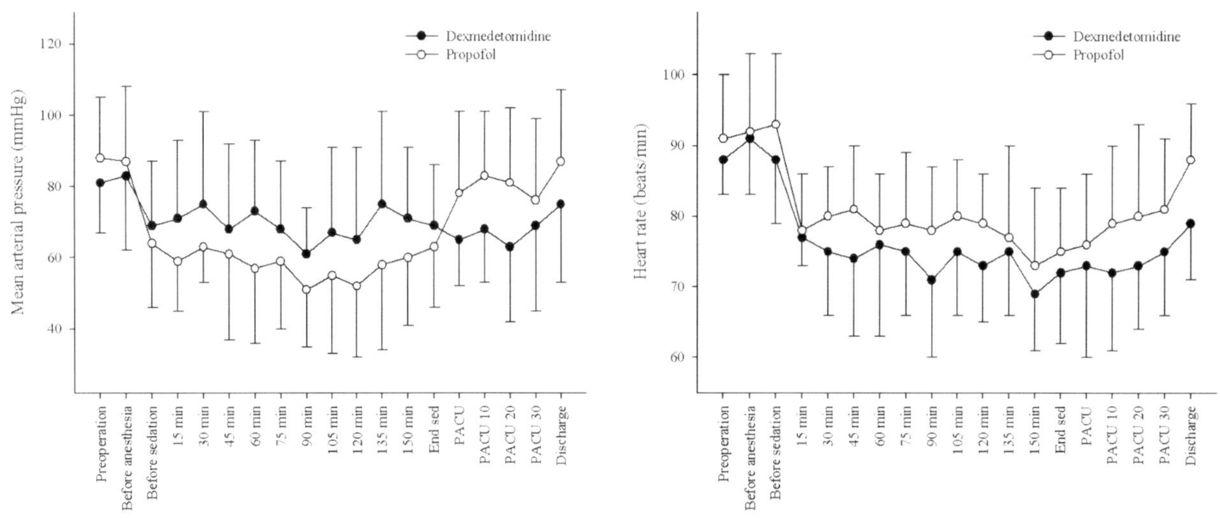

Fig. 3 Changed of mean arterial pressure and heart rate during sedation and postoperative period, PACU, post-anesthetic care unit

propofol group. As expected, dexmedetomidine has a longer half-life than propofol; therefore, mean arterial pressure was maintained at a lower level by continuously blocking central sympathetic outflow in the PACU in the dexmedetomidine group.

The present study had several limitations. The main drawback was the composition of the patients enrolled. We only recruited patients with mild OSA based on Watch-PAT 200 analyses. Thus, it is uncertain whether dexmedetomidine sedation is advantageous to patients with moderate or severe OSA. In addition, patients with a body mass index ≥35 kg/m^2 were excluded from our study. Morbid obesity is a major risk factor for OSA during sedation; hence, intraoperative sedation should be carefully performed for patient safety. Until now, it is not known which drugs are most suitable for sedation of morbid obese patients. Those with a body mass index ≥35 kg/m^2 should be included in future studies. Next, the number of patients was insufficient to draw a conclusion with sufficient power regarding the issue of artificial airway insertion. In our study, an artificial airway was used for patients whose airway obstruction was not solved by a positioning aid. Therefore, these patients can be considered to be at higher risk, and their characteristics need to be evaluated separately. Further studies include larger populations will be required. Finally, the investigator assessing the outcomes could not be blinded to the group arrangement because of the characteristics of propofol and dexmedetomidine. However, the primary outcome- upper airway obstruction- was the objective sign presented on the patient's monitor. Therefore, a bias toward dexmedetomidine or propofol did not appear to be involved in this study.

Conclusion

Dexmedetomidine sedation was shown to be associated with a reduced incidence of obstructive airway events in patients with mild OSA compared with propofol sedation. We recommended dexmedetomidine as a first-line sedative for adult patients with mild OSA. In future studies, this beneficial effect of dexmedetomidine on airway patency during sedation should be investigated in patients with moderate to severe OSA patient and/or morbidly obese patients.

Abbreviations

$ETCO_2$: End-tidal carbon dioxide; OAA/S: Observer's assessment of alertness/sedation; OSA: Obstructive sleep apnea; PACU: Post-anesthetic care unit

Funding

This work was supported by a grant [No. 02–2014-044] from the research fund of Seoul National University Bundang Hospital, South Korea. The role of the funding body is none.

Authors' contributions

H-JS: concept/design, data collection, drafting article, approval of article. E-YK: data collection, critical revision of article, approval of article. J-WH: data collection, critical revision of article, approval of article. S-HD: data analysis/interpretation, critical revision of article, approval of article. H-SN: concept/design, critical revision of article, approval of article. All authors read and approved the final manuscript.

Competing interests

The authors declare that they have no competing interests.

Author details

[1]Department of Anesthesiology and Pain Medicine, Seoul National University Bundang Hospital, 82, Gumi 173, Bundang, Seongnam, Gyeonggi 13620, South Korea. [2]Department of Anesthesiology and Pain Medicine, Daerim St. Mary's Hospital, Seoul, South Korea.

References

1. Becker DE, Haas DA. Management of complications during moderate and deep sedation: respiratory and cardiovascular considerations. Anesth Prog. 2007;54(2):59–68.
2. Becker DE, Haas DA. Recognition and management of complications during moderate and deep sedation part 1: respiratory considerations. Anesth Prog. 2011;58(2):82–92.
3. Liao P, Yegneswaran B, Vairavanathan S, Zilberman P, Chung F. Postoperative complications in patients with obstructive sleep apnea: a retrospective matched cohort study. Can J Anaesth. 2009;56(11):819–28.
4. Mador MJ, Goplani S, Gottumukkala VA, El-Solh AA, Akashdeep K, Khadka G, Abo-Khamis M. Postoperative complications in obstructive sleep apnea. Sleep Breath. 2013;17(2):727–34.
5. Hall JE, Uhrich TD, Barney JA, Arain SR, Ebert TJ. Sedative, amnestic, and analgesic properties of small-dose dexmedetomidine infusions. Anesth Analg. 2000;90(3):699–705.
6. Na HS, Song IA, Park HS, Hwang JW, Do SH, Kim CS. Dexmedetomidine is effective for monitored anesthesia care in outpatients undergoing cataract surgery. Korean J Anesthesiol. 2011;61(6):453–9.
7. Ryu JH, Lee SW, Lee JH, Lee EH, Do SH, Kim CS. Randomized double-blind study of remifentanil and dexmedetomidine for flexible bronchoscopy. Br J Anaesth. 2012;108(3):503–11.
8. Nishizawa T, Suzuki H, Sagara S, Kanai T, Yahagi N. Dexmedetomidine versus midazolam for gastrointestinal endoscopy: a meta-analysis. Dig Endosc. 2015;27(1):8–15.
9. Huupponen E, Maksimow A, Lapinlampi P, Sarkela M, Saastamoinen A, Snapir A, Scheinin H, Scheinin M, Merilainen P, Himanen SL, et al. Electroencephalogram spindle activity during dexmedetomidine sedation and physiological sleep. Acta Anaesthesiol Scand. 2008;52(2):289–94.
10. Hsu YW, Cortinez LI, Robertson KM, Keifer JC, Sum-Ping ST, Moretti EW, Young CC, Wright DR, Macleod DB, Somma J. Dexmedetomidine pharmacodynamics: part I: crossover comparison of the respiratory effects of dexmedetomidine and remifentanil in healthy volunteers. Anesthesiology. 2004;101(5):1066–76.

11. Lee MH, Yang KH, Lee CS, Lee HS, Moon SY, Hwang SI, Song JH. The effect-site concentration of propofol producing respiratory depression during spinal anesthesia. Korean journal of anesthesiology. 2011;61(2):122–6.
12. Peacock JE, Luntley JB, O'Connor B, Reilly CS, Ogg TW, Watson BJ, Shaikh S. Remifentanil in combination with propofol for spontaneous ventilation anaesthesia. Br J Anaesth. 1998;80(4):509–11.
13. Mahmoud M, Ishman SL, McConnell K, Fleck R, Shott S, Mylavarapu G, Gutmark E, Zou Y, Szczesniak R, Amin RS. Upper airway reflexes are preserved during Dexmedetomidine sedation in children with Down syndrome and obstructive sleep apnea. J Clin Sleep Med. 2017;13(5):721–7.
14. Pang KP, Gourin CG, Terris DJ. A comparison of polysomnography and the WatchPAT in the diagnosis of obstructive sleep apnea. Otolaryngol Head Neck Surg. 2007;137(4):665–8.
15. Hohener D, Blumenthal S, Borgeat A. Sedation and regional anaesthesia in the adult patient. Br J Anaesth. 2008;100(1):8–16.
16. Mingir T, Ervatan Z, Turgut N. Spinal Anaesthesia and perioperative anxiety. Turk J Anaesthesiol Reanim. 2014;42(4):190–5.
17. Vasu TS, Grewal R, Doghramji K. Obstructive sleep apnea syndrome and perioperative complications: a systematic review of the literature. J Clin Sleep Med. 2012;8(2):199–207.
18. Kaw R, Pasupuleti V, Walker E, Ramaswamy A, Foldvary-Schafer N. Postoperative complications in patients with obstructive sleep apnea. Chest. 2012;141(2):436–41.
19. Peng K, Li J, Ji FH, Li Z. Dexmedetomidine compared with propofol for pediatric sedation during cerebral angiography. J Res Med Sci. 2014;19(6):549–54.
20. Mahmoud M, Gunter J, Donnelly LF, Wang Y, Nick TG, Sadhasivam S. A comparison of dexmedetomidine with propofol for magnetic resonance imaging sleep studies in children. Anesth Analg. 2009;109(3):745–53.
21. Mahmoud M, Radhakrishman R, Gunter J, Sadhasivam S, Schapiro A, McAuliffe J, Kurth D, Wang Y, Nick TG, Donnelly LF. Effect of increasing depth of dexmedetomidine anesthesia on upper airway morphology in children. Paediatr Anaesth. 2010;20(6):506–15.
22. Watt S, Sabouri S, Hegazy R, Gupta P, Heard C. Does dexmedetomidine cause less airway collapse than propofol when used for deep sedation? J Clin Anesth. 2016;35:259–67.
23. Mathru M, Esch O, Lang J, Herbert ME, Chaljub G, Goodacre B, vanSonnenberg E. Magnetic resonance imaging of the upper airway. Effects of propofol anesthesia and nasal continuous positive airway pressure in humans. Anesthesiology. 1996;84(2):273–9.
24. Sundman E, Witt H, Sandin R, Kuylenstierna R, Boden K, Ekberg O, Eriksson LI. Pharyngeal function and airway protection during subhypnotic concentrations of propofol, isoflurane, and sevoflurane: volunteers examined by pharyngeal videoradiography and simultaneous manometry. Anesthesiology. 2001;95(5):1125–32.
25. Mahmoud M, Jung D, Salisbury S, McAuliffe J, Gunter J, Patio M, Donnelly LF, Fleck R. Effect of increasing depth of dexmedetomidine and propofol anesthesia on upper airway morphology in children and adolescents with obstructive sleep apnea. J Clin Anesth. 2013;25(7):529–41.
26. Eastwood PR, Szollosi I, Platt PR, Hillman DR. Comparison of upper airway collapse during general anaesthesia and sleep. Lancet (London, England). 2002;359(9313):1207–9.
27. Arain SR, Ebert TJ. The efficacy, side effects, and recovery characteristics of dexmedetomidine versus propofol when used for intraoperative sedation. Anesth Analg. 2002;95(2):461–6. table of contents
28. Shah PJ, Dubey KP, Sahare KK, Agrawal A. Intravenous dexmedetomidine versus propofol for intraoperative moderate sedation during spinal anesthesia: a comparative study. J Anaesthesiol Clin Pharmacol. 2016;32(2):245–9.
29. Bloor BC, Ward DS, Belleville JP, Maze M. Effects of intravenous dexmedetomidine in humans. II Hemodynamic changes. *Anesthesiology.* 1992;77(6):1134–42.
30. Goodchild CS, Serrao JM. Propofol-induced cardiovascular depression: science and art. Br J Anaesth. 2015;115(4):641–2.

3

Minimal effective weight-based dosing of ondansetron to reduce hypotension in cesarean section under spinal anesthesia: a randomized controlled superiority trial

Maliwan Oofuvong*, Thitikan Kunapaisal, Orarat Karnjanawanichkul, Nussara Dilokrattanaphijit and Jaranya Leeratiwong

Abstract

Background: The weight-based dosing of ondansetron to reduce hypotension has never been investigated. The aim of this study is to determine the optimal dose of ondansetron required based on the patient's weight to reduce hypotension following spinal anesthesia for cesarean section.

Methods: In this prospective, triple-blinded, parallel group, randomized controlled trial, a total of 228 pregnant women were randomized to receive either normal saline (group NS) or ondansetron 0.05 mg/kg (group O1) or ondansetron 0. 1 mg/kg (group O2) intravenously 5 min before induction of spinal anesthesia. The incidence of hypotension, mean arterial pressure, heart rate, vasopressor requirements, and blood loss between the three groups were compared. Maternal and neonatal complications were also assessed. Changes in blood pressure and heart rate were compared using the generalized estimating equations method.

Results: Thirteen patients were excluded from the analysis because of no intervention ($n = 12$) and protocol violation ($n = 1$). Two hundred and fifteen patients remained for the intention-to-treat analysis. The incidence of hypotension in groups NS ($n = 72$), O1 ($n = 71$), and O2 ($n = 72$) were 81.9%, 84.5%, and 73.6%, respectively ($P = 0.23$). The episodes of hypotension before delivery (first 14 min after spinal anesthesia) were significantly higher in group O1 compared to NS (5 vs 2, $P = 0.02$). The overall heart rates throughout the operations were not different among the three groups. The ephedrine requirements and amount of blood loss were also similar among the three groups. The metoclopramide requirement was significantly lower in group O2 compared to group NS (2.8% vs 16.7%, $P = 0.01$). There were no serious adverse events in terms of maternal or neonatal complications.

Conclusions: Ondansetron 0.05 mg/kg or 0.1 mg/kg administered before spinal anesthesia did not reduce the incidence of hypotension in this study.

Keywords: Weight-based dosing, Ondansetron, Hypotension, Spinal anesthesia, Cesarean section

* Correspondence: oomaliwa@gmail.com
Department of Anesthesiology, Faculty of Medicine, Prince of Songkla University, 15 Kanjanavanich Road, Songkhla 90112, Thailand

Background

Spinal anesthesia is now the technique of choice for women undergoing cesarean section. However, hypotension is a common problem after surgery with reported incidences varying from 53 to 85% worldwide [1, 2]. The Bezold–Jarisch reflex, which occurs after spinal anesthesia, induces vasodilatation and decreases venous return which results in bradycardia and hypotension [3]. A systematic review reported that neither intravenous fluid preload nor vasoconstriction given before spinal anesthesia is effective in preventing hypotension [4]. One factor known to influence the Bezold–Jarisch reflex is serotonin. Ondansetron is a serotonin receptor blocker. It decreases serotonin induced by the Bezold–Jarisch reflex by suppressing venodilatation [5]. Two studies found that ondansetron given at a dose of 8 mg before spinal anesthesia could reduce hypotension by 86% in general surgery [6] and by 33% in cesarean section [7]. However, another study showed that the same dose of ondansetron could not significantly reduce hypotension in pregnant women [8]. Fattahi et al. [9] showed that the mean arterial pressure after spinal anesthesia in patients who had a cesarean section was significantly higher in women given ondansetron 0.15 mg/kg compared to the control group. Sahoo et al. [10] reported the lower dose of ondansetron (4 mg) compared to control group could reduce hypotension in parturients in cesarean section. In terms of safety, Pasternak et al. [11] and Einarson et al. [12] showed that ondansetron administered in over 600,000 pregnant women had no significant effect on the newborn.

All of these studies used a fixed dose of ondansetron. To our knowledge, the optimal dose based on the patient's weight has never been investigated. Using a weight-based dose of ondansetron might maximize its effect and prevent suboptimal dose or overdose in some parturients since they have a larger volume of distribution compared to normal patients. Hence, this study aims to determine the minimal weight-based dose of ondansetron required to reduce hypotension after spinal anesthesia in women undergoing cesarean section.

Methods

This was a prospective triple-blinded parallel randomized controlled superiority trial. The study was approved by the Institutional Ethics Committee of The Faculty of Medicine, Prince of Songkla University, Songkhla, Thailand on March 3, 2016 (EC 58382081), Clinicaltrials.in.th number TCTR 20160323001 on March 22, 2016.

Participants

A written informed consent was obtained from all participants. The eligible participants were singleton pregnant women at a gestational age of 37–42 weeks who underwent elective cesarean section under spinal anesthesia and had no abnormal signs on electrocardiography. The study was carried out between May 2016 and February 2017 at Songklanagarind Hospital which is an 853–bed tertiary care hospital in southern Thailand. The exclusion criteria included the inability to communicate, history of hypertension, history of being allergic to ondansetron, congenital abnormality or acquired heart disease, coagulopathy, morbid obesity (body mass index > 35 kg/m^2), abnormal pregnancy with intrauterine growth retardation, congenital anomalies, poly- or oligo-hydramnios, and placenta previa. These criteria were meant to exclude patients who had a high risk of hemodynamic instability.

Standard operating procedures

After obtaining written informed consent from the participants by TK, baseline electrocardiography was performed and the women were randomized with a 1:1:1 allocation ratio to receive intravenously either normal saline (group NS) or ondansetron 0.05 mg/kg (group O1) or ondansetron 0.1 mg/kg (group O2) (maximal dose of 8 mg). Block randomization was performed in blocks of three by computer generated tables by a hospital research assistant who was not involved in the trial. A 4 mL clear solution was prepared for all study participants in sequential numbers by a nurse anesthetist in the recovery room who was not involved in the operation. The vial containing the solution was put into a concealed envelope for the nurse anesthetist who was in charge in the operating room. The syringes had no identifying markers indicating group allocation. The patient, anesthesiologist in charge, and the investigators were blinded to the group allocation. The intention-to-treat protocol was applied in this study. Premedication by ranitidine or metoclopramide or both could be given according to the decision of the anesthesiologist in charge.

In the operating room, 1000 mL of isotonic crystalloid was given to every patient. Philips IntelliVue MX700 was used to monitor non-invasive blood pressure, pulse oximetry, and electrocardiography during the period of anesthesia. Before spinal anesthesia was performed, the 4 mL clear solution containing the allocated treatment was administered intravenously five min before spinal anesthesia. Spinal anesthesia was performed at level L2–L3 or L3–L4 in the vertebral space with 2.0 mL of 0.5% hyperbaric bupivacaine and 0.2 mg of intrathecal morphine at a rate of 0.2 mL/sec by an experienced resident anesthetist. After spinal anesthesia was performed, systolic blood pressure (SBP), diastolic blood pressure (DBP), and mean arterial blood pressure (MAP) were recorded every one min for 15 min and then every five minutes, while the heart rates were recorded every five minutes until the end of the operation by a nurse anesthetist who was masked to the group allocation. Left uterine displacement of 15 to 20 degrees was performed after spinal anesthesia by placing a wedge under the right hip until the baby was delivered. After the baby was delivered, oxytocin (20 units per 1000 mL of isotonic crystalloid) was routinely given while methylergometrine would be given only upon request of the gynecologist surgeon. The doses of oxytocin and methylergometrine were measured.

Outcomes of the study

The primary outcomes of the study were the incidence of hypotension and the change in MAP. Hypotension was defined as a decrease in MAP > 30% from baseline. If hypotension occurred, 6 mg of ephedrine or 5 mcg of norepinephrine was administered intravenously according to the discretion of the anesthesiologist in charge.

The secondary outcomes were maternal complications during the intraoperative period and in the post-anesthetic care unit and neonatal complications 24 h postoperatively. If itching occurred, 10 mg of chlorpheniramine was given intravenously. Metoclopramide (10 mg) was given intravenously for treatment of nausea and vomiting during the intraoperative period. Any side effects from ondansetron such as burning and QT prolongation were evaluated. The QT prolongation was determined by a QT interval more than half of the preceding RR interval in 3-lead electrocardiogram monitoring intraoperatively and at post-anesthetic care unit. The well-being of the newborn baby was evaluated as well as any adverse events 24 h postoperatively.

Sample size determination

The sample size calculation was based on a difference in the incidence of hypotension between the control group (0.85) and the ondansetron group (8 mg) from a previous study which reported the incidence as 0.6 [7]. For a power of 90% to detect this difference and a type I error rate of 0.05, 73 patients per group were required under the assumption that 10% of the study participants would withdraw from the study.

Statistical analysis

Continuous variables are presented as median and interquartile range for non-normally distributed data or mean and standard deviation for normally distributed data. Categorical variables are presented as frequency and percentage. Continuous variables were compared using two-way analysis of variance and the Kruskal–Wallis test for normally and non-normally distributed data, respectively. Categorical variables were compared using Pearson's Chi square test or Fisher's exact test for normally and non-normally distributed data, respectively. Post-hoc analysis was performed for multiple comparisons between groups when the overall differences were significant. Changes in SBP, DBP, MAP, and heart rate were compared using the generalized estimating equations method. A P value < 0.05 was considered statistically significant. Group allocation was also blinded to the statistician who analyzed the data.

Results

Two hundred and twenty-eight women were enrolled in the study with details shown in the consort diagram in Fig. 1. Data collection was completed in 215 patients for the intention-to-treat analysis. Patient characteristics and anesthetic data are presented in Table 1. No differences among the groups were observed in demographic data and anesthetic data. The overall incidence of maternal hypotension was 80%. There were no differences in the incidence of hypotension between the three groups either before or after delivery except episodes of hypotension before delivery were significantly higher in group O1 compared to NS (5 vs 2, $P = 0.02$) (Table 2). The arterial pressures (SBP, MAP, and DBP) are shown in Fig. 2. MAP levels at 4 and 9 min after spinal anesthesia were significantly lower in group O1 compared to the NS group ($P = 0.024$ and $P = 0.034$, respectively). The overall heart rates throughout the operations were not different among the three groups (Fig. 3). Ephedrine requirements were similar among the three groups: group NS (6 mg), group O1 (12 mg), and group O2 (6 mg) ($P = 0.21$). There were also no differences in blood loss among the three groups: group NS (447.9 ± 201.3 mL), group O1 (490.8 ± 241.2 mL), and group O2 (440.3 ± 198.2 mL) ($P = 0.32$). Table 3 shows the surgical and anesthetic parameters for the three groups. The metoclopramide requirement in the post-hoc analysis in group O2 was significantly lower than in group NS ($P = 0.01$). Table 4 compares the incidence of maternal and newborn adverse events between the three groups. No significant differences were found although tachypnea was slightly higher among newborns of women who received low dose ondansetron (7.0%, $n = 5$) compared to the control group (2.8%, $n = 2$) ($P = 0.28$). There were no reports of burning or QT prolongation in mothers and no reports of bradycardia or hypothermia in newborns in any group.

Discussion

In this study, we found that a weight-based dose of prophylactic ondansetron did not influence the incidence of maternal hypotension. The results of this study were consistent with two other studies [8, 13] but were in contrast with others [6, 7, 9, 10]. Two recent systematic reviews [14, 15] showed ondansetron reduced the incidence of hypotension (relative risk ratio [RR] = 0.63, 95% confidence interval [CI]: 0.45–0.88 and RR = 0.67, 95% CI: 0.54–0.83, respectively) and bradycardia (RR = 0.31, 95% CI: 0.19–0.50 and RR = 0.49,

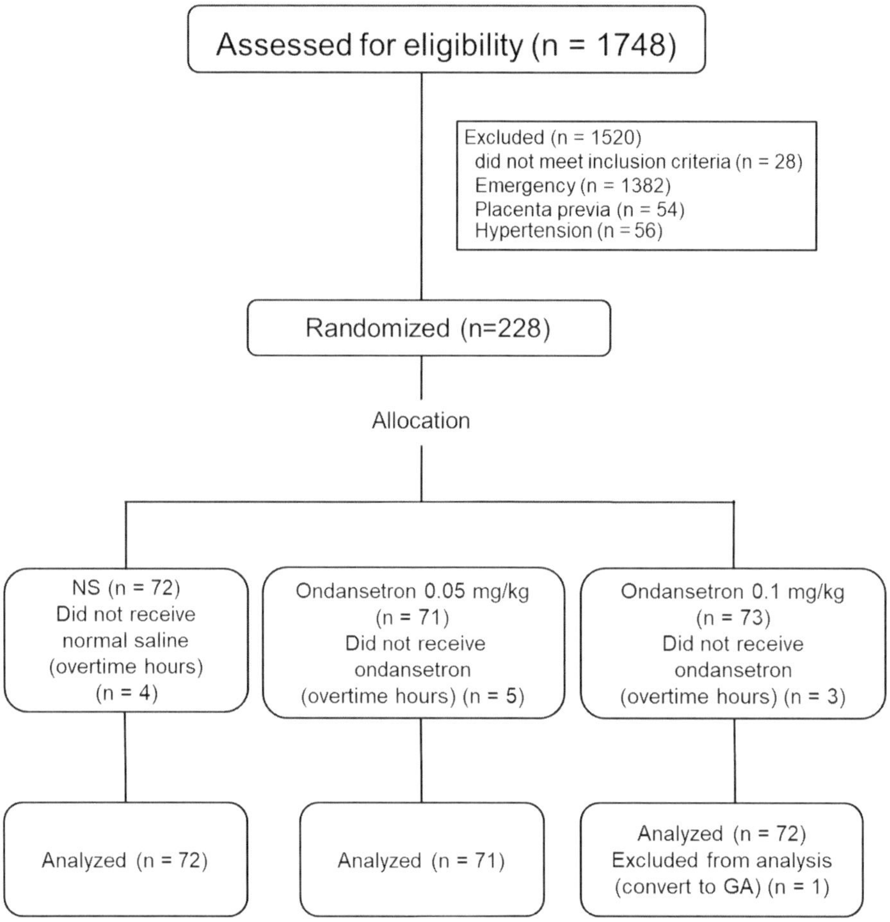

Fig. 1 Consort flow diagram. *GA* general anesthesia

95% CI: 0.28–0.87, respectively) after spinal anesthesia in cesarean section even though a low quality of evidence was reported [15]. However, the minimal effective weight-based dosing of ondansetron in parturients was not determined [9, 10, 14, 15].

In our study, ondansetron had little effect on hemodynamic stability after subarachnoid block in parturients. Factors that impact the level of anesthesia and analgesia given to the patient might also affect the patient's arterial pressure as well as the way to measure arterial pressure. There are some possible reasons for the difference in the incidence of hypotension compared to other reports. First, we did not monitor invasive arterial blood pressure or cardiac output. Real time arterial pressure monitoring may be better at detecting actual variations of blood pressure than noninvasive blood pressure monitoring although we measured blood pressure every minute during the first 15 min after spinal anesthesia. A noninvasive blood pressure measurement might not be sufficiently sensitive to notice hemodynamic changes to promptly treat hypotension in parturients, especially in preeclamptic patients [16]. Langesaeter et al. [17] and Rosseland et al. [18] showed that continuous invasive arterial pressure monitoring during cesarean section under subarachnoid block provided hemodynamic stability in parturients, especially when vasopressor was given. Second, vasodilatation from subarachnoid block might have a stronger influence on blood pressure than the Bezold–Jarisch reflex in our study. From the results, 0.05 mg of ondansetron caused more episodes of hypotension before delivery compared to the control group ($P = 0.02$), especially at 4 and 9 min after spinal anesthesia (Fig. 2) which led to failure to prevent the Bezold–Jarisch reflex. Therefore, ondansetron may have little effect on preventing hypotension in these cases since we administered a vasopressor to treat vasodilatation immediately after hypotension occurred causing no differences in the incidence of hypotension among the three groups. We recorded blood pressure after a subarachnoid block was performed every minute for 15 min. If hypotension occurred, ephedrine or norepinephrine was administered instantly until the MAP reached the lower limit of baseline level. The peak onset of ephedrine or norepinephrine is approximately 1–2 min [19] and repeated

Table 1 Comparison of demographic and anesthesia related data between the three groups

Parameter	Normal saline (*n* = 72)	Ondansetron 0.05 mg/kg (*n* = 71)	Ondansetron 0.1 mg/kg (*n* = 72)	*P*-value
Age (years)[a]	31.8 (4.5)	32.2 (5.5)	32.7 (4.8)	0.55
Weight (kg)[a]	67.5 (9.6)	68.7 (9.1)	69.6 (8.9)	0.39
Height (cm)[a]	157.2 (5.5)	156.9 (5.7)	157.9 (5.2)	0.48
Body mass index (kg/m^2)[a]	27.3 (3.5)	27.9 (3.0)	27.9 (3.2)	0.47
Type of operation				
CS only	49 (68.1)	49 (69)	46 (63.9)	0.79
CS with tubal resection	23 (31.9)	22 (31)	26 (36.1)	
Site of spinal anesthesia				
L2–3	2 (2.8)	0 (0)	0 (0)	0.33
L3–4	70 (97.2)	71 (100)	72 (100)	
Number of blocks				
1	70 (97.2)	70 (98.6)	69 (95.8)	0.87
2	2 (2.8)	1 (1.4)	3 (4.2)	
Anesthesia level[b]	T7 (T6–T8)	T6 (T6–T8)	T6 (T6–T8)	0.33
Analgesia level[b]	T4 (T3–T4)	T3 (T3–T4)	T4 (T3–T4)	0.43
Premedication with metoclopramide	25 (34.7)	21 (29.6)	21 (29.2)	0.73
Premedication with ranitidine	25 (34.7)	21 (29.6)	21 (29.2)	0.73

Data are presented as frequency (%) unless stated otherwise
[a]mean (SD)
[b]median (IQR)
CS cesarean section

Table 2 Comparison of incidence and episodes of hypotension between the three groups

Parameter	Normal saline (*n* = 72)	Ondansetron 0.05 mg/kg (*n* = 71)	Ondansetron 0.1 mg/kg (*n* = 72)	*P*-value
Total incidence,				
n (%)	59 (81.9)	60 (84.5)	53 (73.6)	0.23
(95% CI)	(73.1–90.8)	(76.1–92.9)	(63.4–83.8)	
Episodes, median (IQR)	2 (0–4.0)	3 (0.5–5.0)	1 (0–3.2)	0.07
Before delivery				
Incidence,				
n (%)	57 (79.2)	59 (83.1)	50 (69.4)	0.13
(95% CI)	(69.8–88.5)	(74.4–91.8)	(58.8–80.1)	
Episodes, median (IQR)	2 (1–6.0)[a]	5 (1.5–8.0)[b]	2 (0–5.0)[ac]	0.015
After delivery				
Total incidence,				
n (%)	37 (52.1)	41 (57.7)	39 (54.9)	0.80
(95% CI)	(40.5–63.7)	(46.3–69.2)	(43.4–66.5)	
Episodes, median (IQR)	0 (0–2.0)	1 (0–3.0)	1 (0–1.5)	0.64

IQR interquartile range, *CI* confidence interval
[ac]Groups sharing the same superscript were not significantly different, [b]Group was significantly different compared to the others

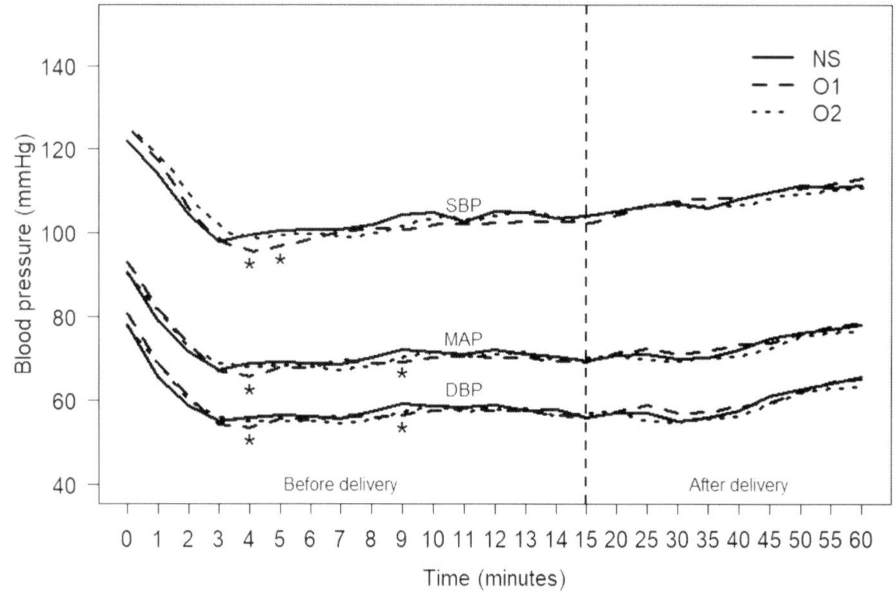

Fig. 2 Changes in maternal systolic blood pressure (SBP), diastolic blood pressure (DBP) and mean arterial pressure (MAP) for the three groups. *NS* normal saline, *O1* ondansetron 0.05 mg/kg, *O2* ondansetron 0.1 mg/kg. Spinal anesthesia was performed between Time 0–1, Time 0 = baseline blood pressure, Time 1–60 = 1 to 60 min after spinal anesthesia, *$P < 0.05$ compared group O1 to NS at a certain time compared to Time 0

doses were given as needed. Third, the weight-based dosing of 0.1 mg/kg of ondansetron might not be adequate to maximize the effect to prevent the Bezold–Jarisch reflex. A high dose of ondansetron (12 mg) or 0.15 mg/kg of ondansetron was reported to increase MAP in patients who had a cesarean section under spinal anesthesia compared to the control group [9, 20]. In our study, the mean dose of 3 to 7.9 mg of ondansetron was given which might not be adequate to prevent the Bezold–Jarisch reflex even though some studies found a lower dose of ondansetron (4 or 6 mg) could significantly prevent hypotension in the same setting [10, 20]. However, we were concerned that the dose of 0.15 mg/kg of ondansetron might be harmful to the fetus in terms of possible umbilical arterial vasoconstriction due to ondansetron acting on the 5-HT1B receptor [21]. Fourth, our analysis was based on an intention-to-treat principle which included repeat administration of subarachnoid blocks following failure of the first spinal anesthesia. A repeat dose of subarachnoid block can affect the level of anesthesia and analgesia, although there were no significant differences in the number of blocks given between the three groups ($P = 0.87$).

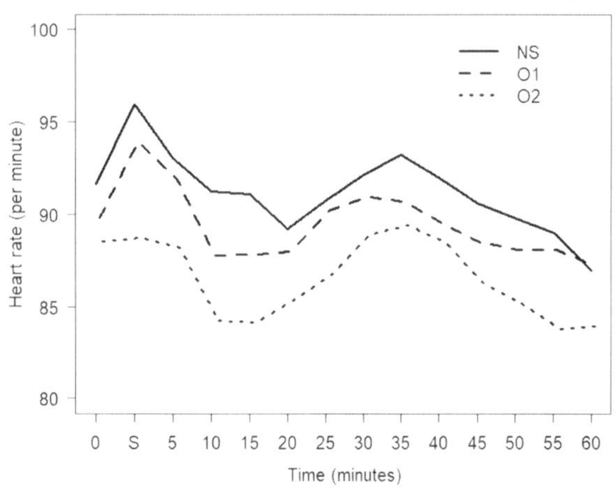

Fig. 3 Changes in heart rate for the three groups. *NS* normal saline, *O1* ondansetron 0.05 mg/kg, *O2* ondansetron 0.1 mg/kg. Time 0 = baseline heart rate, Time S = spinal anesthesia and 5 min after received intervention, Time 5–60 = 5 to 60 min after spinal anesthesia

The definition of hypotension used in this study was a decrease in the MAP by 30% from the baseline level which was quite similar to many studies [7, 8, 22, 23]. MAP was used instead of SBP to define hypotension because MAP provides a physiologically more appropriate measurement of hypotension than SBP [24]. The overall incidence of hypotension among women undergoing cesarean section following spinal anesthesia in our study (80%) was lower than reported in a previous study done in Songklanagarind Hospital (85%) [2]. One-third of each intervention group received metoclopramide as premedication. Even though a case report showed 10 mg of metoclopramide could cause severe hypotension [25], the baseline blood pressure before spinal anesthesia was not different among the three groups (Fig. 2).

Ondansetron did not cause any adverse events in our study. The parturients experienced neither QT

Table 3 Comparison of surgical and anesthetic parameters between the three groups

Parameter	Normal saline (*n* = 72)	Ondansetron 0.05 mg/kg (*n* = 71)	Ondansetron 0.1 mg/kg (*n* = 72)	*P*-value
Duration of surgery (min)	56.6 (18.1)	58.9 (22.3)	55.2 (16.5)	0.52
Ephedrine (mg), median (IQR)	6 (0–18)	12 (0–18)	6 (0–18)	0.21
Norepinephrine (mcg), median (IQR)	0 (0–10)	0 (0–10)	0 (0–10)	0.47
Oxytocin (unit)	22.7 (8.5)	21.3 (9.1)	22.4 (9.7)	0.62
Methylergometrine (mg), median (IQR)	0 (0–0.2)	0 (0–0.2)	0 (0–0.2)	0.77
Blood loss (mL)	447.9 (201.3)	490.8 (241.2)	440.3 (198.2)	0.32
Crystalloid (mL)	1934.7 (303.3)	1884.5 (346.2)	1891.7 (284.8)	0.58
Packed red cells (mL)	0 (0)	2.8 (23.9)	0 (0)	0.36
Metoclopramide, n (%)	12 (16.7)^{a}	6 (8.5)^{ab}	2 (2.8)^{b}	0.02

Data are presented as mean (SD) unless stated otherwise
^{ab}Groups sharing the same superscript were not significantly different
IQR interquartile range

abnormalities nor burning sensation during the injection and the newborns did not experience bradycardia or hypothermia 24 h postoperatively. The incidence of urticaria or arrhythmia was not higher in the two ondansetron groups. Although the incidence of vomiting was lower in the high dose ondansetron (0.1 mg/kg) group, the incidence was not statistically different ($P = 0.09$). However, postoperative metoclopramide requirement was significantly lower in the high dose ondansetron compared to the normal saline group ($P = 0.01$). Therefore, the effect of ondansetron to prevent or treat nausea and vomiting was achieved as expected. There were no significant differences in terms of hypotension or tachypnea in newborns between the three groups. The incidence of tachypnea was slightly higher among the newborns of women who received the low dose of ondansetron compared to the control group (7% vs 2.8%). Tachypnea resolved within 2–3 h after oxygen therapy was administered. Although ondansetron can transfer across the placenta to newborn babies [26], adverse events related to ondansetron in newborns have not been reported.

Strengths and limitations

The strengths of this study were reduced selection bias due to the randomized treatment allocation and the triple-blind design (patients, investigators, and statistician). We used the intention-to-treat principle in the analysis which helped decrease the bias and ensure a balance of patients between the three groups. There are two weaknesses of this study. First, several resident anesthetists performed the spinal block which might have affected the level of anesthesia and incidence of hypotension in the study participants. However, these residents had a high level of experience (> 20 spinal blocks) and a fixed rate of subarachnoid injection (0.2 mL/s) was used in all participants. Second, we did not monitor invasive arterial blood pressure because invasive monitoring is not routinely used in healthy parturients in our setting and it is also costly. However, the

Table 4 Comparison of maternal and newborn adverse events between the three groups

Adverse event	Normal saline (*n* = 72)	Ondansetron 0.05 mg/kg (*n* = 71)	Ondansetron 0.1 mg/kg (*n* = 72)	*P*-value
Mother				
Urticaria	1 (1.4)	0 (0)	2 (2.8)	0.78
Arrhythmia	2 (2.8)	0 (0)	1 (1.4)	0.78
Vomiting	10 (13.9)	10 (14.1)	3 (4.2)	0.09
Itching	10 (13.9)	4 (5.6)	7 (9.7)	0.25
Newborn				
Apgar 1, median (IQR)	9 (8–9)	9 (8–9)	9 (8–9)	0.94
Apgar 5, median (IQR)	9 (9–9)	9 (9–9)	9 (9–9)	0.14
Hypotension	0 (0)	1 (1.4)	0 (0)	0.33
Tachypnea	2 (2.8)	5 (7.0)	0 (0)	0.04*

Data are presented as frequency (%) unless stated otherwise
*no differences for multiple comparisons between groups ($P > 0.05$)

accuracy of the study is high and reproducibility of the results for a similar setting (a tertiary care hospital) should be achievable even though the study was conducted in a single hospital.

Conclusions

Ondansetron administered at a dose of 0.05 mg/kg or 0.1 mg/kg before spinal anesthesia was not effective in reducing the incidence of hypotension in pregnant women undergoing cesarean section. Higher weight-based dosing of ondansetron should be examined keeping the safety issues in mind.

Abbreviations

CI: Confidence interval; DBP: Diastolic blood pressure; MAP: Mean arterial blood pressure; RR: Relative risk ratio; SBP: Systolic blood pressure

Acknowledgements

We would like to thank Assistant Professor Edward McNeil for editing the manuscript and Glenn Shingledecker for correcting some grammatical errors in the manuscript.

Funding

This work was funded by the Faculty of Medicine, Prince of Songkla University, Hat Yai, Songkhla, Thailand.

Authors' contributions

All those listed as authors contributed to the preparation of the manuscript. Each listed author participated in the work and they can defend its content. MO coordinated the study, participated in the study design, undertook the statistical analysis and wrote the draft manuscript. TK participated in its design, collected the data and wrote the draft manuscript. OK participated in its design and revised the draft manuscript. ND participated in its design, and collected the data. JL participated in its design, and collected the data. All authors have read and approved the final version.

Competing interests

The authors declare that they have no competing interests.

References

1. Somboonviboon W, Kyokong O, Charuluxananan S, Narasethakamol A. Incidence and risks factors of hypotension and bradycardia after spinal anesthesia for cesarean section. J Med Assoc Thail. 2008;91:181–7.
2. Loetwiriyakun W, Chanchayanon T. Optimal dose of intravenous ephedrine for prevention of hypotension during spinal Anaesthesia for caesarean delivery. ASEAN J of Anaesth. 2004;5:3–9.
3. Birnbach DJ, Browne IM. Anesthesia for obstetric. In: Miller RD, Eriksson LI, Fleisher LA, Weiner-Kronish JP, Young WL, editors. Miller's anesthesia. 7th ed. New York: Churchill Living-Stone; 2010. p. 2203–40.
4. Cyna AM, Andrew M, Emmett RS, Middleton P, Simmons SW. Techniques for preventing hypotension during spinal anaesthesia for cesarean section. Cochrane Database Syst Rev. 2006;4:CD002251.
5. Aviado DM, Guevara AD, The Bezold-Jarisch reflex. A historical perspective of cardiopulmonary reflexes. Ann N Y Acad Sci. 2001;940:48–58.
6. Owczuk R, Wenski W, Polak-Krzeminska A, Twardowski P, Arszułowicz R, Dylczyk-Sommer A, Wujtewicz MA, Sawicka W, Morzuch E, Smietanski M, Wujtewicz M. Ondansetron given intravenously attenuates arterial blood pressure drop due to spinal anesthesia: a double- blind, placebo-controlled study. Reg Anesth Pain Med. 2008;33:332–9.
7. Wang M, Zhuo L, Wang Q, Shen M, Yu YY, Yu JJ, Wang ZP. Efficacy of prophylactic intravenous ondansetron on the prevention of hypotension during cesarean delivery: a dose-dependent study. Int J Clin Exp Med. 2014;7:5210–6.
8. Marciniak A, Owczuk R, Wujtewicz M, Preis K, Majdylo K. The influence of intravenous ondansetron on maternal blood haemodynamics after spinal anaesthesia for caesarean section: a double-blind, placebo-controlled study. Ginekol Pol. 2015;86:461–7.
9. Fattahi Z, Hadavi R, Sahmeddini A. Effect of ondansetron on post-dural puncture headache (PDPH) in parturients undergoing cesarean section: a double- blind randomized placebo – controlled study. J Anesth. 2015;29: 702–7.
10. Sahoo T, SenDasgupta C, Goswami A, Haza A. Reduction in spinal-induced hypotension with ondansetron in parturients undergoing cesarean section: a double-blind randomized, placebo-controlled study. Int J Obstet Anesth. 2012;21:24–8.
11. Pasternak B, Svanstrom H, Hviid A. Ondansetron in pregnancy and risk of adverse fetal outcomes. N Engl J Med. 2013;368:814–23.
12. Einarson A, Maltepe C, Navioz Y, Kennedy D, Tan MP, Koren G. The safety of ondansetron for nausea and vomiting of pregnancy: a prospective comparative study. BJOG. 2004;111:940–3.
13. Ortiz-Gomez JR, Palacio-Abizanda FJ, Morillas-Ramirez F, Fornet-Ruiz I, Lorenzo-Jimenez A, Bermejo-Albares ML. The effect of intravenous ondansetron on maternal haemodynamics during elective cesarean delivery under spinal anesthesia: a double-blind, randomized, placebo-controlled trial. Int J Obstet Anesth. 2014;23:138–43.
14. Tubog TD, Kane TD, Pugh MA. Effects of ondansetron on attenuating spinal anesthesia-induced hypotension and bradycardia in obstetric and nonobstetric subjects: a systematic review and meta-analysis. AANA J. 2017;85:113–22.
15. Chooi C, Cox JJ, Lumb RS, Middleton P, Chemali M, Emmett RS, Simmons SW, Cyna AM. Techniques for preventing hypotension during spinal anaesthesia for caesarean section. Cochrane Database Syst Rev. 2017;8:CD002251. https://doi.org/10.1002/14651858.CD002251.pub3. [Epub ahead of print]
16. Dyer RA, Anthony J, Ledeboer Q, James MF. Cardiovascular responses to the change from the left lateral to the upright position in pregnant hypertensives. Int J Gynaecol Obstet. 2004;84:208–13.
17. Langesaeter E, Rosseland LA, Stubhaug A. Continuous invasive blood pressure and cardiac output monitoring during cesarean delivery: a randomized, double-blind comparison of low-dose versus high-dose spinal anesthesia with intravenous phenylephrine or placebo infusion. Anesthesiology. 2008;109:856–63.
18. Rosseland LA, Hauge TH, Grindheim G, Stubhaug A, Langesæter E. Changes in blood pressure and cardiac output during cesarean delivery: the effects of oxytocin and carbetocin compared with placebo. Anesthesiology. 2013; 119:541–51.
19. Glick DB. The autonomic nervous system. In: Miller RD, Eriksson LI, Fleisher LA, Weiner-Kronish JP, Young WL, editors. Miller's anesthesia. 8th ed. Philadelphia: Saunders Elsevier; 2015. p. 346–83.
20. Marashi SM, Soltani-Omid S, Soltani Mohammadi S, Aghajani Y, Movafegh A. Comparing two different doses of intravenous ondansetron with placebo on attenuation of spinal-induced hypotension and shivering. Anesth Pain Med. 2014;4(2):e12055. https://doi.org/10.5812/aapm.12055. eCollection 2014 May.
21. Kaumann AJ, Levy FO. 5-hydroxytryptamine receptors in the human cardiovascular system. Pharmacol Ther. 2006;111:674–706.
22. Rashad MM, Farmawy MS. Effects of intravenous ondansetron and granisetron on hemodynamic changes and motor and sensory blockade induced by spinal anesthesia in parturients undergoing cesarean section. Egypt J Anaesth. 2013;29:369–74.

23. Khalifa OS. A comparative study of prophylactic intravenous granisetron, ondansetron, and ephedrine in attenuating hypotension and its effect on motor and sensory block in elective cesarean section under spinal anesthesia. Ain-Shams J Anesthesiol. 2015;8:166–72.
24. Henry J, Miller M, Kelly K, Champney D. Mean arterial pressure (MAP): an alternative and preferable measurement to systolic blood pressure (SBP) in patients for hypotension detection during hemapheresis. J of Clin Apher. 2002;17:55–64.
25. Nguyen TT, Petzel Gimbar RM. Sustained hypotension following intravenous metoclopramide. Ann Pharmacother. 2013;47:1577–80.
26. Siu SS, Chan MT, Lau TK. Placental transfer of ondansetron during early human pregnancy. Clin Pharm. 2006;45:419–23.

4

Early postoperative recovery in operating room after desflurane anesthesia combined with Bispectral index (BIS) monitoring and warming in lengthy abdominal surgery: a randomized controlled study

Hong Yu[1], Lu Zhang[1], Ye Ma[2] and Hai Yu[1*]

Abstract

Background: This study aimed to determine whether the use of desflurane (DES) anesthesia combined with bispectral index (BIS) monitoring and warming is effective in reducing anesthesia-controlled operating room time (ACT) in patients undergoing lengthy abdominal surgery.

Methods: Seventy patients, 40 years of age or older, undergoing abdominal surgery expected to last three to five hours were randomly assigned to the DES group ($n = 35$) or the control group ($n = 35$). Patients in the DES group were maintained with desflurane anesthesia and received BIS monitoring and warming. Patients in the control group were given non-desflurane anesthesia for maintenance, and the usage of BIS monitoring and warming were not mandatory and determined by anesthesia care providers. Early postoperative recovery times were recorded.

Results: The times to extubation (8.8 ± 8.5 vs 14.7 ± 13.7 min, $P = 0.035$), eye opening (8.4 ± 8.6 vs 14.4 ± 13.4 min, $P = 0.028$), responds on command (8.2 ± 8.5 vs 14.4 ± 13.0 min, $P = 0.022$), and the ACT (23.8 ± 11.4 vs 32.7 ± 15.4 min, $P = 0.009$) were significantly less in the DES group than that in the control group. The postanesthesia care unit (PACU) length of stay, incidence of prolonged extubation, and surgeon and anesthesiologist satisfaction were similar in two groups. Also, the result of multivariable linear regressions showed that patients who were younger, female, lower BMI and non-DES anesthesia regimen resulted in prolonged extubation.

Conclusions: Desflurane anesthesia combined with BIS monitoring and warming is associated with early postoperative recovery in lengthy abdominal surgery.

Keywords: Anesthesia, General, Anesthetics volatile, Desflurane, Anesthetics volatile, Sevoflurane, Recovery, Anesthesia-controlled time, ACT, Warming, Bispectral index monitoring

* Correspondence: yuhaishan117@yahoo.com
[1]Department of Anesthesiology, West China Hospital of Sichuan University, Chengdu 610041, People's Republic of China
Full list of author information is available at the end of the article

Background

Anesthesia-controlled time (ACT) and turnover time are two of the most important factors that regulate operating room (OR) efficiency [1]. Prolonged extubation is an important factor affecting operating room efficiency, which is a concern of surgeons and anesthesia care providers [2, 3]. Prolonged extubation slows work flow and requires OR staff to monitor while waiting for the next operation. Choosing appropriate anesthetic agents or techniques is essential for anesthesia care providers to reduce time of extubation and post-anesthesia recovery.

Desflurane, with the lowest blood-gas partition coefficient of the available halogenated agents, has been suggested be a potential for rapid recovery after discontinuation [4]. Previous meta-analysis found that desflurane reduced the extubation time by 34% relative to isoflurane and by 25% relative to sevoflurane [3, 5]. Compared to propofol, desflurane reduced the mean time to extubation and time to follow commands by 21% and 23%, respectively [2]. However, the time of emergence and extubation between propofol-based total intravenous anesthesia (TIVA) via target-controlled infusion (TCI) system and desflurane are controversial [6].

Besides the use of anesthesia agents, many factors contribute to faster post-anesthesia recovery and extubation. Studies have suggested that intraoperative bispectral index (BIS) monitoring can reduce anesthetic use and recovery times [7, 8]. In addition, inadvertent perioperative hypothermia also impacted recovery quality of general anesthesia by influencing the kinetics and action of various anesthetic and paralyzing agents [9]. The longer anesthesia time, the higher the likelihood the patient would experience hypothermia [10]. Actively warming patients has been demonstrated to offer good conditions for early tracheal extubation [11].

Considering the multiple factors affecting the early extubation, the aim of this study was to explore whether desflurane-based anesthesia combined with BIS monitoring and active warming in lengthy abdominal surgery could reduce the extubation time, improve the quality of post-anesthesia recovery, and satisfaction of surgeons and OR members.

Methods

Study design

This study was a prospective randomized controlled trial with two parallel arms undertaken in West China Hospital of Sichuan University, China. The ethics committee of our institution approved the study protocol. All patients provided written informed consent before inclusion. Randomization was performed using a computer-generated randomization sequence and allocation concealment was maintained until the time of anesthesia induction by using opaque, numbered and sealed envelopes. The trial was prospectively registered at Chictr.org.cn (ID ChiCTR-INR-17013333).

Inclusion and exclusion criteria

Patients were eligible for participation if they met the following criteria: elective abdominal surgery (surgical time > 3 h and < 5 h) and older than 40 years of age. Exclusion criteria were as follows: combined propofol and desflurane anesthesia, combined sevoflurane and desflurane anesthesia, no postanesthesia care unit (PACU) stay, and failure to extubate. Patients who are participating in other interventional studies are also ineligible.

Experimental protocol

Patients who met the enrollment criteria were randomized 1:1 to either the desflurane (DES) or the control group. General anesthesia was induced with midazolam 0.05 mg kg^{-1}, sufentanil 0.3–0.5 $\mu g{\cdot}kg^{-1}$, propofol 1.5–2 mg kg^{-1} and cisatracurium 0.15 mg kg^{-1}. The trachea was intubated with an appropriately sized tracheal tube (Mallinckrodt, COVIDIEN, Mexico). Patients were ventilated with the Datex Ohmeda ventilator (Aestiva/5 Compact Plus, Datex-Ohmeda, Freiburg, Germany) by using volume-controlled ventilation and with an inspired oxygen fraction of 0.6 and a peak inspiratory pressure ≤ 30 cmH_2O. The ventilation rate was adjusted to maintain end-tidal carbon dioxide partial pressure between 35 and 45 mmHg.

In the DES group, anesthesia was maintained with desflurane, continuous infusion of remifentanil 0.1–0.2 $\mu g{\cdot}kg^{-1}{\cdot}min^{-1}$, and repetitive bolus injection of cisatracurium and sufentanil as required throughout the procedure. Maintenance of the effective desflurane concentrations was adjusted according depth of anesthesia monitored by BIS (Aspect Medical Systems, Newton, MA, USA). Patient temperature was maintained by forced-air warming blanket (setting temperature 38 °C) or warming infusion (setting temperature 37 °C) to avoid nasopharyngeal temperature lower than 36 °C.

In the control group, the only absolute criterion was no desflurane inhalation during the procedure. Anesthesia was maintained with propofol, sevoflurane, or both, and the concentrations were adjusted according BIS or clinical signs. Repeated dose of cisatracurium, sufentanil and continuous infusion of remifentanil 0.1–0.2 $\mu g{\cdot}kg^{-1}{\cdot}min^{-1}$ were prescribed throughout the procedure. Unlike the DES group, the usage of BIS monitoring and warming were not mandatory and decided by anesthesia care providers.

At the end of the operation, desflurane, sevoflurane or propofol and remifentanil were discontinued, and the lungs were ventilated with 100% oxygen at a fresh gas flow of 8 L/min. Reversal of neuromuscular block was achieved by administrating neostigmine (0.04 mg/kg) with atropine (0.02 mg/kg) once spontaneous breathing returned. After the patient regained consciousness, with spontaneous and smooth respiration, the endotracheal tube was removed and the patient was transferred to the PACU for further care.

Outcomes

The following times were calculated: 1) extubation time: completion of surgery to extubation; 2) eye opening time: completion of surgery to patients' eye opening; 3) time to respond on command: completion of surgery to the time when patients can respond on command to squeeze fingers; 4) surgical time: incision to surgical completion and application of dressing; 5) anesthesia time: initiation of anesthesia to extubation; 6) exit from OR time: extubation to exit for OR; 7) total OR time: arrival in the OR to departure from the OR; 8) ACT: the combination of anesthesia induction time, extubation time and exit from OR time; 9) PACU length of stay (LOS): time from arrival in the PACU to meeting the PACU discharge criteria (post anesthesia recovery score ≥ 9 according activity, respiration, circulation, consciousness and color) [12]. Also, the anesthetist and surgeon satisfaction and the incidence of prolonged extubation were recorded. The anesthetist was asked to express the satisfaction with the anesthesia type while the surgeon judged the turnover time of each procedure scored on a scale from 1 to 5 (1 = poor to 5 = excellent). Prolonged extubation is defined as an extubation time equal to or longer than 15 min [5].

Statistical analysis

We hypothesized that desflurane would cause a 25% reduction of extubation time compared with that in the control group. At 90% power and significance at the two-sided 5% level, this required a sample size of 60 subjects (30 per group), which we increased by 33% to accommodate withdrawal or missing data points. All analyses were performed by an independent expert unaware of the allocated treatment groups.

Data are expressed as mean ± standard deviation (SD) or number (percentage). Comparisons between the two groups were performed using unequal-variance student t test for continuous variables. Chi-square or Fisher exact tests were used as appropriate for categorical variable comparisons between groups. Multivariable linear regression analyses were performed to assess the association between variables contributed to prolonged extubation. Results were considered statistically significant at a P value less than 0.05. Statistical analyses were performed using statistical software SPSS 17.0.

Results

Characteristics of the study population

A total of 218 patients undergoing abdominal surgery were recruited. Among them, 80 were included and randomly assigned to the DES group ($n = 40$) or the control group ($n = 40$). After randomization, 10 patients were excluded and 35 patients (DES) vs. 35 patients (control) were included for final analysis (Fig. 1). No significant difference was found between two groups in terms of baseline characteristics. In the control group, sixteen patients received warming, nine received BIS monitoring and two received both (Table 1).

Comparison of postoperative recovery between the DES group and the control group

Patients from the DES group were found to have shorter time to extubation, eye opening, and respond on command than patients from the control group (extubation, 8.8 ± 8.5 vs 14.7 ± 13.7 min, $P = 0.035$; eye opening, 8.4 ± 8.6 vs 14.4 ± 13.4 min, $P = 0.028$; responds on command, 8.2 ± 8.5 vs 14.4 ± 13.0 min, $P = 0.022$). Additionally, the ACT in the DES group was significantly shorter than that in the control group (23.8 ± 11.4 vs 32.7 ± 15.4 min, $P = 0.009$). There was no significant difference found in the PACU LOS, incidence of prolonged extubation, and surgeon and anesthetist satisfaction between two groups (Table 2).

Multivariable linear regressions

The result of multivariable linear regressions comparing prolonged extubation time between several variants in all patients is shown in Table 3. Age, gender, body mass index (BMI) and group were factors that contribute to extubation time. The results showed that patients with younger age, female, lower BMI and non-DES anesthesia regimen have longer extubation time.

Discussion

The turnover time and ACT are of particular interest to anesthetists and surgeons, and are affected most by anesthetic agents and anesthesia care during surgery. In this randomized trial, we investigated the effects of desflurane-based anesthesia regimen including BIS monitoring and warming on early postoperative recovery in lengthy abdominal surgery. It was observed that desflurane anesthesia regimen when combined with BIS monitoring and warming is associated with reduced extubation time, eye opening time, response on command time, and ACT in lengthy abdominal surgery. However, the PACU LOS was similar between the two groups.

The results of previous studies comparing the extubation time of desflurane with propofol-based TIVA or sevoflurane have been controversial. For the studies

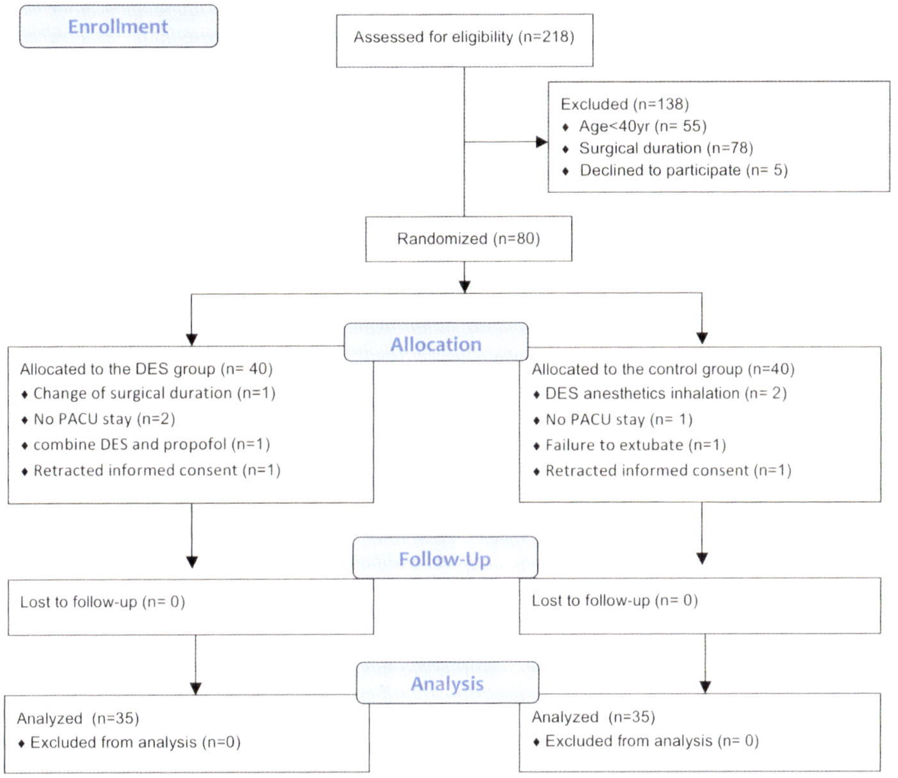

Fig. 1 Flow chart

comparing the desflurane with sevoflurane, most observed a more rapid recovery from desflurane [4, 13, 14], whereas others comparing desflurane with TIVA found no superiority of desflurane [1, 15, 16]. Sevoflurane and desflurane are both widely used inhalation anesthetics, while desflurane has been shown to be associated with shorter emergence time and earlier recovery time in several studies [14]. Desflurane is characterized by a lower solubility coefficient than sevoflurane, particularly after long–duration surgeries [13, 14, 17]. With regards to the studies comparing desflurane and propofol, a recent meta-analysis found desflurane reduced the extubation time by 21% [2]. However, two observational studies found the use of TIVA with TCI system is more effective than desflurane in reducing ACT [1, 18]. In our study, anesthesia agents for the control group were administered as both propofol or sevoflurane according to the anesthetic care providers, i.e., propofol (9 patients), sevoflurane (10 patients), or combined propofol with sevoflurane (16 patients). Hence, our findings suggest that desflurane anesthesia significantly reduces extubation time (average by 5.9 min or 40%) relative to non-desflurane anesthesia.

One factor to be addressed was that the faster postoperative recovery in the DES group was attributed to not only desflurane but also the BIS monitoring and warming. A recent meta-analysis has shown that the use of monitoring with BIS reduced extubation time, orientation time and PACU LOS [19]. Also, warming to prevent perioperative hypothermia has been reported to reduce the extubation time and improve outcomes in the elderly during lengthy surgery [20]. However, it is worth mentioning that the anesthesia care made by the treating anesthetists in the control group was optional. Therefore, a crossover of treatment between two groups concerning the use of warming and BIS monitoring was observed. In the control group, 66% of patients received at least one of these two measures (i.e. sixteen patients received warming, nine received BIS monitoring and two received both). Consequently, it is rational to assume that the BIS monitoring and warming are widely accepted measures to improve anesthesia care.

The result of multivariable linear regressions showed that patients with younger age, female, lower BMI and non-DES anesthesia regimen resulted in prolonged extubation time, which contradicted previous studies [1, 16, 21, 22]. Lai et al. reported that older age, male, higher BMI, and longer anesthesia time contribute to slower emergence in open major upper abdominal surgery [1]. Chan et al demonstrated that surgical time greater than 210 min and older age, contributed to prolonged extubation for open

Table 1 Baseline patient characteristics

Characteristics	DES ($n = 35$)	Control ($n = 35$)	P value
Age (yr)	57.5 ± 10.3	56.2 ± 11.6	0.62
ASA II/III	28/7	27/8	0.77
Gender (M/F)	19/16	24/11	0.22
Body mass index (kg/m^2)	21.85 ± 2.55	22.68 ± 3.03	0.23
Surgical procedure			
stomach	10 (28.6%)	8 (22.9%)	0.77
liver	11 (31.4%)	15 (42.8%)	0.32
pancreas	3 (8.6%)	5 (14.3%)	0.45
colorectum	11 (31.4%)	7 (20%)	0.27
Anesthesia procedure			
warming	35 (100%)	16 (45.7%)	0.0001
depth of anesthesia monitoring	35 (100%)	9 (20%)	0.0001
both	35 (100%)	2 (5.7%)	0.0001
Agents during anesthesia			
desflurane	35 (100%)	0 (0%)	0.001
TIVA	0 (0%)	9 (26%)	0.001
sevoflurane	0 (0%)	10(28%)	0.001
sevoflurane+propofol	0 (0%)	16 (46%)	0.001
sufentanil, μg	37.8 ± 7.1	38.8 ± 8.9	0.64
remifentanil, μg	1399 ± 441	1466 ± 494	0.55
cisatracurium, mg	23.7 ± 5.1	24.2 ± 6.0	0.71

Dichotomous data are presented as number (%); continuous data are presented as mean (standard deviation). No significant difference was found between the two groups

colorectal surgery [22]. The difference may be caused by sufficiently homogeneity in terms of patient population. First, the patients of Lai and Chan et al. were older than those in our study (68 yrs. and 65 yrs. vs. 57 yrs). Also, we excluded the patients with age younger than 40 years instead of 18 years, and the mosre narrow yet older age range might weaken the relevance between older age and prolonged extubation. Second, the patients' BMI of Lai and Chan et al. studies were slightly higher than those in our study

Table 2 Operating room time measurements between DES and control group

Items	DES Group ($n = 35$)	Control Group ($n = 35$)	P value
Extubation time, min	8.8 ± 8.5	14.7 ± 13.7	0.035
Eye opening time, min	8.4 ± 8.6	14.4 ± 13.4	0.028
Time to respond on command, min	8.2 ± 8.5	14.4 ± 13.0	0.022
Anesthesia-controlled time, min	23.8 ± 11.4	32.7 ± 15.4	0.009
Exit From OR after extubation, min	10.6 ± 8.0	11.0 ± 7.3	0.835
Anesthesia induction time, min	6.1 ± 2.4	7.5 ± 4.7	0.132
Surgical time, min	216.2 ± 45.8	221.4 ± 60.2	0.69
Anesthesia time, min	261.2 ± 48.7	262.5 ± 63.2	0.92
Total OR time, min	293.6 ± 50.5	315.5 ± 78.1	0.17
PACU LOS, min	84.0 ± 34.0	92.1 ± 33.4	0.34
Prolonged extubation (≥15 min)	6 (17.1%)	9 (25.7%)	0.38
Anesthetist satisfaction	4.71 ± 0.67	4.54 ± 0.82	0.21
surgeon satisfaction	4.86 ± 0.43	4.71 ± 0.52	0.34

Data are shown as mean ± standard deviation or number (percentage). *DES* desflurane, *OR* operation room, *PACU* postanesthesia care unit, *LOS* length of stay, *SD* standard deviation

Table 3 Multivariable linear regression analyses of variables associated with extubation time

	β	95% CI	*P* value
Age	−0.249	(−0.470, −0.028)	0.001
Gender	−6.369	(−11.19, −1.540)	0.028
BMI	−1.063	(−1.947, − 0.178)	0.019
Group	8.541	(3.768, 13.31)	0.001
Surgery time	0.06	(−0.106, 0.226)	0.474
Anesthesia time	−0.026	(−0.183, 0.131)	0.742

β, difference between each variables using extubation time as dependent variable. *Gender* Female 0, Male 1; *Group* The DES group 0, the control group 1; *BMI* Body mass index, *CI* Confidence interval. *P* value< 0.05 were considered significant

(24.5 kg/m^2 and 23.9 kg/m^2 vs. 22.3 kg/m^2), although the patients involved were both Asian. In the current study, the average extubation time of eight underweight patients (BMI < 18.5 kg/m^2, average 17.33 kg/m^2) were 20 min and that of seven overweight patients (BMI > 25 kg/m^2, average 26.88 kg/m^2) were 8 min, and consequently, the multivariable linear regressions showed a negative correlation between BMI and extubation time. Similarly, Suemitsu et al.. reported a longer extubation time of underweight patients compared with normal-weight patients (25.3 min vs. 22.7 min) [23]. Lee et al reported the "obesity paradox" applies to colorectal cancer, as indicated by decreased hospital LOS of overweight patients and increased hospital LOS of underweight patients [24]. Meyerhardt et al. demonstrated that weight loss after colorectal cancer-diagnosis was associated with worse cancer-specific mortality and overall mortality [25]. In current study, 64 of 70 (91%) patients were cancer patients and majority of them were complicated with weight loss after cancer-diagnosis. Although it is well known that obesity increases the risk of prolonged extubation, few studies investigated the relationship between being underweight and early recovery in the operating room which further studies are needed. Moreover, we showed that neither surgical time and anesthesia time contribute to prolonged extubation, which might be due to the relative small sample size and restrictive surgery duration of 3 to 5 h.

There are several limitations to the present study. First, the sample size was relatively small, which may cause a potential selection bias. Second, although the data collector and analyzer were blinded, the anesthesia care providers were not blinded. Also, the anesthesia providers involved have different clinical experience levels, which might increase the risk of bias as the proficiency of the anesthesiologist can influence the extubation time. Third, there is the crossover of treatment between two groups. Also, BIS and body temperature were monitored to keep them in the normal range in the DES group only while the data were not recorded or compared between two groups. All of them might underestimate the effect of the desflurane regimen.

Conclusions

In conclusion, desflurane anesthesia combined with BIS monitoring and warming was shown to be associated with earlier postoperative recovery in lengthy abdominal surgery when compared to non-desflurane anesthesia and standard practice. This can be an alternative used to contribute to faster turnover time and improved OR efficiency in clinical practice.

Abbreviations

ACT: Anesthesia-controlled time; BIS: Bispectral index; BMI: Body mass index; DES: Desflurane; LOS: Length of stay; OR: Operating room; PACU: Postanesthesia care unit; SD: Standard deviation; TCI: Target-controlled infusion; TIVA: Total intravenous anesthesia

Acknowledgements

We thank the general anesthesiology team in West China Hospital for their continued support, the patients and staff at the Department of General Surgery for their assistance throughout this study. We also thank Taylor Sawyer for proofreading our written paper.

Funding

This work was supported by Scientific research funding of West China Hospital (No. 339140192).

Authors' contributions

HY planned the study. HY, LZ and YM conducted the study. HY and YM took part in the data analysis. HY, HY and LZ took responsibility for the study writing and editing. All authors read and approved the final manuscript.

Competing interests

The authors declare that theye have no competing interest.

Author details

[1]Department of Anesthesiology, West China Hospital of Sichuan University, Chengdu 610041, People's Republic of China. [2]Department of Anesthesiology, China-Japan Friendship Hospital, Beijing 100029, People's Republic of China.

References

1. Lai HC, Chan SM, Lu CH, Wong CS, Cherng CH, Wu ZF. Planning for operating room efficiency and faster anesthesia wake-up time in open major upper abdominal surgery. Medicine. 2017;96(7):e6148.
2. Wachtel RE, Dexter F, Epstein RH, Ledolter J. Meta-analysis of desflurane and propofol average times and variability in times to extubation and following commands. Can J Anaesth. 2011;58(8):714–24.
3. Dexter F, Bayman EO, Epstein RH. Statistical modeling of average and variability of time to extubation for meta-analysis comparing desflurane to sevoflurane. Anesth Analg. 2010;110(2):570–80.
4. Gokcek E, Kaydu A, Akdemir MS, Akil F, Akinci IO. Early postoperative recovery after intracranial surgical procedures. Comparison of the effects of sevoflurane and desflurane. Acta cirurgica brasileira. 2016;31(9):638–44.
5. Agoliati A, Dexter F, Lok J, Masursky D, Sarwar MF, Stuart SB, Bayman EO, Epstein RH. Meta-analysis of average and variability of time to extubation comparing isoflurane with desflurane or isoflurane with sevoflurane. Anesth Analg. 2010;110(5):1433–9.
6. Lai H-C, Chan S-M, Lin B-F, Lin T-C, Huang G-S, Wu Z-F. Analysis of anesthesia-controlled operating room time after propofol-based total intravenous anesthesia compared with desflurane anesthesia in gynecologic laparoscopic surgery: a retrospective study. J Med Sci. 2015;35(4):157.
7. Luginbuhl M, Wuthrich S, Petersen-Felix S, Zbinden AM, Schnider TW. Different benefit of bispectal index (BIS) in desflurane and propofol anesthesia. Acta Anaesthesiol Scand. 2003;47(2):165–73.
8. Punjasawadwong Y, Phongchiewboon A, Bunchungmongkol N. Bispectral index for improving anaesthetic delivery and postoperative recovery. Cochrane Database Syst Rev. 2014;6:CD003843.
9. Doufas AG. Consequences of inadvertent perioperative hypothermia. Best Pract Res Clin Anaesthesiol. 2003;17(4):535–49.
10. Yi J, Lei Y, Xu S, Si Y, Li S, Xia Z, Shi Y, Gu X, Yu J, Xu G, et al. Intraoperative hypothermia and its clinical outcomes in patients undergoing general anesthesia: national study in China. PLoS One. 2017;12(6):e0177221.
11. Vanni SM, Braz JR, Modolo NS, Amorim RB, Rodrigues GR Jr. Preoperative combined with intraoperative skin-surface warming avoids hypothermia caused by general anesthesia and surgery. J Clin Anesth. 2003;15(2):119–25.
12. Heavner JE, Kaye AD, Lin BK, King T. Recovery of elderly patients from two or more hours of desflurane or sevoflurane anaesthesia. Br J Anaesth. 2003; 91(4):502–6.
13. Chen G, Zhou Y, Shi Q, Zhou H. Comparison of early recovery and cognitive function after desflurane and sevoflurane anaesthesia in elderly patients: a meta-analysis of randomized controlled trials. J Int Med Res. 2015;43(5):619–28.
14. Singh PM, Borle A, McGavin J, Trikha A, Sinha A. Comparison of the recovery profile between Desflurane and sevoflurane in patients undergoing bariatric surgery-a meta-analysis of randomized controlled trials. Obes Surg. 2017; 27(11):3031–9.
15. Lu CH, Yeh CC, Huang YS, Lee MS, Hsieh CB, Cherng CH, Wu ZF. Hemodynamic and biochemical changes in liver transplantation: a retrospective comparison of desflurane and total intravenous anesthesia by target-controlled infusion under auditory evoked potential guide. Acta Anaesthesiol Taiwanica : Off J Taiwan Soc Anesthesiol. 2014;52(1):6–12.
16. Wu ZF, Jian GS, Lee MS, Lin C, Chen YF, Chen YW, Huang YS, Cherng CH, Lu CH. An analysis of anesthesia-controlled operating room time after propofol-based total intravenous anesthesia compared with desflurane anesthesia in ophthalmic surgery: a retrospective study. Anesth Analg. 2014; 119(6):1393–406.
17. Jakobsson J. Desflurane: a clinical update of a third-generation inhaled anaesthetic. Acta Anaesthesiol Scand. 2012;56(4):420–32.
18. Lu CH, Wu ZF, Lin BF, Lee MS, Lin C, Huang YS, Huang YH. Faster extubation time with more stable hemodynamics during extubation and shorter total surgical suite time after propofol-based total intravenous anesthesia compared with desflurane anesthesia in lengthy lumbar spine surgery. J Neurosurg Spine. 2015;24(2):268–74.
19. Oliveira CR, Bernardo WM, Nunes VM. Benefit of general anesthesia monitored by bispectral index compared with monitoring guided only by clinical parameters. systematic review and meta-analysis. Brazilian J Anesthesiol (Elsevier). 2017;67(1):72–84.
20. Ma H, Lai B, Dong S, Li X, Cui Y, Sun Q, Liu W, Jiang W, Xu F, Lv H, et al. Warming infusion improves perioperative outcomes of elderly patients who underwent bilateral hip replacement. Medicine. 2017;96(13):e6490.
21. Chan SM, Lee MS, Lu CH, Cherng CH, Huang YS, Yeh CC, Kuo CY, Wu ZF. Confounding factors to predict the awakening effect-site concentration of propofol in target-controlled infusion based on propofol and fentanyl anesthesia. PLoS One. 2015;10(5):e0124343.
22. Chan WH, Lee MS, Lin C, Wu CC, Lai HC, Chan SM, Lu CH, Cherng CH, Wu ZF. Comparison of anesthesia-controlled operating room time between Propofol-based Total intravenous anesthesia and Desflurane anesthesia in open colorectal surgery: a retrospective study. PLoS One. 2016;11(10):e0165407.
23. Suemitsu R, Sakoguchi T, Morikawa K, Yamaguchi M, Tanaka H, Takeo S. Effect of body mass index on perioperative complications in thoracic surgery. Asian Cardiovasc Thorac Ann. 2008;16(6):463–7.
24. Lee S. The obesity paradox in colorectal Cancer surgery: an analysis of Korean healthcare big data, 2012-2013. Nutr Cancer. 2017;69(2):248–53.
25. Meyerhardt JA, Kroenke CH, Prado CM, Kwan ML, Castillo A, Weltzien E, Cespedes Feliciano EM, Xiao J, Caan BJ. Association of Weight Change after colorectal Cancer diagnosis and outcomes in the Kaiser Permanente northern California population. Cancer Epidemiol, Biomarkers Prev: Publi Am Assoc Cancer Res, cosponsored by the Am Soc Prev Oncol. 2017;26(1):30–7.

5

A comparison of two hyperangulated video laryngoscope blades to direct laryngoscopy in a simulated infant airway: a bicentric, comparative, randomized manikin study

Marc Kriege*, Nina Pirlich, Thomas Ott, Eva Wittenmeier and Frank Dette

Abstract

Background: In infants, securing the airway is time-critical because of anatomical and physiological differences related to airway management in children less than 1 year old. The aim of this study was to compare the time to ventilation using two different hyperangulated video laryngoscope blades with the time to ventilation via conventional direct laryngoscopy in a normal airway [NA] and in a simulated difficult airway [DA].

Methods: This study was a comparative, bicentric, open-label, randomized controlled evaluation. An infant high-fidelity simulator (SimBaby™; Laerdal® Medical, Stavanger, Norway) was used, and two scenarios were proposed, as follows: NA and DA evoked with tongue edema and cervical collar. After theoretical and practical briefing, each participant compared in the two airway scenarios the novel King Vision™ Pediatric aBlade (KV) (Ambu® A/S, Bad Nauheim, Germany) video laryngoscope and the C-MAC™ D-blade Ped (DB) (Karl Storz® SE & Co. KG, Tuttlingen, Germany) video laryngoscope to conventional laryngoscopy using the Miller Blade (MiB) and the Macintosh Blade (MaB) in a random sequence.

Results: Eighty physicians (65 AN and 15 PCCM staff) were included. In the NA scenario, the median [IQR] time to successful time to ventilation (TTV) was significantly shorter for the KV at 13 s [12–15 s] than for the MaB at 14.5 s [13–16 s], DB at 14.5 s [13–16] and MiB at 16 s [14–19] ($p < 0.001$). In DA, the KV also shortened TTV to 14 s [13–16], whereas TTV was 23 s with the MaB [20–26], 19 s with the DB [16–21], and 27 s with the MiB [22–31] ($p < 0.001$). There were no differences in first-pass intubation success rates (FPAs) between hyperangulated blades and direct laryngoscopes in NA. In DA, the hyperangulated blades enabled 92 (DB) to 100% (KV) FPAs compared with 65 (MiB) to 76% (MaB) for conventional laryngoscopy ($p < 0.001$).

Conclusion: Video laryngoscopes with hyperangulated blades were associated with shorter TTV in normal and difficult infant airway situations. The higher FPAs of hyperangulated blades in DA may avoid desaturations and decrease adverse events in pediatric airway management.

Keywords: Infant, Airway, Intratracheal intubation, Video laryngoscopy, Pediatric

* Correspondence: makriege@uni-mainz.de
Department of Anesthesiology, University Medical Center of the Johannes Gutenberg-University, Langenbeckstraße 1, 55131 Mainz, Germany

Background

Securing a pediatric airway is a critical skill for the anesthesiologist and pediatric intensive care physician [1]. Problems in airway management can lead to severe hypoxemia and are associated with prolonged mechanical ventilation in pediatric intensive care units (PICUs) [2]. Infants are significantly different from older children or adults with regard to their anatomical and physiological characteristics. The major anatomical differences in infants are large occiputs, larger tongues relative to their pharyngeal space, omega-shaped floppy epiglottises, and, most significantly, more cranially located larynges. Furthermore, the ranges of pathological processes typically seen in the pediatric population present unique anatomical or functional difficulties in airway management [3]. Consecutively, anesthesiologists and pediatric critical care medicine choose different airway tools to provide safe and effective control of the airway. Physiological differences include limited pulmonary reserve due to hemodynamic and respiratory compensation and urgent situations necessitating tracheal intubation place infants at increased physiological risk for adverse events. To optimize the time required for successful tracheal intubation during elective and urgent airway management, physicians can choose between direct or indirect laryngoscopy using the video laryngoscopy technique. Direct laryngoscopy requires alignment of the oropharyngeal-laryngeal axes, and these differences restrict optimal visualization of the glottis. The management of a difficult airway in infants with a weight of less than 10 kg has always been a challenge [4]. Fortunately, an unanticipated difficult airway is extremely rare in infants; however, the overall incidence of difficult laryngoscopy (Cormack & Lehane Class ≥ III) is significantly higher in patients < 12 months of age (4.7% vs. 0.7%) than in older children [1, 4].

Over the last 10 years, several studies have shown that video laryngoscopy is useful in pediatric anesthesia and critical care medicine [5, 6]. In contrast to conventional direct laryngoscopy, the video laryngoscopy technique enables visualization of the glottis without alignment of the oropharyngeal-laryngeal axes. The video laryngoscope blade offers field of vision of laryngeal structures similar to a Macintosh or Miller blade and provides 15- to 30-degree views to 60- to 90-degree views when used with a hyperangulated blade. Lifting the tongue and laryngeal structures using the direct laryngoscope may require a force up to approximately 1.5–3.0 kg [7]; in contrast, the force required when using a video laryngoscope with a hyperangulated blade design is only 0.4–1.3 kg, as measured in adult patients [7]. These advantages yield a smaller upward lifting force with less neck movement and alleviate stimulation of the oropharyngeal structures during laryngoscopy [7]. Selection of an adequate blade type may provide advantages of visualization of the glottis, higher first-pass intubation success rate (FPA) and optimization of the time to successful ventilation. The use of hyperangulated blades and conventional laryngoscope blades has not been extensively compared in pediatric patients to date, and such studies have been limited to a few small trials using these devices in normal pediatric airways in children aged approximately less than 1 year of age [6–8].

We designed a randomized controlled study involving a normal airway (NA) and simulated difficult airway (DA) with an infant high-fidelity simulator. We aimed to compare the performance of the novel King Vision™ Pediatric aBlade (KV) to that of the C-MAC™ D-Blade Ped (DB), both of which use hyperangulated video laryngoscopy blades, and two types of conventional direct laryngoscopes. The purpose of this study was to evaluate whether KV and DB can improve the time to successful ventilation over that achieved using conventional laryngoscopy in a simulated infant airway. As secondary endpoints, we collected the time to view, time to tracheal tube placement, FPA, glottis visualization and degree of ease or difficulty of tracheal intubation based on the Likert scale. We hypothesized that the use of hyperangulated blades would be superior to direct laryngoscopy in terms of time to ventilation in NA and DA.

Methods

This study was a bicentric (Department of Anesthesiology and Center of Pediatric and Adolescent Medicine), comparative randomized study performed in the operating room (OR) and PICU at a tertiary university hospital. The ethics committee of the Medical Association of the state of Rhineland Palatine (Germany) approved this study (Registration No.: 837.384.14 (9623)). The order of devices used by the participants was determined by computerized randomization (http://www.random.org).

Selection of participants

In all, 65 anesthesiologists and 15 practitioners of pediatric critical care medicine (PCCM) participated in this study. All were previously trained with video laryngoscopes and had sufficient clinical experience using the device (Table 1), with a lack of experience with the novel King Vision Pediatric aBlade. The expertise of the participating anesthesiologists and faculty of pediatric critical care medicine (PCCM) ranged from "beginner" (residents) to "expert" (consultants). Each physician was introduced to the study devices separately via a standardized instructional video by the principal investigator. After an introduction including handling as well the specifics of the device in NA, an intubation procedure was demonstrated. Subsequently, the participants had five attempts with each device to familiarize themselves and obtain an adequate learning curve (8) with each device before the evaluation started. As there were four devices

Table 1 Demographics and level of experience

Provider analysis	Anesthesiologists ($n = 65$)	PCCM staff ($n = 15$)	p-value
Status			
Residents/Fellows/Consultants	51/11/3	6/4/5	0.33
Experience			
Practice experience (months)	30 (6–180 [21–48])	36 (6–180 [24–96])	0.43
Airway management in children (< 6 y)			
< 10 applications	6 (9%)	0	0.22
< 50 applications	21 (32%)	4 (26%)	0.67
< 100 applications	26 (40%)	2 (13%)	0.05
> 100 applications	12 (19%)	9 (61%)	0.001
Airway management in infants/children			
< 5 kg	37 (57%)	15 (100%)	0.001
< 10 kg	62 (95%)	15 (100%)	0.39
< 20 kg	65 (100%)	15 (100%)	1.0
Experience in VL (applications)			
< 10	0	0	
< 25	4 (6%)	5 (33%)	0.002
< 50	13 (22%)	1 (7%)	0.22
> 100	48 (74%)	9 (60%)	0.28
Experience in DL (applications)			
< 50	0	0	
< 100	2 (3%)	4 (27%)	0.001
< 500	15 (23%)	5 (33%)	0.4
< 1000	31 (48%)	4 (27%)	0.14
> 1000	17 (26%)	2 (13%)	0.29

Data are presented as medians (range [IQR] and absolute numbers (proportion)

and two airway scenarios, each participant performed a total of 8 intubations.

Setting and interventions

The study was conducted in an antechamber of the OR PICU with the high-fidelity simulator positioned at the head of a stretcher (Fig. 1). Participants were allowed to adjust the stretcher or chair to a comfortable height. A pediatric high-fidelity Simulator SimBaby™ (Laerdal® Medical, Stavanger, Norway) was built to resemble a 65-cm long healthy baby and was capable of creating easy and difficult airway situations. The SimBaby is a realistic airway that includes crying and gurgling sounds, cyanosis, tongue edema, pharyngeal obstruction, chest excursion, and breath sounds. In relation to a real infant derived from growth charts of the WHO, this length corresponds to that of a 6- to 8-month-old infant when looking at the area between the 5th and 95th growth percentile [9, 10]. We evaluated the devices under two airway scenarios as follows: (i) normal (NA) and (ii) difficult intubation condition (DA) created through tongue edema and a cervical collar (Fig. 1; SAM® Splint™, SAM Medical Products, Wilsonville, OR, USA) to

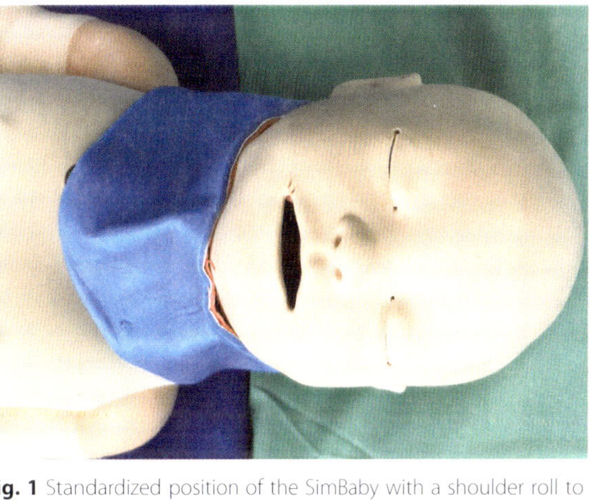

Fig. 1 Standardized position of the SimBaby with a shoulder roll to elevate the shoulders and a soft donut to stabilize the head

reduce the mouth opening from 2.6 mm before to 1.5 mm after adjustment of an extrication collar to inhibit neck movement.

We chose to compare two video laryngoscopes that use a hyperangulated blade with two conventional direct laryngoscopes. The King Vision™ Pediatric aBlade (KV) (Ambu® GmbH, Bad Nauheim, Germany) is a novel video laryngoscope used in a clinical setting in pediatric patients and has not been evaluated under various airway conditions. The KV has a built-in video screen and is available in three pediatric sizes, #1–3 (≥ #2 has a channeled and standard disposable blade with a 37.8-degree angulated blade). In this study, we used a KV #2 standard blade (Fig. 2). The C-MAC™ D-Blade Ped (DB) (Karl Storz®, Tuttlingen, Germany) is a compact system consisting of a monitor, electronic module and interchangeable video laryngoscope blade. The DB has an increased curvature with a 75-degree blade angulation. The manufacturer recommends its use in infants or small children weighing 9.8 to 22 kg. The DB was specifically developed to manage anatomically difficult airway conditions such as those encountered in Down syndrome or Pierre-Robin syndrome. The conventional direct laryngoscopes included the Miller straight blade #1 (MiB) and a Macintosh curved blade #2 (MaB) with a standard laryngoscope handle for pediatric patients. All sizes of the blades were tested prior to the study; they are shown in Fig. 2.

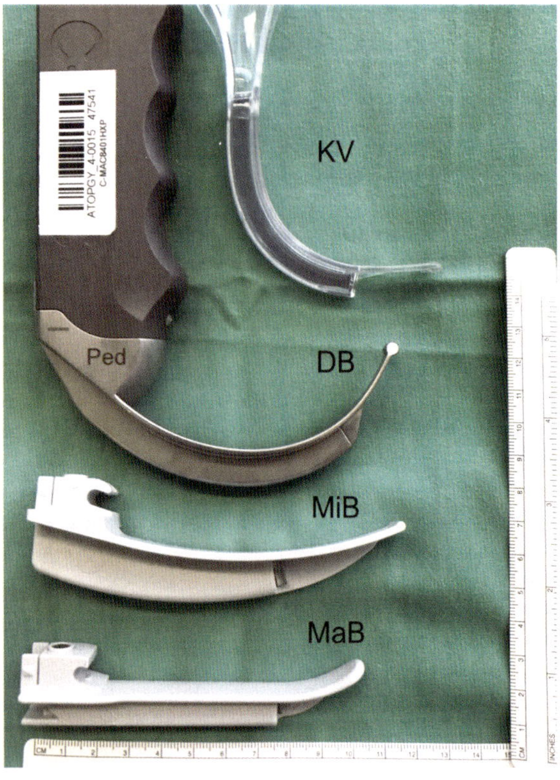

Fig. 2 In order from top to bottom: KV #2 standard blade, DB, Macintosh blade #2 and Miller blade #1

Per the recommendation of the manufacturer of the SimBaby, all intubations were performed with a 3.5-mm internal diameter cuffed endotracheal tube (ET). During intubation using one of the video laryngoscopes, a malleable stylet was inserted into the ET, which was angulated into a hockey-stick shape (distal end of ET angulated 90°). When using a conventional direct laryngoscope, the rigidity of the ET was provided by a malleable stylet (Mallinckrodt® satin slip, 2.6 mm). The SimBaby was placed in a standardized position, and a shoulder roll and a soft donut-shaped foam headrest were used to support the head in all cases (Fig. 1).

Methods of measurements

Demographic analysis was collected for all participants concerning the clinical level of airway management experience with children ≤5 years of age, the time since their most recent intubation in each age group (newborns, infants, and small children) and experience with video laryngoscopy (VL) and conventional direct laryngoscopy in real patients [11]. Experienced users (consultants) were defined as those with performance experience in pediatric tracheal intubation exceeding 100 infants. Inexperienced users were defined as those with experience in less than 100 tracheal intubations in infants [6].

The time interval between the blades passing the gums to confirmation of the best glottic view was recorded as the time to best view (TTBV). The participant announced the Cormack & Lehane Classification (C&L) and the percentage of glottic opening (POGO) score once the best glottic exposure was obtained [12, 13]. External laryngeal manipulations (ELMs) [14], such as the BURP (backwards, upwards and rightwards pressure) maneuver, can be applied to improve the view of the glottis to achieve a C&L I or II. The time to place (TTP) the ET was defined as the time when the first black mark on the ET was threaded between the vocal cords. The time to ventilation (TTV) in seconds (s) was defined as the time from when the blade tip passed the gums of the SimBaby to the point of confirmation of the first visible chest rise of the simulator. Time was measured using a stopwatch. Study personnel were positioned on the right site of the SimBaby.

Failed intubation was defined as follows: a) an elapsed intubation time of more than 40 s in accordance with the current recommendations and in the time period of previously published data [6, 15, 16]; b) failed tracheal placement of the ET (i.e., esophageal); and c) removal of the device/repositioning from the oral cavity without advancing the ET. If the first attempt failed, the provider made a second laryngoscopy attempt with the same device. A total of two laryngoscopy attempts were allowed.

If DL failed, the clinician changed to a prescribed rescue technique with KV. If VL failed after two attempts, the clinician was advised to proceed with DL. The limitation of two intubation attempts and choice of an alternative technique has been recommended in several studies and was chosen in accordance with clinical standards [17]. After each intubation, the physician was asked to rate the degree of difficulty of intubation using a 5-point Likert scale (1 = very easy to 5 = very difficult) for each blade [18].

Outcome measures

Our primary study objective was to determine whether there was a difference in TTV, demonstrated by bilateral lung inflation of the manikin with positive pressure via bag-valve ventilation, between the KV and the DB, MiB and MaB. Secondary outcomes were the TTBV and the TTP, visualization of laryngeal structures using the C&L Classification and the POGO score, FPA, the use of ELMs and the degree of difficulty.

Statistical analysis

A statistical analysis of the data was subsequently undertaken. The Shapiro-Wilk test was used to test the assumption of normal distribution ($p > 0.1$). Normally distributed data are presented as the means (SD) and were analyzed using an independent t-test for unequal variances. Non-normally distributed interval and ordinal data are reported as medians (interquartile range [IQR]); results were compared among groups using the Wilcoxon-Mann-Whitney test. Categorical variables are presented as counts; results were evaluated using the chi-square test. TTV data were compared between groups using the log-rank test. All recorded data were documented using a controlled case report form. Devices were randomized to treatment groups using the GraphPad QuickCalcs Web site: http://www.graphpad.com/quickcalcs/randmenu (accessed January 2015). GraphPad Prism (Vers. 6.0 for MAC; GraphPad Software, San Diego, CA, USA) was used for all statistical analyses. Differences in TTV were considered statistically significant if the *p*-value was less than 0.05.

Results

Characteristics of study subjects

From July to August 2017, a total of 80 physicians (anesthesiologists, $n = 65$; PCCM staff, $n = 15$) eligible to participate in this study were included (Table 1). These 80 participants performed 640 intubation attempts. The faculty of PCCM had more experience in airway management in children less than 6 years of age ($p < 0.001$) and infants with a weight < 5 kg ($p < 0.001$). Otherwise, the anesthesiologists had more overall experience in VL (> 25 applications prior to the study; $p = 0.002$) and DL (> 100 applications prior the study; $p < 0.001$) compared to PCCM. Demographics and the level of experience of all subjects are presented in Table 1.

Main results

For the primary outcome, the median duration for TTV was shorter for the KV at 13 s [12–15] than for the MaB at 14.5 s [13–16], the DB at 14.5 s [13–16], and the MiB at 16 s [14–19]; $p < 0.001$) in the NA scenario. In DA, the KV similarly significantly shortened TTV to 14 s [13–16], whereas TTV was 23 s using the MaB [20–26], 19 s using the DB [16–21], and 27 s using the MiB [22–31]; $p < 0.001$). Both groups (anesthesiologists and PCCM staff) were similar with respect to the time required to obtain TTV with all four devices ($p = 0.5$). Furthermore, TTV was shorter when using the hyperangulated blades for both experienced and inexperienced physicians in the NA/DA scenario ($p < 0.001$). Study outcomes for the various blades are outlined in Table 2 for the NA scenario and in Table 3 for the DA scenario. Figure 3 present the Kaplan-Meier plots of the TTV with all four devices in the NA scenario and DA scenario, respectively.

The overall intubation success rates were higher for the KV 80/80 (100%) in both airway scenarios performed by anesthesiologists and PCCM staff ($p < 0.001$). The number of attempts with each device is listed in Table 2 for the NA scenario and in Table 3 for the DA scenario. A proportion of 8/320 (2.5%) participants had > 2 failed attempts with the DL in the DA scenario ($p < 0.001$). All were successfully intubated with the KV. The reason for a second attempt in the NA scenario was a timeout > 40 s in 3/320 (0.9%) cases, and the reasons for a second attempt in the DA scenario were a timeout in 28/320 (9%) of the trials and removal of the blade in 17/320 (5.3%) of the trials ($p = 0.1$).

In the NA scenario, we obtained a better view of the glottis with hyperangulated blades than with the conventional laryngoscopes ($p < 0.001$). In the DA scenario, the KV enabled a better glottic view (C&L I) 80/80 (100%) than was achieved using the DB 74/80 (92%), MaB 61/80 (76%) and MiB 52/80 (65%; $p < 0.001$).

After completing the series of simulated intubations, the participants rated the degree of difficulty in the NA scenario as lower for the DB than for the MaB, MiB and KV ($p < 0.001$). In contrast, in the DA scenario, the KV was rated easier to use compared with the DB, MaB or MiB ($p = 0.001$).

Discussion

In the present study, a shorter TTV was achieved using video laryngoscopes with a hyperangulated blade in a group of 640 intubation attempts in an infant DA. In particular, TTV was shorter in both airway situations when applying the novel KV. The FPA, visualization of

Table 2 Study results by laryngoscope blades in the NA scenario

					p-values of Pairwise Differences				
Outcomes	MaB	DB	MiB	KV	DB vs. MaB	DB vs. MiB	KV vs. MaB	KV vs. MiB	KV vs. DB
Time [a] Sequences (s)									
TTBV	5.5 [5–7]	5 [4–6.5]	7 [5–8]	5 [3.5–6]	0.01	< 0.001	< 0.001	< 0.001	0.02
TTP	10.25 [9–11.5]	10 [9–11.5]	12 [10–14.5]	9.5 [8.5–11]	0.85	< 0.001	0.02	< 0.001	0.002
TTV	14.5 [13–16]	14.5 [13–16]	16 [14–19]	13 [12–15]	0.75	0.001	0.002	< 0.001	< 0.001
No. attempts[b]									
1st	80/80 (100%)	79/80 (98%)	78/80 (97%)	80/80 (100%)	0.31	0.56	> 0.99	0.15	0.31
2nd	0	1/80 (2%)	2/80 (3%)	0		0.56			
Failed	0	0	0	0					
Glottic view									
C&L 1/2/3[b]	67/13/0	78/2/0	57/23/0	79/1/0	0.007	< 0.001	0.001	< 0.001	> 0.99
POGO (%)[a]	90 [90–100]	100 [100]	95 [80–100]	100 [100]	< 0.001	< 0.001	< 0.001	< 0.001	0.84
ELM[b]	5/80 (6%)	0/80 (0%)	11/80 (14%)	1/80 (1%)	0.02	< 0.001	0.09	0.002	0.32
BURP	0	0	6/11 (54%)	1/1 (100%)					
Neck extension	5/5 (100%)	0	7/11 (63%)	0					
Degree of [a] difficulty (1–5)	1 [1–2]	1 [1–1]	1 [1–2]	1 [1–2]	0.44	< 0.001	< 0.001	0.9	< 0.001

[a]Medians and [IQR] are shown. Pairwise differences among devices were evaluated using the signed-rank test
[b]Absolute numbers (proportion) are shown. Pairwise differences among devices were evaluated using the chi-square test

the glottis and subjective assessment in this comparative study were superior to those of conventional direct laryngoscopy. To date, only one study compared the novel KV with the traditional MiB in elective surgeries performed in children < 2 y of age [19]. This study is one of the first studies comparing the KV with another hyperangulated blade and direct laryngoscopy in a simulated infant airway.

The demographics of the participants were comparable to those in other studies investigating the MaB, DB or MiB [6, 10, 12, 20–22] in pediatric airways. In contrast to other studies comparing experienced and inexperienced practitioners [6, 9–11, 19, 21, 22], this study demonstrated that TTV was similar between the groups. However, in this study, there were no institutional differences in FPA or TTV among the blades or airway scenarios. This likely

Table 3 Study results by laryngoscope blades in the DA scenario

					p-values of Pairwise Differences				
Outcomes	MaB	DB	MiB	KV	DB vs. MaB	DB vs. MiB	KV vs. MaB	KV vs. MiB	KV vs. DB
Time [a] Sequences (s)									
TTBV	11 [8.5–14]	8 [6.5–9]	13.5 [9–15.5]	6.5 [5–7]	< 0.001	< 0.001	< 0.001	< 0.001	< 0.001
TTP	17.5 [15–20]	14 [11–15]	20.5 [16.5–24]	10 [9.5–12]	< 0.001	< 0.001	< 0.001	< 0.001	< 0.001
TTV	23 20–26]	19 [16–21]	27 [22–31]	14 [13–16]	< 0.001	< 0.001	< 0.001	< 0.001	< 0.001
No. attempts[b]									
1st	61/80 (76%)	74/80 (92%)	52/80 (65%)	80/80 (100%)	0.004	< 0.001	< 0.001	< 0.001	0.01
2nd	16/80 (20%)	6/80 (8%)	23/80 (29%)	0	0.29	0.26			
Failed	3/80 (4%)	0	5/80 (6%)	0					
Glottic view									
C&L 1/2/3[b]	19/60/1	61/19/0	7/70/3	77/3/0	< 0.001	< 0.001	< 0.001	< 0.001	< 0.001
POGO (%)[a]	40 [30–60]	90 [90–100]	40 [30–60]	100 [90–100]	< 0.001	< 0.001	< 0.001	< 0.001	< 0.001
ELM[b]	3/80 (4%)	1/80 (1%)	4/80 (5%)	0/80 (0%)	0.31	0.17	0.08	0.04	0.32
BURP	0	0	0	0					
Neck extension	3/3 (100%)	1/1 (100%)	4/4 (100%)						
Degree of[a] difficulty (1–5)	2 [2–3]	1 [1–2]	3 [3–3]	1 [1–1]	< 0.001	< 0.001	< 0.001	< 0.001	0.001

[a]Medians and [IQR] are shown. Pairwise differences among devices were evaluated using the signed-rank test
[b]Absolute numbers (proportion) are shown. Pairwise differences among devices were evaluated using the chi-square test

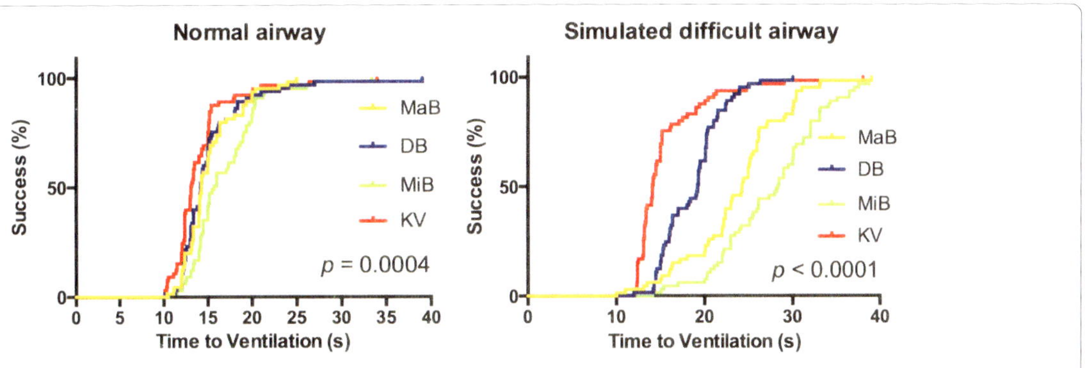

Fig. 3 Kaplan-Meier plots of the time to ventilation for all four devices in (left) the normal airway situation and (right) a difficult airway

reflects a familiarity with the direct and video laryngoscopy techniques. Furthermore, every participant only had 5 attempts with the novel KV or DB prior to the study.

A number of new devices have been introduced to facilitate tracheal intubation in pediatric patients with normal and difficult airways, with reports describing varying success rates and experience in pediatric airway management [10, 11, 22]. In these experiments, manikins were used in various simulation scenarios, including tracheal intubation. In addition to their use in training, they have also been used in various clinical research projects to demonstrate the efficacy of one device over another. SimBaby™ has been used to teach clinical and decision-making skills while mimicking patient care scenarios [9, 10, 23]. Tracheal intubation using a video laryngoscope might be easier to learn than conventional direct laryngoscopy [8, 9]. The success rates vary considerably, and the proportion of patients in whom the glottic opening can be visualized but the ET cannot be inserted into the trachea is high [20, 21, 24]. Several study results have noted that intubation time is longer when using a video laryngoscope with a hyperangulated blade [6, 9, 21]. Surprisingly, TTV was significantly shorter for the novel KV blade in the NA (1.5 s) and DA (13 s) scenarios than for the other devices, which influence the occurrence of systemic complications (e.g., hypoxemia). TTV was longer for the MaB and MiB than for hyperangulated blades relative to the results of studies looking at two conventional blades; however, the values were within the range of published data [6, 9, 23]. In two studies that evaluated children aged < 2 years of age, TTV was shorter for the MiB [19, 22] than for the KV. Straight blades are often recommended for use in neonates and infants to lift the relatively large and floppy epiglottis [22]. These blades avoid a situation in which the hyoid bone cannot be displaced forward and the epiglottis continues to obstruct a view of the larynx. In summary, a good laryngeal view with the intubating device did not equate with ease of intubation. Otherwise, a curved MaB provides more room in the oropharynx to maneuver the ET. The time to visualization of the glottis and successful ventilation were also comparable to the results reported in another study [19]. However, the measurements differed between these studies in which the practitioner took hold of the handle of the device until the cuff of the ET was inflated [9, 20, 24] or until confirmation of the first inflection of the end-tidal capnogram on the anesthesia respirator [6, 19]. In three studies, time measurement stopped when successful lung expansion occurred [9, 20, 21]. All intubations were successfully performed using the KV on FPAs. Comparing TTV or FPA using the DB is difficult because the literature is quite sparse with regard to the use of the DB in pediatric patients or in a suitable manikin. The prolonged intubation time and lower success rate in DB and conventional direct laryngoscopes might be explained as follows: first, the anterior view angle of 55 degrees achieved using the KV differs from the half-moon shaped DB (embedded optical lens with aperture angle of 80°); furthermore, the length differs between the two hyperangulated blades (KV, 7 cm vs. DB, 10 cm). Additionally, it is generally thought that the position of the head has an influence on the laryngeal view [6]. We used a standardized position for the SimBaby in which a shoulder roll elevated the shoulders and a small donut was used to support the head. The goal was to align the oral, pharyngeal, and tracheal axes to facilitate tracheal intubation.

As a secondary outcome, visualization of the glottis was significantly easier with VL in both scenarios. These data are consistent with previously published data in simulated pediatric patients in whom the laryngeal view was found to be better with VL [6, 9, 10, 19]. In contrast to other studies comparing hyperangulated blades with DL, we found a higher FPA and overall success rate when using the KV or DB [11, 15, 21]. In fact, a higher FPA was shown with the KV in DA compared to the first study that evaluated the KV in a normal pediatric airway [19]. These data are comparable to that in study with manikins where the results vary with the operator's prior experience and familiarity with the equipment, institutional preferences, and how well the manikin simulates a real patient [11, 20]. Finally, when considering the number of ELMs, which were slightly higher with direct laryngoscopy, and the participants' subjective difficulty scores, which were also higher for these devices, our data agree with those reported on the management of adult patients [18]. This fact may be derived from the absence of prior experience of the subjects with the DB and KV or with the specific characteristics of the conventional blades and the infant manikin's airway anatomy.

Study limitations

Our study has several limitations. First, we used two different conventional and two different hyperangulated video laryngoscopy blade sizes in an infant simulator. We cannot assure that the simulated clinical conditions truly reproduce the real patient's conditions. Second, this comparative study might have been limited by the heterogeneous experiences of the providers (e.g., experiences in anesthesia practice or pediatric critical care medicine and in video laryngoscopy techniques). We feel, however, that this approach is more clinically relevant than are the study results, reflecting the experience of a small team of anesthesiologists who are highly skilled in airway management. Because of the design of this study, the protocol did not allow blinding of the operators using the different blades. We compared the KV and DB video laryngoscopes (hyperangulated blades) to two direct laryngoscopes with the straight blade (MiB) or a curved blade (MaB) that are used by practitioners with various levels of experience with the four devices. We chose to compare a curved to a straight standard laryngoscope for the following reasons: The most popular curved Macintosh blade differs in angulation from the KV/DB blade, and comparing the two represents a comparison of three disparate blades. Traditional clinical teaching suggests that the straight blade offers the best glottis exposure in infants because of the higher location of the glottis. The lower peak lifting force on the base of the tongue using the hyperangulated video laryngoscopy blades might be associated with a higher success rate in the SimBaby. Finally, TTV might differ in real infants because the retroglossal airspace volume of the SimBaby is 5.3 ± 0.4 cm^3 instead of the 1.9 ± 0.8 cm^3 observed in infants [25].

Conclusion

Use of a hyperangulated video laryngoscope blade, especially the novel King Vision Pediatric aBlade, resulted in significantly faster TTVs and higher FPAs than were achieved using conventional direct laryngoscope blades. VL in general may offer promise for intubation of NA and DA in children. The use of a hyperangulated blade optimizes the placement of ETs by anesthesiologists and PCCM staff in simulated infant airways. Further studies aimed at comparing various video-based laryngoscope blade designs used in infants or children with different types of airway problems will be useful for assisting anesthesiologists and pediatricians in selecting the most appropriate device to use in each individual clinical scenario.

Acknowledgements

The authors wish to thank Gerrit Toenges (Institute of Medical Biostatistics, Epidemiology and Informatics, University Medical Center of the Johannes Gutenberg University, Mainz, Germany).

Authors' contributions

All studies were performed at the Department of Anesthesiology and Center of Pediatric and Adolescent Medicine, University Medical Center of the Johannes Gutenberg-University Mainz, Germany. MK designed and conducted the study, analyzed the data, and wrote the manuscript. TO, EW, NP and FD helped design the study and revised the manuscript. All authors read and approved the final manuscript.

Competing interests

Neither the Department of Anesthesiology of the University Medical Center of the Johannes Gutenberg University-Mainz, Germany nor any of its employees received any compensation for this work. No funding or competing interests are declared. None of the authors have financial interests, received honoraria or provided paid expert testimony. None of the authors have any personal relationships with people or organizations that could inappropriately influence this work. The authors alone are responsible for the content and writing of the paper.

References

1. Graciano AL, Tamburro R, Thompson AE, et al. Incidence and associated factors of difficult tracheal intubations in pediatric ICUs: a report from National Emergency Airway Registry for children: NEAR4KIDS. Intensive Care Med. 2014;40:1659–69.
2. Nishisaki A, Turner DA, Brown CA 3rd, Walls RM, Nadkarni VM. A National Emergency Airway Registry for children: landscape of tracheal intubation in 15 PICUs. Crit Care Med. 2013;41:874–85.
3. Kerrey BT, Rinderknecht AS, Geis GL, Nigrovic LE, Mittiga MR. Rapid sequence intubation for pediatric emergency patients: higher frequency of failed attempts and adverse effects found by video review. Ann Emerg Med. 2012;60:251–9.
4. Fiadjoe JE, Nishisaki A, Jagannathan N, et al. Airway management complications in children with difficult tracheal intubation from the pediatric difficult intubation (PeDI) registry: a prospective cohort analysis. Lancet Respir Med. 2016;4:37–48.
5. Heinrich S, Birkholz T, Ihmsen H, et al. Incidence and predictors of difficult laryngoscopy in 11,219 pediatric anesthesia procedures. Paediatr Anaesth. 2012;22:729–36.
6. Fiadjoe JE, Gurnaney H, Dalesio N, et al. A prospective randomized equivalence trial of the GlideScope cobalt(R) video laryngoscope to traditional direct laryngoscopy in neonates and infants. Anesthesiology. 2012;116:622–8.
7. Russel T, Khan S, Elman R et al. Measurement of forces applied during Macintosh direct laryngoscopy compared with Glidescope® videolaryngoscopy. Anaesthesia. 2012;67:626–31.
8. Orliaguet GA, Blot RM, Bourdaud N, et al. Endotracheal intubation with the GlideScope®, the Airtraq®, the McGrath® videolaryngoscope and direct laryngoscopy: a comparative study on an infant manikin Ann Fran Anesth Reanim. 2013;32:844–9.
9. Fonte M, Oulego-Erroz I, Nadkarni L, et al. A randomized comparison of the GlideScope videolaryngoscope to the standard laryngoscopy for intubation by pediatric residents in simulated easy and difficult infant airway scenarios. Pediatr Emerg Care. 2011;27:398–402.

10. Donoghue AJ, Ades AM, Nishisaki A, Deutsch ES. Videolaryngoscopy versus direct laryngoscopy in simulated pediatric intubation. Ann Emerg Med. 2013;61:271–7.
11. Balaban O, Hakim M, Walia H, et al. A comparison of direct laryngoscopy and Videolaryngoscopy for endotracheal intubation by inexperienced users: a pediatric manikin study. Pediatr Emerg Care. 2017;18:477–85.
12. Levitan RM, Ochroch EA, Kush S, Shofer FS, Hollander JE. Assessment of airway visualization: validation of the percentage of glottic opening (POGO) scale. Acad Emerg Med. 1998;5:919–23.
13. Cormack RS, Lehane J. Difficult tracheal intubation in obstetrics. Anaesthesia. 1984;39:1105–11.
14. Vlatten A, Aucoin S, Litz S, Macmanus B, Soder C. A comparison of the STORZ video laryngoscope and standard direct laryngoscopy for intubation in the pediatric airway--a randomized clinical trial. Paediatr Anaesth. 2009;19: 1102–7.
15. Riveros R, Sung W, Sessler DI, et al. Comparison of the Truview PCD and the GlideScope® video laryngoscopes with direct laryngoscopy in pediatric patients: a randomized trial. Can J Anaesth. 2013;60:450–7.
16. Wozniak M, Arnell K, Brown M, et al. The 30 second rule: the effects of prolonged intubation attempts on oxygen saturation and heart rate in preterm infants in the delivery room. Minerva Pediatr. 2016;70:127–32.
17. Lee JH, Turner DA, Kamat P, et al. The number of tracheal intubation attempts matters! A prospective multi-institutional pediatric observational study. BMC pediatrics. 2016;16:58.
18. Weiss M, Schwarz U, Gerber AC. Difficult airway management: comparison of the Bullard laryngoscope with the video-optical intubation stylet. Can J Anaesth. 2000;47:280–4.
19. Jagannathan N, Hajduk J, Sohn L, et al. Randomized equivalence trial of the king vision aBlade videolaryngoscope with the miller direct laryngoscope for routine tracheal intubation in children <2 yr of age. Brit J Anaesth. 2017; 118:932–7.
20. White M, Weale N, Nolan J, Sale S, Bayley G. Comparison of the cobalt Glidescope video laryngoscope with conventional laryngoscopy in simulated normal and difficult infant airways. Paediatr Anaesth. 2009;19:1108–12.
21. Hippard HK, Kalyani G, Olutoye OA, Mann DG, Watcha MF. A comparison of the Truview PCD and the GlideScope cobalt AVL video-laryngoscopes to the miller blade for successfully intubating manikins simulating normal and difficult pediatric airways. Paediatr Anaesth. 2016;26:613–20.
22. Passi Y, Sathyamoorthy M, Lerman J, Heard C, Marino M. Comparison of the laryngoscopy views with the size 1 miller and Macintosh laryngoscope blades lifting the epiglottis or the base of the tongue in infants and children <2 yr of age. Brit J Anesth. 2014;113:869–74.
23. Vlatten A, Aucoin S, Litz S, MacManus B, Soder C. A comparison of bonfils fiberscope-assisted laryngoscopy and standard direct laryngoscopy in simulated difficult pediatric intubation: a manikin study. Paediatr Anaesth. 2010;20:559–65.
24. Platts-Mills TF, Campagne D, Chinnock B, et al. A comparison of GlideScope video laryngoscopy versus direct laryngoscopy intubation in the emergency department. Acad Emerg Med. 2009;16:866–71.
25. Schebesta K, Hüpfl M, Ringl H, et al. A comparison of paediatric airway anatomy with the SimBaby high-fidelity patient simulator. Resuscitation. 2010;82:468–72.

6

Nefopam downregulates autophagy and c-Jun N-terminal kinase activity in the regulation of neuropathic pain development following spinal nerve ligation

Seon-Hee Oh[1], Myung Ha Yoon[2], Kyung Joon Lim[3], Byung Sik Yu[3], In Gook Jee[4] and Ki Tae Jung[3*]

Abstract

Background: Neurodegeneration is associated with changes in basal cellular function due to the dysregulation of autophagy. A recent study introduced the involvement of autophagy during spinal nerve ligation (SNL). Nefopam has shown potential for reducing neuropathic pain, but the underlying mechanisms are unknown. Here, we investigated the effects of nefopam on neuropathic pain development following SNL, focusing on the involvement of autophagy.

Methods: The functional role of nefopam in capsaicin-induced autophagy was assessed by human glioblastoma M059 K cells. The neuropathic pain model was used to determine whether the effect of nefopam on pain control was mediated through autophagy control. Neuropathic pain was induced by L5 and L6 SNL in male rats randomized into three groups: Group S (sham-operated), Group C (received normal saline), and Group E (received nefopam). A behavioral test using a von Frey was examined. Expression changes of autophagy in response to nefopam was analyzed in spinal cord tissues (L4-L6) by immunoblotting and immunohistochemistry.

Results: The paw withdrawal threshold examined on days 3, 5, 7, and 14 post-SNL was significantly higher in Group E than in Group C. SNL increased the levels of microtubule-associated protein 1 light chain 3B (LC3B-1), with concomitant reduction of sequestosome 1 (SQTSM1/p62), compared with Group S, indicating that SNL induced autophagy. These effects were reversed by nefopam injection, and the results were confirmed by immunohistochemistry for LC3-I/II. Furthermore, SNL-mediated JNK activation was markedly decreased following nefopam injection. Hematoxylin and eosin staining on Day 14 post-SNL revealed that SNL caused lymphocyte infiltration and oligodendrocyte localization in the substantia gelatinosa of the dorsal gray horn, which were reduced by nefopam injection.

Conclusion: Collectively, the mode of action of nefopam on neuropathic pain appears to be associated with downregulation of phospho-JNK and autophagy, as well as modulation of the immune response.

Keywords: Autophagy, JNK, Nefopam, Neuropathic pain, Rat

* Correspondence: mdmole@chosun.ac.kr
[3]Department of Anesthesiology and Pain Medicine, School of Medicine, Chosun University, Chosun University Hospital, 365 Pilmun-daero, Dong-gu, Gwangju 61453, South Korea
Full list of author information is available at the end of the article

Background

Neuropathic pain was previously thought to be the consequence of changes in the activity of neuronal systems, immune cells, and immune cell-derived inflammatory cytokines [1]. However, a recent study reported that an imbalance in the autophagic process following nerve injury can lead to changes in basal cell functions closely associated with neurodegeneration [2].

According to Berliocchi et al. [2], completion of basal autophagy and autophagosome turnover are blocked as a consequence of spinal nerve ligation (SNL), and this may be associated with neurodegeneration and the development of neuropathic pain. When programmed cell death is functionally disordered, various apoptotic stimuli activate autophagy and c-Jun N-terminal kinase (JNK), resulting in the induction of autophagic cell death, which can lead to neurodegeneration [3, 4]. JNK activation is closely related to the development of neuropathic pain. Following nerve injury, JNK is rapidly activated primarily in small diameter C-fiber neurons [5, 6]. Furthermore, JNK inhibitors prevent the development of mechanical allodynia after SNL [5, 7]. A recent study on the effects of curcumin also demonstrated the prevention of chronic neuropathic pain by suppression of JNK phosphorylation [8].

Nefopam is a centrally acting analgesic that has similar action to triple neurotransmitter reuptake inhibitors and anticonvulsants. Recently, nefopam has been suggested for the treatment of neuropathic pain because it has analgesic properties [9–13]. Prophylactic administration of nefopam had a preventive effect on the development of neuropathic pain after chronic constriction injury of the sciatic nerve [14]. However, the molecular mechanisms through which nefopam exerts these anti-neuropathic pain effects are not completely understood. Therefore, we investigated the preventive effects of nefopam on the development of neuropathic pain following SNL, focusing on the involvement of autophagy and JNK activation.

Methods

Cell culture and chemicals for in vitro experiments

Human glioblastoma M059 K cells (ATCC® CRL-2365™) were maintained in DMEM (Gibco BRL, Grand Island, NY) supplemented with heat-inactivated 10% fetal bovine serum, 50 μg/ml penicillin, and 50 μg/ml streptomycin at 37 °C in a 5% CO_2–95% air humidified incubator. Capsaicin, SP600125, and thapsigargin were obtained from Sigma (St. Louis, MO) and Calbiochem (La Jolla, CA USA), respectively. Other chemicals used were of the purest grade available from Sigma (St. Louis, MO).

Animal preparation

This study was approved by the Institutional Animal Care and Use Committee of Chonnam National University (CNU IACUC-H-2015-26) and followed the International Association for the Study of Pain guidelines on ethical standards for the investigation of experimental pain in animals [15]. Experiments were performed on male Sprague–Dawley rats (specific pathogen free) weighing 100–120 g. Rats were purchased from Damul Science (Daejeon, Korea). The animals were raised in cages in a temperature-controlled room (20 to 23 °C) with a 12-h light/dark cycle and free access to food and water.

Groups and induction of neuropathic pain

Rats were randomized into three groups (total $n = 36$, $n = 12$ in each group) according to the random numbers generated by a computer. Rats in the sham group (group S) underwent a sham operation without SNL. While, rats in the control and experimental groups (groups C and E) received SNL for the induction of neuropathic pain Groups and induction of neuropathic pain [16, 17]. Experiments were carried out after confirming that the rats had no neurological abnormality. After sevoflurane anesthesia, L5–S2 spine were dissected and the left L5 and L6 spinal nerves were tightly ligated.

Drug administration

Those in group S had just sham operation. Rats in the group C were administered normal saline for 7 days following the SNL procedure. Those in group E were administered 30 mg/kg of nefopam hydrochloride (Acupan®, Pharmbio, Seoul, Korea) intraperitoneally for 3 days immediately following the SNL procedure [13, 14].

Spinal cord sampling

On the 14th day, rats were euthanized by decapitation under sevflurane overdose anesthesia. Then, the spinal cord was isolated by flushing with ice-cold phosphate-buffered saline from the caudal end of the vertebral column. After obtaining the ipsilateral dorsal spinal cord at L4–L6 by a cut in the spinal cord at the midline, the tissue was immediately stored at − 70 °C by liquid nitrogen until homogenization.

Western blotting

Tissue samples were homogenized in a lysis buffer with a Dounce homogenizer, further lysed with RIPA buffer containing protease inhibitor cocktail (Sigma). Cell lysates was quantified for protein content, and separated by SDS-PAGE in 12–15% acrylamide gels, transferred to polyvinylidene difluoride membranes (Millipore, Billerica, MA, USA), and then immunoblotted with corresponding antibodies. Phospho-JNK (#9251), JNK (#9258), mammalian target of rapamycin (mTor, #2972), and phospho-mTor (#2971) were obtained from Cell Signaling (Danvers, MA, USA). Anti-rabbit polyclonal atg8/LC3 antibody (#3868) was obtained from Cell Signaling (Irvine, CA, USA). TNF-α (sc-52,746) and β-actin (sc-70,319) were purchased from Santa Cruz Biotechnology (Santa Cruz, CA, USA).

The bands were visualized using chemiluminescence Western Blotting Detection Reagents (Millipore), and quantified with ImageJ densitometry software (National Institutes of Health, Bethesda, MD).

Immunohistochemistry

After conventional dewaxing and microwave antigen retrieval in 10 mM sodium citrate buffer (pH 6) for 10 min, sections were incubated with microtubule-associated protein 1 light chain (LC3) antibody (1:50) (#3868) overnight at 4 °C. A negative control without primary antibody was performed for each specimen. Endogenous peroxidase activity was prevented by incubating the sections for 15 min in 0.3% H_2O_2. Immunohistochemistry procedures were performed using the Polink-2 AP broad detection kit according to the supplier's protocol (Life Science Division, WA, USA). The slides were counterstained with hematoxylin and mounted with an immunohistomounting medium (Abcam, Cambridge, MA, USA). Histological changes in spinal cord tissues were observed under a microscope (Nikon, TE300, Japan).

Hematoxylin and eosin staining of paraffin-embedded tissues

Spinal cord tissues were cut into approximately 0.5 cm length pieces vertically in the center of L5 and were fixed in neutral buffered formalin, dehydrated, embedded in paraffin, and sectioned. The sections were deparaffinized in xylene, rehydrated in an ethanol gradient, and stained with hematoxylin and eosin (H & E). Pathological changes in spinal cord tissues were observed under an optical microscope (Nikon, TE300, Japan).

Assessment of mechanical allodynia

Mechanical allodynia was assessed by paw withdrawal threshold (PWT) measured with von Frey filaments (Stoelting, Wood Dale, IL, USA). After acclimation in the laboratory environment for 30 min, mechanical stimulation was applied to the plantar surface of the hind paw vertically for 5 s with a series of eight von Frey filaments (0.4, 0.7, 1.2, 2.0, 3.6, 5.5, 8.5, and 15 g). Abrupt withdrawal or flinching of the hind paw were regarded as a positive response and PWT was calculated by the up and down method [18]. The cut-off value was a negative response to 15 g. A series of tests were conducted on the 3rd, 5th, 7th, and 14th day following SNL.

Statistical analysis

Data were expressed as the mean ± standard error of the mean. The results of the behavioral experiments were analyzed by a repeated measures one-way analysis of variance and Scheffe's post-hoc test. The differences between groups were analyzed by t-test. Non-parametric data were analyzed by the Kruskal-Wallis test followed by Scheffe's post-hoc test. Results with p-values < 0.05 were considered statistically significant. A two tailed t test was performed for comparisons of densitometry between the groups.

Results

Nefopam suppressed JNK-mediated autophagy induced by capsaicin

Capsaicin, the pungent ingredient in hot chili peppers, is a selective agonist of transient receptor potential cation channel subfamily V member 1 (TRPV1), which is involved in pain sensation [19]. Capsaicin exposure induced autophagy in M059 K cells, which was confirmed by reduction of p62 (SQTSMI/sequestosome 1), an autophagy adaptor molecule, which was upregulated by nefopam pretreatment. Furthermore, capsaicin exposure induced downregulation of mTor, and that was upregulated by nefopam pretreatment, indicating that nefopam might suppress capsaicin-induced autophagy via mTor activation. Additionally, capsaicin activated the mitogen-activated protein kinase (MAPK) JNK, which was suppressed by pretreatment with nefopam (Fig. 1a). Next, we examined whether JNK activation is involved in autophagy induction in capsaicin-exposed cells. For this purpose, we used a pharmacological JNK inhibitor, SP600125. As expected, pretreatment with SP600125 before adding capsaicin suppressed capsaicin-induced LC3-II, an autophagy marker (Fig. 1b). To further substantiate the inhibitory role of nefopam in JNK-mediated autophagy we performed additional experiment by using a selective endoplasmic reticulum stress inducer, thapsigargin (Tg) in normal kidney cells (MES13E: SV40 MES 13, ATCC® CRL-1927™). Treatment with Tg induced JNK activation and autophagy, which were suppressed by pretreatment with nefopam (Fig. 1c). Collectively, these results indicat that nefopam may suppress autophagy by regulating signaling pathway implicated with mTor and MAPK JNK.

Nefopam reduced mechanical allodynia and lymphocyte infiltration following SNL

Mechanical allodynia was confirmed in all rats from Group C (received normal saline) and Group E (received nefopam) 3 days after the SNL procedure. Rats from Group S (sham-operated) showed no mechanical allodynia ($n = 12$). The PWT was significantly reduced in rats from Groups C and E compared with those in Group S. The PWT of rats from Group E was higher than that of rats from Group C during the observation period ($n = 12$ for each group). However, significant differences were recorded on Day 5 post-SNL (Fig. 2a). These results indicate that nefopam decreased pain sensation induced by SNL.

To observe histopathological changes on Day 14 after surgery, spinal cord tissue sections were subjected to hematoxylin and eosin staining, and histological changes were observed in the dorsal gray matter region (Fig. 2b, I, II, and III, large circles). In sections from Group S, only a small number of lymphocytes were observed (Fig. 2b, IV, small

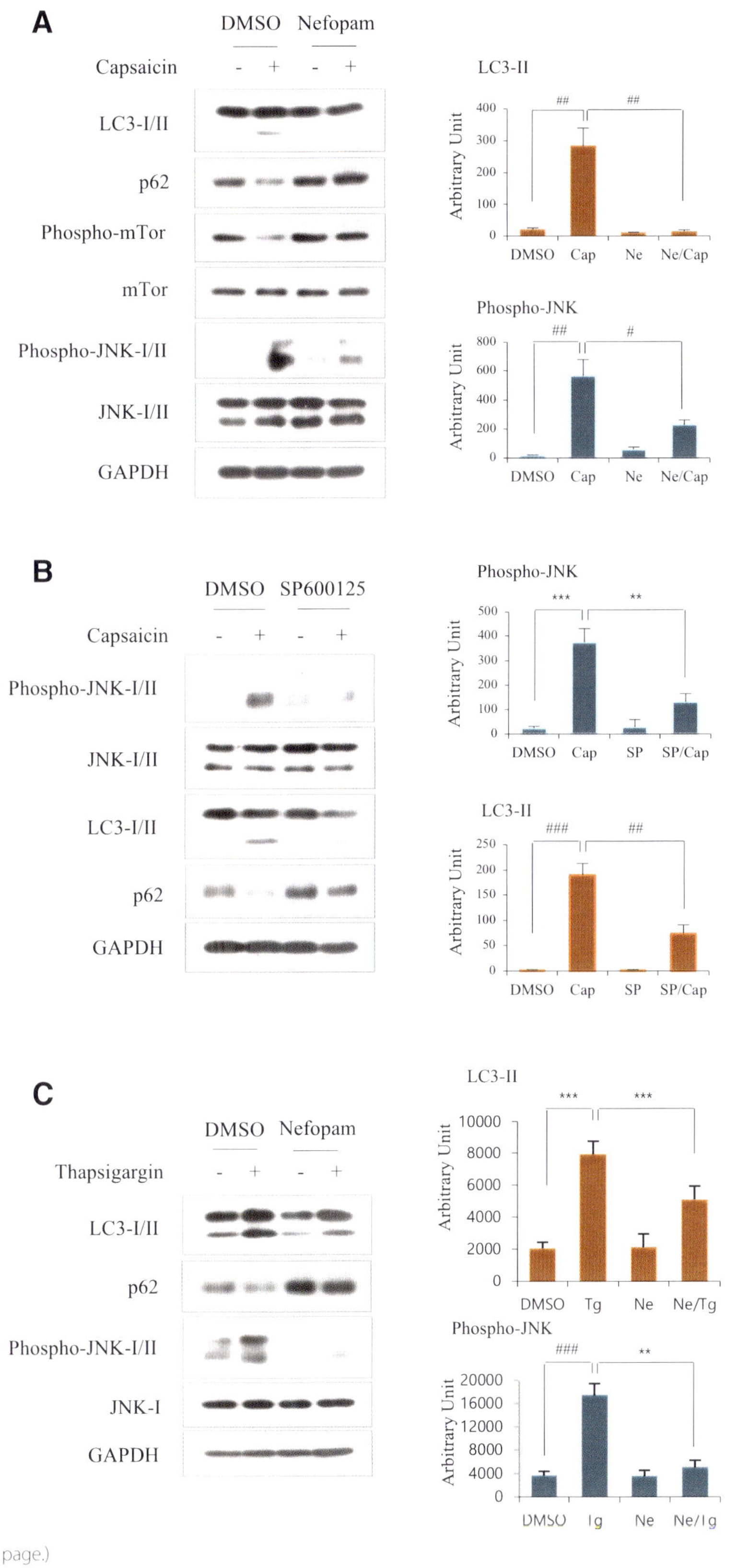

Fig. 1 (See legend on next page.)

(See figure on previous page.)

Fig. 1 Nefopam downregulates capsaicin-induced LC3-II and phospho-JNK in M059 K cells. **a** Cells were pretreated with nefopam (50 μM) and continuously exposed capsaicin (250 μM) for 18 h. Cell lysates were immunoblotted for indicated proteins. **b** M059 K cells were pretreated with SP600125 (10 μM) and continuously exposed capsaicin (250 μM) for 18 h. GAPDH was used as the loading control. **c** Cells were pretreated with nefopam (50 μM) and continuously exposed thapsigargin (Tg, 4 μg/ml) for 18 h. Cell lysates were immunoblotted for indicated proteins. All immunoblot data are representative of at least three independent experiments. Bar graphs show densitometrical analysis for LC3-II and phospho-JNK-II. A two tailed t test was performed for comparisons between groups ($n = 3$). $^{\#}p < 0.01$, $^{\#\#}p < 0.002$, $^{\#\#\#}p < 0.0002$ $^{**}p < 0.005$, $^{***}p < 0.0005$

circles). Normal oligodendrocytes (arrows) with prominent perinuclear halos were also identified. Furthermore, vacuoles containing poorly stained material were observed (Fig. 2, IV, V, and VI, stars). In contrast, tissues from Group C showed lymphocyte infiltration and many oligodendrocytes localized mainly in the substantia gelatinosa of the posterior gray horn (Fig. 2b, V). Tissues from Group E had reduced numbers of lymphocytes and oligodendrocytes compared to those in the SNL group; however, this was still higher than the numbers of these cells in Group S (Fig. 2, VI). Collectively, these data indicate that nefopam suppressed pain-mediated immune responses.

Immunoreactivity of LC3-I/II in spinal cord tissue sections

To examine whether autophagy is involved in the actions of nefopam in pain mitigation, we analyzed the immunoreactivity of LC3-I/II via immunostaining. Cells positive for the LC3-I/II antibody were localized mainly in gray matter across all sections. Strong positive signals were localized in the cell bodies of the neurons residing in the ventral horn. Furthermore, immunoreactivity revealed differences between the dorsal gray horn and the ventral gray horn. We thus compared LC3-I/II immunoreactivity in the dorsal gray matter of the spinal cord ipsilateral with the ligation side. In Group S, the immunoreactivity of LC3-I/II was observed in most cells (polygonal or ovoid) localized in the dorsal gray matter (Fig. 3, I and IV), which was further enhanced in the tissues from Group C (Fig. 3, II and V), but was suppressed by nefopam injection (Fig. 3, III and VI). Antibody diluents, used as a negative control for LC3-I/II, did not exhibit LC3-I/II immunoreactivity (Fig. 3, VII). These results suggest the involvement of LC3-I/II in nefopam action on neuropathic pain.

LC3-I/II expression and JNK activation in nefopam-mediated pain

Our in vitro experiments revealed that the expression of phospho-JNK and LC3-II induced by capsaicin, a pain sensation inducer, were suppressed by nefopam (Fig. 1). We thus investigated the action of nefopam on JNK and autophagy activation with an in vivo experiment. Tumor necrosis factor alpha (TNF-α) is known to play a pivotal role in neuropathic pain [20]. Consistently, SNL resulted in TNF-α production, which was suppressed by nefopam injection. The immunohistochemical staining for LC3-I/II expression was further confirmed by western blot analysis (Fig. 4a), and LC3-I expression was evaluated by densitometry (Fig. 4b). We did not detect membrane-bound LC3-II with the antibodies used. However, on Day 14 post-SNL, we observed an increase in LC3-I with a concomitant decrease in the autophagy adaptor molecule, p62, indicating that autophagy was increased by SNL. Furthermore, SNL-mediated LC3-I levels decreased, and p62 levels increased following nefopam injection (Fig. 4a and c), indicating that SNL-mediated autophagy was inhibited by nefopam.

We then examined MAPK JNK, which is known to be related to neuropathic pain following SNL [7]. SNL resulted in JNK activation compared with rats from Group S, as demonstrated by western blotting with phospho-antibody on Day 14 post-SNL, and JNK was markedly suppressed by nefopam, as evaluated by densitometry (Fig. 4a, d). However, the levels of phospho-JNK in one of the rats demonstrated less change. The level of phospho-JNK in Group S was high, indicating that JNK may play a role at the non-stressed basal level.

Discussion

In the present study, we demonstrated that nefopam injection following SNL downregulated JNK activation and autophagy and increased PWT. To the best of our knowledge, this is the first study to demonstrate the effects of nefopam on the regulation of MAPK JNK activation and autophagy.

Recently, there was a suggestion about the possibility of nefopam in the treatment of neuropathic pain [9], because the analgesic mechanisms of nefopam are related to not only the inhibition of monoamine reuptake but also the inhibition of NMDA receptors [21]. The excitatory neurotransmitter, glutamate, acts via N-methyl-D-aspartate receptors (NMDARs). NMDARs might control the neurochemical axis involved in neuronal function through MAPK activation [22]. When NMDA receptors are stimulated, MAPK is activated by tyrosine phosphorylation [22]. In stressful conditions such as nerve injury, JNK activating Jun transcription factor and the p38 MAPK are stimulated [22]. Previous reports showed that neuropathic pain following SNL may be associated with autophagic activity [2, 23], and neurodegeneration in a results of JNK-mediated autophagic cell death [3, 4]. Therefore, we attempted to determine the role of nefopam in the prevention of

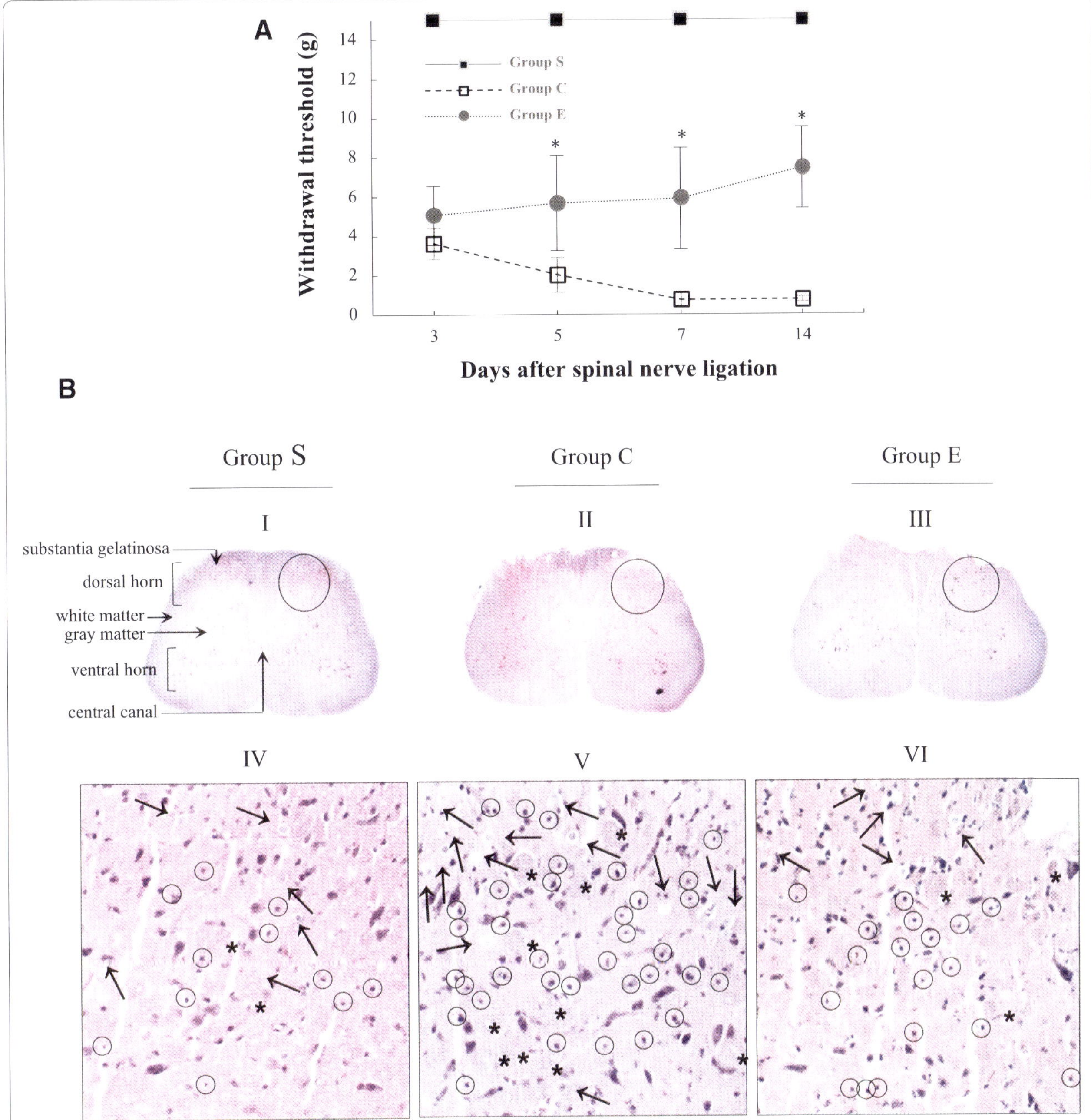

Fig. 2 Mechanical allodynia and histological changes following SNL. **a** Paw withdrawal threshold over time. The paw withdrawal thresholds were observed on the 3rd, 5th, 7th, and 14th day post spinal nerve ligation (SNL). The development of neuropathic pain was confirmed with decreased withdrawal thresholds of the rats from group C and E compared to the group S throughout the observation periods ($p < 0.001$). The withdrawal thresholds are significantly higher in rats from group E than in those from group C from the 5th day post SNL ($p < 0.001$). $^*p < 0.05$ compared with group C. **b** Hematoxylin and eosin staining in the the spinal cord sections. Sections from group S (I, IV) show only a small number of lymphocytes (small circles), normal oligodendrocytes (arrows) with prominent perinuclear halos, and vacuoles containing poorly stained material (stars). Sections from group C (II, V) show lymphocytes infiltration and many oligodendrocytes localized in the substantia gelatinosa of the posterior gray horn. Sections from group E (III, VI) show a reduced number of lymphocytes and oligodendrocytes than those in group C. Group S, Sham-operated; Group C, saline-treated after SNL; Group E, nefopam-treated after SNL. Original magnification, X200. →, Oligodendrocytes; o, Lymphocytes; *, Vacuoles

neuropathic pain development in relation to autophagy and JNK activation.

For this purpose, we conducted the study using M059 K cells which can demonstrate the capsaicin induces autophagy which is involved in pain sensation, firstly [24]. Pain could act as a stress to cells, and a variety of stresses induce autophagy and stress-activated MAPK JNK activation [24]. We used capsaicin, an agonist of the non-selective cation channel

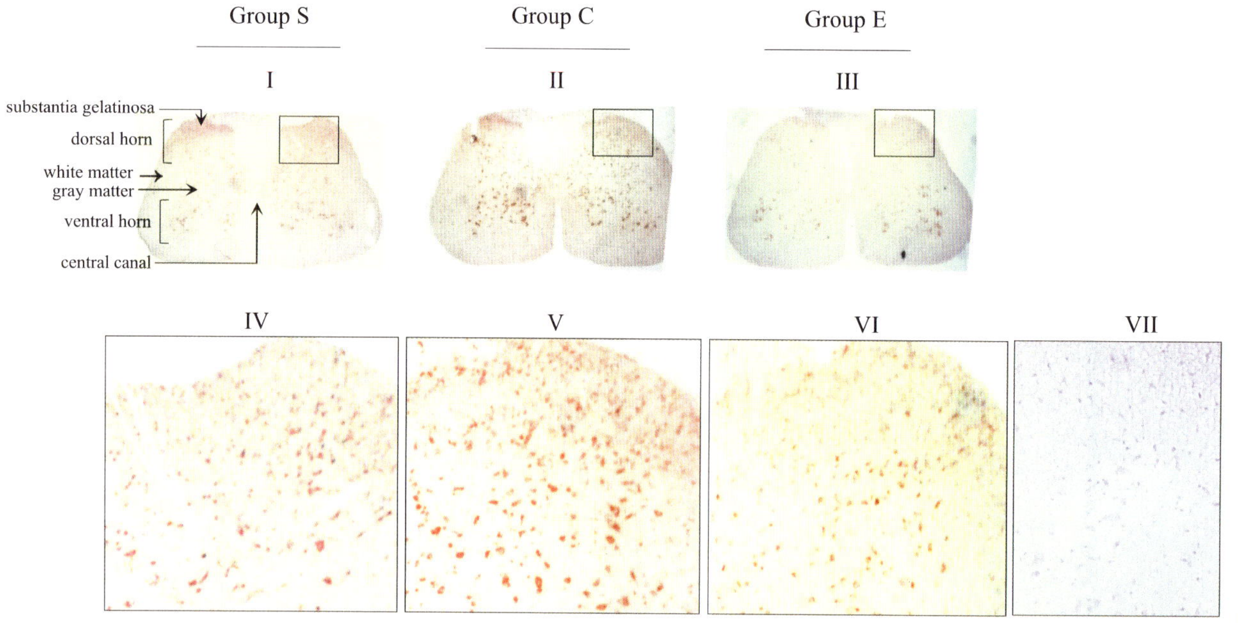

Fig. 3 Immunohistochemical study for LC3-I/II expression in the spinal cord sections. In group S (I, IV), the immunoreactivity of LC3-I/II is visible in most cells (polygonal or ovoid) localized in the dorsal gray matter of ipsilateral spinal cord sections, which is further enhanced in group C (II, V), but suppressed in group E (III, VI). Antibody diluents, used as a negative control for LC3-I/II (VII). Group S, sham-operated; Group C, saline-treated after SNL; Group E, nefopam-treated after SNL. Original magnification, X 200

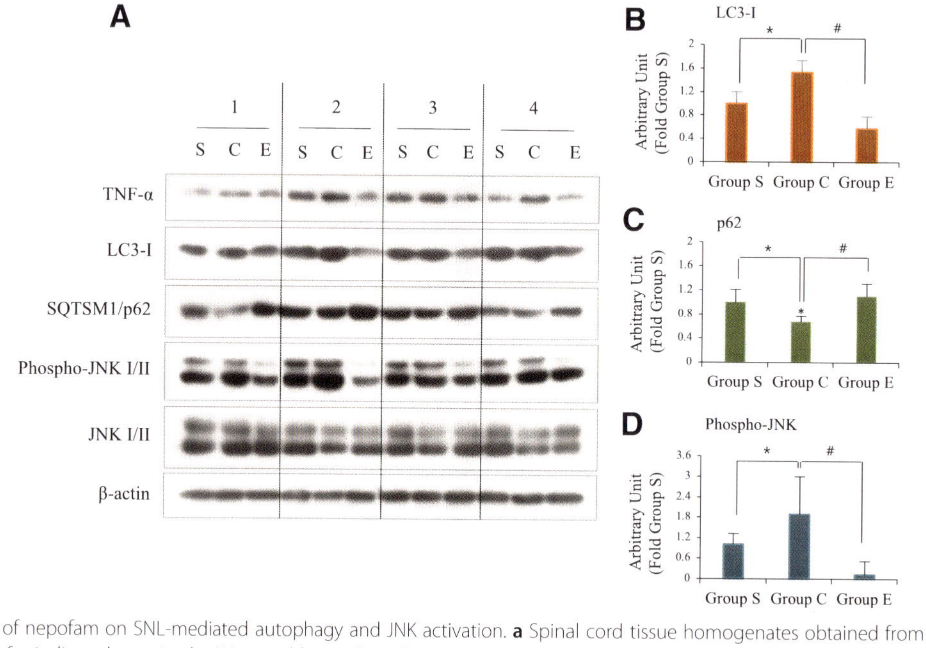

Fig. 4 The effects of nepofam on SNL-mediated autophagy and JNK activation. **a** Spinal cord tissue homogenates obtained from on 14 day after SNL, and analyzed for indicated proteins by Western blot analysis. β-actin was used as the loading control. Group S, sham-operated; Group C, saline-treated after SNL; Group E, nefopam-treated after SNL. **b**-**d** Densitometrical analysis for LC3-I, p62, and phospho-JNK-II. A two tailed t test was performed for comparisons between groups ($n = 4$). * $p < 0.05$, $^{\#}p < 0.01$

TRPV1, which depolarizes cells and leads to a painful sensation when activated [25]. Furthermore, capsaicin is known to induce autophagy via JNK activation [24]. In the present study, we found that capsaicin induced autophagy and mTor inhibition in neuronal blastoma M059 K cells, indicating that capsaicin-induced autophagy might be dependent on mTor pathway, which was inhibited by nefopam. Moreover, capsaicin activated JNK, which was associated with autophagy induction, as determined by a pharmacological inhibitor of JNK. The causative relationship between autophagy and nefopam was tested by using autophagy inducer, Tg; nefopam suppressed Tg-mediated autophagy and JNK activation. Therefore, nefopam may suppress autophagic activation by inhibiting the mTor signaling pathway and JNK. These in vitro data suggested the possibility that pain mitigation by nefopam may depend on JNK-mediated autophagy. Therefore, our present results suggest a possibility that nefopam may act on pain relief via suppression of JNK-mediated autophagy.

Then, the effect of nefopam on the development of neuropathic pain was confirmed in vivo study. Administration of intraperitoneal nefopam (30 mg/kg, 3 days post SNL) increased the withdrawal threshold and downregulated activation of JNK and autophagy. Immunohistochemistry for LC3-I/II, an autophagy marker, revealed that SNL-induced LC3-I/II immunoreactivity decreased following nefopam injection. Strong positive staining was localized in the cell body of the neurons, indicating that the action of nefopam might occur via affecting on function of neuron. Furthermore, a change in the immunoreactivity of LC3-I/II was revealed in the dorsal horn of the gray matter, indicating that autophagy may affect sensory neurons rather than motor neurons. However, our hypothesis requires further clarification. Western blot analysis of spinal cord tissue lysates revealed that SNL activated JNK and autophagy, which were mitigated by nefopam. Therefore, our in vitro results are consistent with previous reports showing that SNL-mediated JNK activation was inhibited by nefopam [5, 6].

Glial cells including oligodendrocytes, astrocytes, and microglia, are known to play important roles in the pathology of neuroinflammation and neuropathic pain [26]. In the present study, histological analysis revealed that the number of oligodendrocytes in the substantia gelatinosa of the dorsal gray horn of rat underwent SNL increased than in sham-operated rats, which reduced by treatment with nefopam, indicating that oligodendrocytes might respond to the peripheral nerve injury. However, less is known about the involvement of oligodendrocytes than astrocytes and microglial cells in neuroinflammation. A recent study demonstrated an important role of oligodendrocyte-derived interleukin (IL)-33 in neuropathic pain [27]. Oligodendrocytes in the spinal cord release IL-33 after chronic constriction injury, and IL-33 acts on IL-33 receptors (ST2) and the IL-1 receptor accessory protein (IL-1RAcP) expressed by endothelial cells, microglia, astrocytes, and neurons. Activation of the receptor complex triggers intracellular molecular signaling pathways such as phosphoinositide-3-kinase–protein kinase B (PI3K-PKB), mTOR, MAPKs (ERK, JNK, and p38), and nuclear factor κB (NF-κB), which are implicated in the production of IL-1β and TNF-α, and in development of neuropathic pain. TNF-α is implicated in the development of pro-inflammatory processes and neuropathic pain after nerve injury [28, 29]. We found that nefopam suppressed SNL-induced TNF-α production. Furthermore, lymphocytes infiltration into the spinal cord response to the SNL was found, indicating that immune responses might be involved in development of neuropathic pain. Indeed, in the spared nerve injury model of peripheral neuropathic pain, T-cell infiltration and activation in the dorsal horn of the spinal cord following peripheral nerve injury contribute to the evolution of neuropathic pain-like hypersensitivity [30]. Therefore, our present results suggest that nefopam may reduce proinflammatory cytokines by inhibiting oligodendrocyte activation and the immune response. However, further research is required to validate these findings.

Although, autophagic responses are known to help cells avoid death by offering an alternative cell-death pathway as a stress adaptation [31], the role of autophagy in the development of neuropathic pain is controversial. Shi et al. [32] reported that miRNAs regulate neuroinflammation and neuropathic pain through controlling autophagy. The level of miR-195 increased after SNL, which leads to change in autophagy and proinflammatory cytokine production in microglia, suggesting that miR-195/autophagy signaling involves in regulating neuroinflammation and neuropathic pain, and offering a new target for therapy of neuropathic pain. Recent report also showed blocking of basal autophagic turnover in the upregulated condition of autophagy after SNL may result in a degenerative pathway through the accumulation of dysfunctional macromolecules and organelles. Berliocchi et al. [2] suggested neuropathic pain after SNL is associated with disruption of autophagy by blocking autophagosome turnover. According to their results, the levels of LC3 and p62 has increased, and this accumulation of p62 represent impairment of normal autophagic process and blockade in the autophagic flux. On the contrary, the LC3-I levels has increased but p62 levels has decreased in our study, which represent increased activity of autophagy, not dysregulation. It is not clear why this discrepancy has developed, but the difference of the timing of harvesting spinal nerve (7 days from SNL vs. 14 days in our study), the species of animal used (mouse vs. SD rat in our study), or the methodology would be the reasons. Even though, autophagic activity inversely correlate with expression levels of p62, but it is not clear how p62 levels correlate with autophagy induction in vivo [33]. Moreover, autophagy may be upregulated as a response for stresses, but there is no clear evidence whether autophagic activity might be transcriptionally upregulated [33]. Because autophagic activity does not only depend on increased LC3-II, as well as on the coordination of regulatory proteins [2], confirmation through independent experiments such as morphologic evaluation is recommended to overcome these potential limitations [33]. In the present study, immunohistochemistry data show that increased autophagic activity by SNL was reduced by nefopam treatment, which was consistent with Western blot data. Suppression of autophagy may protect cells against neuroinflammation and relieve neuropathic pain development.

Based on our in vitro and in vivo studies, we speculate that the inhibitory effect of nefopam on neuropathic pain following SNL might be associated with regulation of the JNK-mediated autophagy signaling by nefopam. Although our present results show a relationship between autophagy and the effects of nefopam, however, it need to be improved the precise mechanisms of nefopam molecular regulation on autophagic processes and proinflammatory cytokines to ensure our hypothesis on the causal relationship between nefopam and autophagy.

Conclusions

In conclusion, SNL increased autophagy and JNK activation, and also increased lymphocyte infiltration into the dorsal gray matter. Consequently, PWT significantly increased and neuropathic pain developed. However, nefopam injection markedly decreased autophagy and JNK activation. Nefopam increased PWT after SNL, and its mode of action appeared to be associated with the downregulation of phospho-JNK and autophagy.

Abbreviations

H & E: Hematoxylin and eosin; IL: Interleukin; IL-1RAcP: IL-1 receptor accessory protein; JNK: C-Jun N-terminal kinase; LC3: Microtubule-associated protein 1 light chain; MAPK: Mitogen-activated protein kinase; mTor: Mammalian target of rapamycin; NMDARs: N-methyl-D-aspartate receptors; PI3K-PKB: Phosphoinositide-3-kinase–protein kinase B; PWT: Paw withdrawal threshold; SNL: Spinal nerve ligation; TNF-α: Tumor necrosis factor alpha; TRPV1: Transient receptor potential cation channel subfamily V member 1

Acknowledgements

The present study was supported by grants from the Clinical Medicine Research Institute at Chosun University Hospital, (2014).

Funding

The present study was supported by grants from the Clinical Medicine Research Institute at Chosun University Hospital, (2014).

Authors' contributions

SH participated in study design, and performed cell culture and chemicals for in vitro experiments, spinal cord sampling, western blotting, HE staining, immunohistochemistry, statistical analysis, and was a major contributor in writing the manuscript. MH participated in study design, neuropathic pain modeling, and performed drug administration, assessment of mechanical allodynia, spinal cord sampling, acquisition of data, analysis and interpretation of data. KJ participated in study design, interpretation of data and revising the manuscript for important intellectual content. BS participated in interpretation of data and revising the manuscript for important intellectual content. IG performed interpretation of data, analysis and interpretation of data, statistical analysis, and participated in writing the initial draft of manuscript.KT performed study design, spinal cord sampling, and performed neuropathic pain modeling, drug administration, assessment of mechanical allodynia, acquisition of data, analysis and interpretation of data, statistical analysis, and drafting/revising the manuscript. All authors read and approved the final manuscript.

Competing interests

The authors declare that they have no competing interests.

Author details

[1]School of Medicine, Chosun University, 309 Pilmundaero, Dong-gu, Gwangju 501-759, South Korea. [2]Department of Anesthesiology and Pain Medicine, Medical School, Chonnam National University, 42 Jebongro, Donggu, Gwangju 501-757, South Korea. [3]Department of Anesthesiology and Pain Medicine, School of Medicine, Chosun University, Chosun University Hospital, 365 Pilmun-daero, Dong-gu, Gwangju 61453, South Korea. [4]Department of Anesthesiology and Pain Medicine, Chosun University Hospital, 365 Pilmun-daero, Dong-gu, Gwangju 61453, South Korea.

References

1. Austin PJ, Moalem-Taylor G. The neuro-immune balance in neuropathic pain: involvement of inflammatory immune cells, immune-like glial cells and cytokines. J Neuroimmunol. 2010;229(1–2):26–50.
2. Berliocchi L, Russo R, Maiaru M, Levato A, Bagetta G, Corasaniti MT. Autophagy impairment in a mouse model of neuropathic pain. Mol Pain. 2011;7:83.
3. Shimizu S, Yoshida T, Tsujioka M, Arakawa S. Autophagic cell death and cancer. Int J Mol Sci. 2014;15(2):3145–53.
4. Shimizu S, Konishi A, Nishida Y, Mizuta T, Nishina H, Yamamoto A, Tsujimoto Y. Involvement of JNK in the regulation of autophagic cell death. Oncogene. 2010;29(14):2070–82.
5. Gao YJ, Ji RR. Activation of JNK pathway in persistent pain. Neurosci Lett. 2008;437(3):180–3.
6. Manassero G, Repetto IE, Cobianchi S, Valsecchi V, Bonny C, Rossi F, Vercelli A. Role of JNK isoforms in the development of neuropathic pain following sciatic nerve transection in the mouse. Mol Pain. 2012;8:39.
7. Zhuang ZY, Wen YR, Zhang DR, Borsello T, Bonny C, Strichartz GR, Decosterd I, Ji RR. A peptide c-Jun N-terminal kinase (JNK) inhibitor blocks mechanical allodynia after spinal nerve ligation: respective roles of JNK activation in primary sensory neurons and spinal astrocytes for neuropathic pain development and maintenance. J Neurosci. 2006;26(13):3551–60.
8. Jeon Y, Kim CE, Jung D, Kwak K, Park S, Lim D, Kim S, Baek W. Curcumin could prevent the development of chronic neuropathic pain in rats with peripheral nerve injury. Curr Ther Res Clin Exp. 2013;74:1–4.
9. Kim KH, Abdi S. Rediscovery of nefopam for the treatment of neuropathic pain. Korean J Pain. 2014;27(2):103–11.
10. Nam JS, Cheong YS, Karm MH, Ahn HS, Sim JH, Kim JS, Choi SS, Leem JG. Effects of nefopam on streptozotocin-induced diabetic neuropathic pain in rats. Korean J Pain. 2014;27(4):326–33.

11. Gregori-Puigjane E, Setola V, Hert J, Crews BA, Irwin JJ, Lounkine E, Marnett L, Roth BL, Shoichet BK. Identifying mechanism-of-action targets for drugs and probes. Proc Natl Acad Sci U S A. 2012;109(28):11178–83.
12. Lee HG, Kim WM, Kim JM, Bae HB, Choi JI. Intrathecal nefopam-induced antinociception through activation of descending serotonergic projections involving spinal 5-HT7 but not 5-HT3 receptors. Neurosci Lett. 2015;587:120–5.
13. Zanjani TM, Saghaei E, Ameli H, Sabetkasaei M. Anti-allodynic effect of Nefopam and morphine in a rat model of neuropathic pain. Novelty Biomed. 2013;1(1):16–22.
14. Biella GE, Groppetti A, Novelli A, Fernandez-Sanchez MT, Manfredi B, Sotgiu ML. Neuronal sensitization and its behavioral correlates in a rat model of neuropathy are prevented by a cyclic analog of orphenadrine. J Neurotrauma. 2003;20(6):593–601.
15. Zimmermann M. Ethical guidelines for investigations of experimental pain in conscious animals. Pain. 1983;16(2):109–10.
16. Kim SH, Chung JM. An experimental model for peripheral neuropathy produced by segmental spinal nerve ligation in the rat. Pain. 1992;50(3):355–63.
17. Chung JM, Kim HK, Chung K. Segmental spinal nerve ligation model of neuropathic pain. Methods Mol Med. 2004;99:35–45.
18. Chaplan SR, Bach FW, Pogrel JW, Chung JM, Yaksh TL. Quantitative assessment of tactile allodynia in the rat paw. J Neurosci Methods. 1994; 53(1):55–63.
19. Caterina MJ, Leffler A, Malmberg AB, Martin WJ, Trafton J, Petersen-Zeitz KR, Koltzenburg M, Basbaum AI, Julius D. Impaired nociception and pain sensation in mice lacking the capsaicin receptor. Science. 2000;288(5464):306–13.
20. Leung L, Cahill CM. TNF-alpha and neuropathic pain--a review. J Neuroinflammation. 2010;7:27.
21. Verleye M, Andre N, Heulard I, Gillardin JM. Nefopam blocks voltage-sensitive sodium channels and modulates glutamatergic transmission in rodents. Brain Res. 2004;1013(2):249–55.
22. Dobrek L, Thor P. Glutamate NMDA receptors in pathophysiology and pharmacotherapy of selected nervous system diseases. Postepy Hig Med Dosw (Online). 2011;65:338–46.
23. Zhang E, Yi MH, Ko Y, Kim HW, Seo JH, Lee YH, Lee W, Kim DW. Expression of LC3 and Beclin 1 in the spinal dorsal horn following spinal nerve ligation-induced neuropathic pain. Brain Res. 2013;1519:31–9.
24. Oh SH, Lim SC. Endoplasmic reticulum stress-mediated autophagy/apoptosis induced by capsaicin (8-methyl-N-vanillyl-6-nonenamide) and dihydrocapsaicin is regulated by the extent of c-Jun NH2-terminal kinase/extracellular signal-regulated kinase activation in WI38 lung epithelial fibroblast cells. J Pharmacol Exp Ther. 2009;329(1):112–22.
25. Caterina MJ, Schumacher MA, Tominaga M, Rosen TA, Levine JD, Julius D. The capsaicin receptor: a heat-activated ion channel in the pain pathway. Nature. 1997;389(6653):816–24.
26. Mika J, Zychowska M, Popiolek-Barczyk K, Rojewska E, Przewlocka B. Importance of glial activation in neuropathic pain. Eur J Pharmacol. 2013; 716(1–3):106–19.
27. Zarpelon AC, Rodrigues FC, Lopes AH, Souza GR, Carvalho TT, Pinto LG, Xu D, Ferreira SH, Alves-Filho JC, McInnes IB, et al. Spinal cord oligodendrocyte-derived alarmin IL-33 mediates neuropathic pain. FASEB J. 2015;30(1):54–65.
28. Schafers M, Svensson CI, Sommer C, Sorkin LS. Tumor necrosis factor-alpha induces mechanical allodynia after spinal nerve ligation by activation of p38 MAPK in primary sensory neurons. J Neurosci. 2003;23(7):2517–21.
29. Xu JT, Xin WJ, Zang Y, Wu CY, Liu XG. The role of tumor necrosis factor-alpha in the neuropathic pain induced by lumbar 5 ventral root transection in rat. Pain. 2006;123(3):306–21.
30. Costigan M, Moss A, Latremoliere A, Johnston C, Verma-Gandhu M, Herbert TA, Barrett L, Brenner GJ, Vardeh D, Woolf CJ, et al. T-cell infiltration and signaling in the adult dorsal spinal cord is a major contributor to neuropathic pain-like hypersensitivity. J Neurosci. 2009;29(46):14415–22.
31. Mizushima N, Levine B, Cuervo AM, Klionsky DJ. Autophagy fights disease through cellular self-digestion. Nature. 2008;451(7182):1069–75.
32. Shi G, Shi J, Liu K, Liu N, Wang Y, Fu Z, Ding J, Jia L, Yuan W. Increased miR-195 aggravates neuropathic pain by inhibiting autophagy following peripheral nerve injury. Glia. 2013;61(4):504–12.
33. Mizushima N, Yoshimori T, Levine B. Methods in mammalian autophagy research. Cell. 2010;140(3):313–26.

7

Incidence of tolerance in children undergoing repeated administration of propofol for proton radiation therapy: a retrospective study

RyungA Kang[1,2†], Byung Seop Shin[1†], Young Hee Shin[1], Nam-Su Gil[1], Ye Na Oh[1] and Ji Seon Jeong[1*]

Abstract

Background: Propofol is an excellent hypnotic drug for use in repeated radiation procedures in young children. To date, tolerance to propofol generally does not develop in pediatric patients undergoing radiation therapy. However, several studies have suggested that there may be potential for development of tolerance to propofol. The aim of this study was to evaluate the development of a tolerance to propofol used for repeated deep sedation in children undergoing proton radiation therapy (PRT).

Methods: All children undergoing PRT at our institution between December 2015 and January 2018 were eligible for inclusion in this study. Sedation was induced by a bolus dose of propofol (2.0 $mg.kg^{-1}$) followed by a continuous infusion of 250 $\mu g.kg^{-1}.min^{-1}$ via an infusion pump to achieve deep sedation. Sedation was maintained with the propofol infusion of 200 $\mu g.kg^{-1}.min^{-1}$, which was adjusted in 25 $\mu g.kg^{-1}.min^{-1}$ increments up or down as necessary to ensure deep sedation. The primary outcome was mean doses of propofol over time.

Results: Fifty-eight children were analyzed. The mean (SD) age was 4.5 (2.1) years. The mean (SD) number of treatment sessions was 19 (7). Fifteen patients (26%) developed tolerance to propofol. However, there were no significant differences between the children who developed tolerance and the children who did not develop tolerance in mean propofol dose and awakening time over time ($p = 0.887$ and $P = 0.652$, respectively). Age, the number of PRT, and attending anesthesiologists was not significantly associated with the incidence of tolerance to propofol.

Conclusion: Repeated prolonged deep sedation for PRT elicited multiple times over several weeks in young children using propofol did not develop tolerance in 74% of patients. Although the incidence of 26% tolerance to propofol may still be present, the increase in propofol dose was minimal. Therefore, the use of repeated propofol for children was safe.

Keywords: Propofol, Tolerance, Proton radiation therapy, Children, Deep sedation, Anesthesia

* Correspondence: jiseon78.jeong@samsung.com
[†]RyungA Kang and Byung Seop Shin contributed equally to this work.
[1]Department of Anesthesiology and Pain Medicine, Samsung Medical Center, Sungkyunkwan University school of Medicine, 81 Irwon-ro, Gangnam, Seoul 06352, South Korea
Full list of author information is available at the end of the article

Background

Proton radiation therapy (PRT), which destroys abnormal tissues in the body via delicate control of the range of a proton beam, requires deep sedation in children to avoid movement and maintain a precise position during irradiation. [1–3] Since the total duration of treatment is several weeks, children undergoing PRT are repeatedly exposed to anesthetic agents. Repeated exposure to some anesthetic drugs can lead to the development of drug tolerance, which is defined as a decrease in a drug's effect over time or the need to increase the drug's dose over time to achieve the same effect. [4]

Propofol is an excellent hypnotic drug for use in repeated radiation procedures in young children because of its unique pharmacologic properties, such as rapid onset, fast recovery from anesthesia, and low incidence of nausea and vomiting. [5] To date, tolerance to propofol generally does not develop in pediatric patients undergoing radiation therapy. However, several studies have suggested that there may be potential for development of tolerance to propofol, either by increased clearance of the drug [6, 7] or by changes in the body's sensitivity to the drug's effects. [8, 9] Taken together, the data on tolerance to propofol seem to be controversial. Therefore, in this retrospective study, we aimed to evaluate the tolerance to propofol for repeated deep sedation in children undergoing PRT.

Methods

All children aged 16 years or younger who underwent deep sedation for PRT at our institution (Samsung Medical Center in Seoul, Korea) between December 2015 and January 2018 were eligible for inclusion in this study. Among them, children who underwent only a simulation session and did not experience sedation with anesthetic agents were excluded. The Institutional Review Board of Samsung Medical Center approved this retrospective study (SMC 2018–02-121) and waived the requirement for written informed consent. All data were retrospectively collected from the computerized medical records. The collected data included patient baseline characteristics; site of irradiation; total number of treatments; total amount of propofol required; hemodynamic parameters including mean arterial blood pressure, heart rate, respiratory rate, and oxygen saturation; and the patient's recovery profile in the post-anesthesia care unit (PACU).

The sedation procedure for radiation therapy was performed daily, with the exception of weekends or holidays, according to our standardized institutional protocol. Each session can last between 30 and 90 min depending on the complexity of the treatment set-up and delivery. Patients came to the treatment room having fasted according to the current American Society of Anesthesiologists guidelines and did not receive premedication before induction. All patients had a permanent pre-existing indwelling central venous catheter. Before induction, we administered a bolus of intravenous fluid (10 $ml.kg^{-1}$) to decrease the incidence of hypotension. [10] Standard monitoring including electrocardiogram, non-invasive arterial blood pressure measurement, pulse oximetry, and a facial mask for delivering supplemental oxygen and for end-tidal CO_2 monitoring were installed and were continuously monitored in three-minutes intervals during radiation therapy. Prior to the PRT, we performed airway optimization in all patients. Sedation was induced by a bolus dose of propofol (2.0 $mg.kg^{-1}$) based on body weight. Subsequently, attending anesthesiologist evaluated the effect of the initial bolus dose of propofol and followed by a continuous infusion of 250 $\mu g.kg^{-1}.min^{-1}$ via an infusion pump to achieve deep sedation [Richmond agitation-sedation scale (RASS) [11] score: − 4] while maintaining spontaneous breathing. During maintenance of sedation, every patient received 200 $\mu g.kg^{-1}.min^{-1}$ of propofol, and the infusion rate was adjusted in 25 $\mu g.kg^{-1}.min^{-1}$ increments up or down at the discretion of the anesthesiologists in order to maintain deep sedation. [12] If involuntary movement was present, a supplemental dose of propofol (1.0 $mg.kg^{-1}$) was administered to sustain deep sedation. Patients were observed by means of video cameras for inadvertent movements in the treatment room, and vital sign data were transmitted to a monitor screen in the control room. During sedation, airway interventions were performed when patients demonstrated apnea (> 10 s), oxygen desaturation ($SpO_2 < 90\%$), and/or airway obstruction, which included checking for equipment malfunctions, airway repositioning, performing the chin lift/jaw thrust maneuver, or establishing bag-mask ventilation as needed. If there was no improvement, other airway devices such as an oral/nasal airway, a laryngeal mask airway (LMA), or an endotracheal tube (ET) were applied. [12] However, if a head mask was used during the PRT, oral airway, LMA, and ET could not be applied, and only nasal airway could be used. Despite management with an airway device, in the case of airway obstruction, treatment was discontinued, and computed tomography (CT) simulation was considered. After the end of PRT, all patients were transferred to a pediatric PACU adjacent to the treatment room, and standard monitoring was continued until the patient was discharged. [13] Recovery was assessed using the RASS score. Awakening time was defined as the time from the end of propofol infusion to the patient displaying alertness and calmness (RASS score: 0).

Statistical analysis

The primary objective of this study was to evaluate the development of tolerance to propofol during the course of repeated deep sedation for PRT. Tolerance to propofol was determined by statistical significance of the slope by regression analysis of propofol dose over time for every patient. For the primary outcome, the binary logistic regression analysis was performed with potential confounding variables such as age, number of repeated PRT, and an attending anesthesiologist and was adjusted during multivariable analysis. Secondary outcomes included the awakening time, frequency of airway intervention, and sedation-related adverse events. Since treatment was not provided on the weekends, the treatment period was divided into intervals of five days, with an overall number of four weeks. For the descriptive statistics in all patients, all parameters were averaged for each week. An analysis of variance with repeated measures using the mixed model was applied to each parameter, because the numbers of treatments were not the same for all of the patients. To examine the shape of a time-related trend, linear and quadratic equations were applied to the data and tested using contrast analysis. Contrast analysis was used to examine whether the overall significant trend in time was also expressed by a significant difference in the study period. The levels of each session were compared with the level of the first session for each parameter. Continuous variables are expressed as mean ± standard deviation and analyzed by t-test. Categorical variables are expressed as number (percentage) and analyzed by the chi - square test. For the regression analysis, odds ratio with a 95% confidence interval was presented. Analyses were performed using SAS version 9.2 (SAS Institute, Cary, NC, USA), SAS PROC MIXED version 6.1, or SPSS version 20.0 (SPSS Inc., Armonk, NY, USA), and $p < 0.05$ was considered to be statistically significant.

Results

Sixty-five children were treated with PRT at our institution during the study period. Of these, children who underwent only a simulation session ($n = 5$) and/or those who did not experience sedation with anesthetic agents ($n = 2$) were excluded. All 58 of the enrolled patients (29 males and 29 females) received propofol alone as the sedation anesthetic. The mean (SD) age was 4.5 (2.1) years (Table 1). The mean (SD) number of treatment sessions was 19 (7). The minimal number of PRT was 6 and the maximal number of PRT was 34. Twenty-six children (44.8%) were treated for brain tumors, and the rest were treated for neuroblastoma ($n = 26$) or facial rhabdomyosarcoma ($n = 6$). All PRT procedures were performed with the patient in the supine position.

Of the 58 patients, 15 patients (26%) developed tolerance to propofol. The proportion of tolerance to propofol was 0.26 and a 95% confidence interval was 0.16 to 0.38. In these 15 patients, the mean (SD) slope of the regression analysis was 0.011 (0.008), indicating that the increase of propofol dosage was minimal. As shown in Fig. 1, there were no significant differences between the children who developed tolerance and the children who did not develop tolerance in mean propofol dose and awakening time over time ($P = 0.887$ and $P = 0.652$, respectively). There were no significant differences in age, height, weight, gender, and the treatment number of PRT between the children who developed tolerance and the children who did not develop tolerance (Table 2).

Table 1 Patients' characteristics

Characteristic	All children ($n = 58$)
Age (years)	4.5 ± 2.1
Height (cm)	102.9 ± 15.0
Weight (kg)	17.4 ± 10.4
Sex (male/female)	29/29
Tumor lesion	
Brain	26 (44.8)
Neuroblastoma, retroperitoneum	16 (27.6)
Neuroblastoma, adrenal gland	8 (13.8)
Neuroblastoma, chest	2 (3.4)
Rhabdomyosarcoma, face	6 (10.3)

Values are mean ± standard deviations or number (%)

In all patients, there were no significant differences in time-related trend and mean propofol dose over time ($P = 0.975$ and $P = 0.369$, respectively), indicating no constant increase or decrease in the requirement of propofol. Awakening time tended to be long over time (time-related trend $P < 0.001$, linear trend $P = 0.051$, and quadratic trend $P = 0.266$), but overall mean differences in awakening time did not reach a level of significance ($P = 0.130$). Other clinical parameters including hemodynamic variables (e.g., mean arterial blood pressure and heart rate); sedation time; procedure time; and PACU stay time between the various intervals showed no statistically significant differences over time (Table 3).

To determine the relationship between the tolerance to propofol and possible confounders, adjust analysis was performed. The results of the univariable analysis indicated that the age, the number of PRT, and attending anesthesiologists was not significantly associated with the occurrence of tolerance to propofol (Table 4).

Two patients (3.4%) received a nasal airway from the sixth treatment onwards because of upper airway obstruction exacerbated by steroid treatment. There were no adverse events requiring airway intervention except for additional airway device use. No serious events including aspiration, increased level of care, cardiac arrest, or death occurred during PRT.

Discussion

In this retrospective study, we demonstrated requirements of propofol were not significantly changed over the PRT period. Also, we did not observe a clear trend in propofol

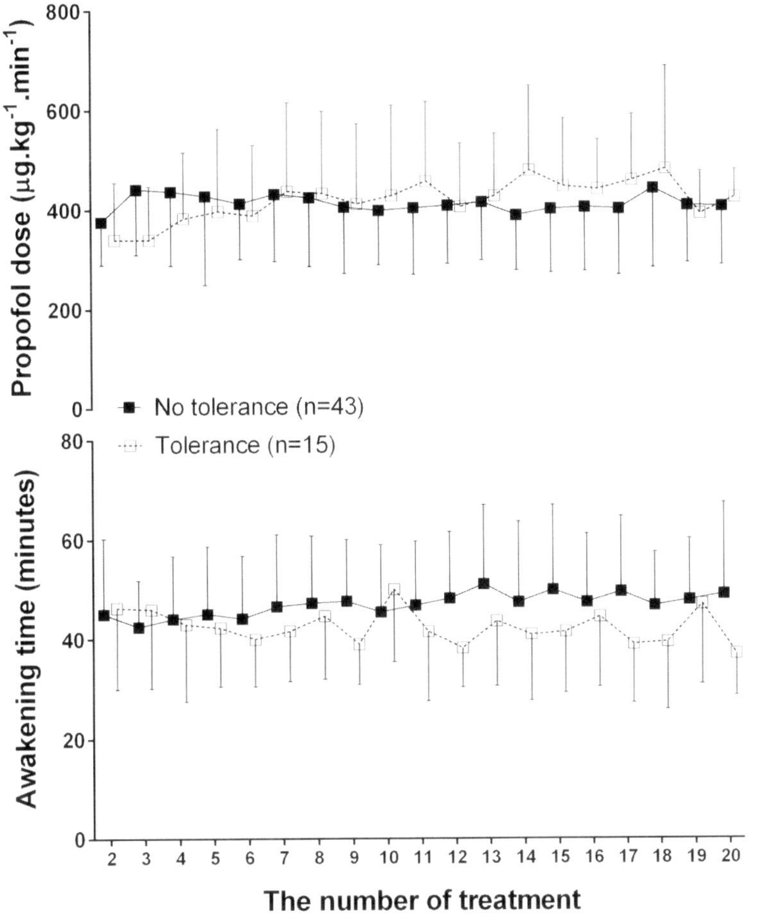

Fig. 1 Mean doses of propofol (upper plane) and mean awakening time (lower plane) in children with tolerance to propofol ($n = 15$) and in children without tolerance to propofol ($n = 43$) during the course of proton radiation therapy. Symbols represent the mean and error bars represent standard deviations

dose over time. Awakening time tended to increase over time, but the overall mean difference was not significant. Thus, based on our findings, we suggest that most of the children undergoing repeated PRT did not develop tolerance to propofol. Although the incidence of 26% tolerance to propofol may still be present, the increase of propofol dosage was minimal and no significant differences in patient characteristics between the children who developed tolerance and the children who did not develop tolerance were found.

Several previous studies have reported that tolerance to propofol does not develop in patients undergoing repeated radiation therapy [1, 14] or electroconvulsive therapy. [15] However, these studies had insufficient data to reach a firm conclusion regarding the nondevelopment of tolerance to propofol. First, the study by Keidan and colleagues

Table 2 Comparison between the children who developed tolerance and the children who did not develop tolerance

	No tolerance ($n = 43$)	Tolerance ($n = 15$)	p value
Age (years)	4.4 ± 2.4	4.7 ± 1.3	0.898
Height (cm)	102.5 ± 16.7	104.2 ± 8.4	0.706
Weight (kg)	17.6 ± 11.8	16.6 ± 4.2	0.739
Sex (male/female)	19/24	10/5	0.230
Treatment number of proton therapy	19 ± 6	19 ± 8	0.718

Values are mean ± standard deviations or number

Table 3 Clinical parameters for each week of proton therapy

Parameters	Week 1	Week 2	Week 3	Week 4	*p* value* for mean differences during study period
Mean arterial blood pressure during procedure, mmHg	61.6 ± 9.9	61.0 ± 10.5	61.0 ± 9.9	62.9 ± 10.5	0.655
Mean heart rate during procedure, bpm	90.3 ± 13.9	89.0 ± 13.0	89.6 ± 14.8	86.1 ± 14.5	0.496
Sedation time, min	32.6 ± 17.2	30.2 ± 14.7	28.4 ± 12.6	25.4 ± 12.5	0.361
Procedure time, min	25.3 ± 16.7	23.3 ± 14.4	21.2 ± 12.6	18.7 ± 12.3	0.217
PACU stay time, min	68.3 ± 13.5	70.3 ± 18.6	71.7 ± 18.3	67.8 ± 14.7	0.387

Data are presented as mean ± standard deviations. *PACU,* post-anesthesia care unit. *Analysis of variance with repeated measures using the mixed model

[1] did not identify a development of tolerance to propofol during PRT using a bispectral index parameters. However, in their report, the number of patients was too small ($n = 15$) to make this conclusion. The study of Setlock and colleagues [14] also included a small number of children ($n = 6$). Also, propofol was used in conjunction with ketamine or midazolam during PRT, and the authors failed to exclude the possibility of an interaction between propofol and other anesthetics. Third, Soyka and Fischer [15] did not find tolerance to propofol during repeated electroconvulsive therapy. However, they did not consider trends or mean differences in propofol over time: they compared the average doses of propofol at the first session to the last session, rather than comparing all values of propofol during the entire session. In addition, the patients in this study were given one injection at a time; repeated injections given during the same session or prolonged infusion or treatment for a longer period of time could result in either more pronounced or reduced tolerance to propofol. Compared with these previous studies, our study included a larger number of patients ($n = 58$), used propofol alone as a sedative agent, and compared all values of propofol during the entire session. In particular, by determining the tolerance to propofol for every patient, our results suggest the indidence of tolerance and can determine the degree of association between the repeated number of propofol administration and the occurrence of tolerance.

Table 4 Risk of tolerance to propofol among the age, number of treatments, and anesthesiologists

	Univariable analysis	
	OR [95%CI]	P value
Age	1.004 [0.982–1.027]	0.713
Number of treatments	0.994 [0.909–1.087]	0.896
Anesthesiologists		0.681
Anesthesiologists A	1	
Anesthesiologists B	0.556 [0.138–2.238]	
Anesthesiologists C	0.615 [0.139–2.727]	

CI confidence interval, *OR* odds ratio

In contrast, one case report in children [16] and one prospective study in adults underwent electroconvulsive therapy [6] suggest that tolerance to propofol may develop with repeated administration, and that increasing doses of the propofol may be required or lead to reduced time to wakefulness over the course of treatment. [6, 8] The demonstration of tolerance relies primarily on the need to increase the amount of medication used to achieve the desired level of sedation, analgesia, or hypnosis. [1] Possible mechanisms of tolerance to propofol can be assumed from the pharmacological evidence for abuse to propofol because the tolerance is one of the diagnostic criteria for abuse. [9] The effect of propofol is mediated by the gamma-aminobutyric acid receptor, which is also known to be potentiated by abusive substances such as alcohol, barbiturates, and benzodiazepines. [17] In addition, propofol increases the extracellular dopamine concentrations by increasing the discharge rate and excitability of dopamine neurons by affecting the mesolimbic reward system. [18] Such evidence might contribute to the development of tolerance to propofol. However, in our study, the amount of propofol was slightly increased in 15 patients with tolerance to propofol, but the required dose was not increased in most patients. In addition, increased awakening time was observed instead of reduced awakening time which is the characteristic of patients who developed tolerance to propofol over the course of PRT. Perhaps this might be due to the repeated daily *nil* per os (NPO) time and sleep cycle changes. [19] Although we administered a bolus of intravenous fluid prior to induction, repeated NPO time for several weeks can be exhausting in young children. As a result, the general condition of the children can worsen and can adversely affect the awakening time. However, none of the previous studies or our study measured the plasma concentrations of propofol to confirm their results. Therefore, it is difficult to make a clear conclusion about this.

Although several studies have reported tolerance to propofol, the reason why the majority of patients did not show tolerance to propofol might be due to the low cumulative time for propofol use. In a previous cost-benefit study comparing the sedation duration of propofol and midazolam reported that tolerance to propofol developed in patients who received propofol over 144 h. [20] In contrast, propofol was given for an average of 9.5 h in our study. Another possible reason is the precise titration of the infusion rate of propofol. Regardless of the agent chosen, tolerance can be delayed with the use of sedation scales to allow for appropriate titration of the infusion. In addition, the use of sedation scales allows for the drip to be adjusted according to the specific patient's needs so that a minimal amount of the drug is administered. [4]

The use of propofol alone tends to increase the incidence of sedation-related serious adverse events, because it has a dose-dependent response to upper airway collapse by inhibition of the airway dilator muscle and of the upper airway reflexes. [21] However, in our study, although we used propofol alone, the frequency of airway interventions was 2/58 (3.4%). These two children had no specific findings until the fifth treatment, but soft tissue edema was exacerbated by the use of steroid, and airway intervention was subsequently needed. The reason for the low incidence of airway intervention in this study might be due to the fact that all patients underwent optimal airway positioning using an immobilization device such as a base of the skull frame, neck cast, intracranial mask, or a modified Gill-Thomas-Cosman frame during the CT simulation session before performing PRT. Consequently, deep sedation with propofol alone for PRT did not increase the risk of sedation-related serious adverse events.

Our study has several limitations. First, it was a retrospective study; thus, we cannot establish a cause-and-effect relationship in relation to tolerance to propofol. Second, the depth of sedation was assessed using RAAS score by 3 different anesthesiologists. Thus, it could increase the risk of inter-observer bias. However, all of them were experts in pediatric sedation for more than 4 years and the propofol dose determined by the RASS score were not significantly associated with the development of the tolerance depending on 3 different anesthesiologists. Third, the incidence of 26% tolerance to propofol was observed, but since the plasma concentration of propofol was not measured, it cannot be confirmed whether the tolerance to propofol actually developed. Thus, further prospective studies are recommended including more objective methods of assessing deep sedation and measurement of plasma concentrations of propofol to determine the occurrence of tolerance.

Conclusions

We found that 74% of patients did not develop tolerance after repeated deep sedation using propofol infusion over several weeks. Although the incidence of 26% tolerance to propofol may still be present, the increase in propofol dose was minimal. Therefore, the use of repeated propofol for children was safe. Further large-scale prospective studies are needed before clinical relevance can be defined.

Abbreviations

CT: Computed tomography; ET: Endotracheal tube; LMA: Laryngeal mask airway; NPO: Nil per os; PACU: Post-anesthesia care unit; PRT: Proton radiation therapy; RASS: Richmond agitation sedation scale

Acknowledgements

We would like to thank In-Suk Son and Min-Ji Kim, the statistical team of the Samsung Medical Center.

Authors' contributions

RAK and BSS wrote the manuscript, analyzed the data, and interpretation of data. YHS, NSG, and JSS gave a critical comment, analyzed the data, and designed the study. YNO analyzed the data and interpretation of data. All authors revised the manuscript critically for important intellectual content. All authors read and approved the final manuscript.

Competing interests

The authors declare that they have no competing interests.

Author details

[1]Department of Anesthesiology and Pain Medicine, Samsung Medical Center, Sungkyunkwan University school of Medicine, 81 Irwon-ro, Gangnam, Seoul 06352, South Korea. [2]Department of Anesthesiology and Pain Medicine, Kangwon National University School of Medicine, Chuncheon, South Korea.

References

1. Ilan Keidan AP, Shabtai EL, Pfeffer RM. Children undergoing repeated exposures for radiation therapy do not develop tolerance to Propofol. Anesthesiology. 2004; 100:251–4.
2. McFadyen JG, Pelly N, Orr RJ. Sedation and anesthesia for the pediatric patient undergoing radiation therapy. Curr Opin Anaesthesiol. 2011;24(4):433–8.
3. Oh TK, Lee SJ, Kim JH, Park B, Eom W. The administration of high-dose propofol sedation with manual and target-controlled infusion in children undergoing radiation therapy: a 7-year clinical investigation. Springerplus. 2016;5:376.
4. Tobias JD. Tolerance, withdrawal, and physical dependency after long-term sedation and analgesia of children in the pediatric intensive care unit. Crit Care Med. 2000;28(6):2122–32.
5. Cravero JP, Havidich JE. Pediatric sedation--evolution and revolution. Paediatr Anaesth. 2011;21(7):800–9.
6. Cohen Y, Feldinger E, Ogorek D, Weinbroum AA. Increased propofol requirement during succeeding administrations for electroconvulsive therapy. J Clin Anesth. 2004;16(4):282–5.
7. Buckley PM. Propofol in patients needing long-term sedation in intensive care: an assessment of the development of tolerance. A pilot study. Intensive Care Med. 1997;23(9):969–74.
8. Fassoulaki A, Farinotti R, Mantz J, Desmonts JM. Does tolerance develop to the anaesthetic effects of propofol in rats? Br J Anaesth. 1994;72(1):127–8.
9. Wilson C, Canning P, Caravati EM. The abuse potential of propofol. Clin Toxicol (Phila). 2010;48(3):165–70.
10. Mason KP, Turner DP, Houle TT, Fontaine PJ, Lerman J. Hemodynamic response to fluid management in children undergoing dexmedetomidine sedation for MRI. AJR Am J Roentgenol. 2014;202(6):W574–9.

11. Sessler CN, Gosnell MS, Grap MJ, Brophy GM, O'Neal PV, Keane KA, Tesoro EP, Elswick RK. The Richmond agitation-sedation scale: validity and reliability in adult intensive care unit patients. Am J Respir Crit Care Med. 2002; 166(10):1338–44.
12. Kang R, Shin YH, Gil NS, Kim KY, Yeo H, Jeong JS. A comparison of the use of propofol alone and propofol with midazolam for pediatric magnetic resonance imaging sedation - a retrospective cohort study. BMC Anesthesiol. 2017;17(1):138.
13. Aldrete JA. The post-anesthesia recovery score revisited. J Clin Anesth. 1995; 7(1):89–91.
14. Setlock MA, Palmisano BW, Berens RJ, Rosner DR, Troshynski TJ, Murray KJ. Tolerance to profol generally does not develop in pediatric patients undergoing radiation therapy. Anesthesiology. 1996;85:207–9.
15. Soyka M, Fischer W. No evidence for development of tolerance after repeated use of propofol for electroconvulsive therapy. Pharmacopsychiatry. 2015;48(1):7–10.
16. Deer TR, GFR. Propofol tolerance in pediatric patients. Anesthesiology. 1992; 77:828–9.
17. Weerts EM, Ator NA, Griffiths RR. Comparison of the intravenous reinforcing effects of propofol and methohexital in baboons. Drug Alcohol Depend. 1999;57(1):51–60.
18. Li KY, Xiao C, Xiong M, Delphin E, Ye JH. Nanomolar propofol stimulates glutamate transmission to dopamine neurons: a possible mechanism of abuse potential? J Pharmacol Exp Ther. 2008;325(1):165–74.
19. Oto J, Yamamoto K, Koike S, Imanaka H, Nishimura M. Effect of daily sedative interruption on sleep stages of mechanically ventilated patients receiving midazolam by infusion. Anaesth Intensive Care. 2011;39(3):392–400.
20. Carrasco G, Molina R, Costa J, Soler JM, Cabre L. Propofol vs midazolam in short-, medium-, and long-term sedation of critically ill patients. A cost-benefit analysis. Chest. 1993;103(2):557–64.
21. Eastwood PR, Platt PR, Shepherd K, Maddison K, Hillman DR. Collapsibility of the upper airway at different concentrations of propofol anesthesia. Anesthesiology. 2005;103(3):470–7.

8

Pleth variability index or stroke volume optimization during open abdominal surgery: a randomized controlled trial

Hans Bahlmann[1,2*], Robert G. Hahn[3] and Lena Nilsson[1,2]

Abstract

Background: The impact of Goal Directed Fluid Therapy (GDFT) based on the non-invasive Pleth Variability Index (PVI) on clinical outcome after abdominal surgery has only sparingly been explored. The purpose of this study was to compare the effect of intraoperative GDFT guided by PVI to a control group using esophageal Doppler on the incidence of complications and length of hospital stay after major abdominal surgery. We hypothesized that there would be no difference between the groups.

Methods: This was a randomized controlled trial in a Swedish university hospital between November 2011 and January 2015; 150 patients scheduled for open abdominal surgery lasting 2 h or more were included. Exclusion criteria included hepatic resection or severe cardiac arrhythmia. The patients were randomized 1:1 to either the intervention group or the control group. The intervention group received intraoperative GDFT by administering fluid boluses of 3 ml/kg tetrastarch aiming at a PVI value below 10%, while GDFT in the control group aimed for optimization of stroke volume as assessed with esophageal Doppler. Blinded observers assessed complications until postoperative day 30 using pre-defined definitions, as well as length of hospital stay.

Results: One hundred and-fifty patients were randomized and 146 patients were available for the final data analysis. Median duration of surgery was 3 h. A total of 64 complications occurred in the PVI group ($N = 74$) and 70 in the Doppler group ($N = 72$) ($p = 0.93$). Median (IQR) length of stay was 8.0 (8.0) days in the PVI group and 8.0 (9.5) in the Doppler group ($P = 0.57$).

Conclusions: No difference in clinical outcome, as defined by number of postoperative complications, and length of hospital stay, was found when goal directed fluid therapy was applied using PVI as an alternative to esophageal Doppler. PVI appears to be an acceptable alternative to esophageal Doppler for goal directed fluid therapy during major open abdominal surgery.

Keywords: Doppler ultrasonography, Fluid therapy, Laparotomy, Photoplethysmography, Stroke volume, Complications

* Correspondence: hans.bahlmann@regionostergotland.se
[1]Department of Medical and Health Sciences, Linköping University, University Hospital, 58185 Linköping, Sweden
[2]Department of Anesthesiology and Intensive Care, Linköping University, University Hospital, 58185 Linköping, Sweden
Full list of author information is available at the end of the article

Background

The incidence of postoperative complications after major abdominal surgery is increased by both overly restricted and overly liberal fluid administration [1]. Goal directed fluid therapy (GDFT) aims to determine the optimal amount of fluid for an individual patient, and meta-analyses point out its clinical benefits, especially in patients not participating in an enhanced recovery program [2, 3]. Hemodynamic optimization has mostly been guided by stroke volume, commonly measured via esophageal Doppler, or by dynamic parameters such as stroke volume variation, pulse pressure variation or the pulse oximetric Pleth Variability Index (PVI), which all are based on cardiopulmonary interactions.

The latter techniques have been advocated because they are easier to apply and of similar clinical value as methods aiming at optimization of stroke volume [3] despite certain methodological issues, such as the influence of tidal volume, respiratory and heart rate ratio, spontaneous breathing, chest wall compliance, arrhythmia and abdominal pressure [4, 5]. The impact of PVI on clinical outcome in terms of postoperative complications or length of stay is sparingly described in randomized studies [6–8]. PVI guided bolus doses were compared either to a fluid regimen using bolus doses based on mean blood pressure [6, 7] or on Doppler measured stroke volume changes [8]. Although no difference on the incidence of postoperative complications or length of stay was reported, the studies are small and two of them restricted to colonic surgery. We found it of interest to further evaluate the effect of PVI on clinical outcome in abdominal surgery.

We designed a randomized controlled trial comparing patients treated with fluid optimization guided by PVI with control patients who received stroke volume optimization guided by esophageal Doppler.

This is a planned secondary analysis of a study primarily designed to analyze differences in intraoperative fluid use. Primary outcome measures were the amount of colloid used for optimization of fluid status and the concordance between different methods for assessing preoperative dehydration. These results have been published elsewhere [9, 10] and included the first half of the study cohort (75 patients). The present article focuses on clinical outcome in the whole cohort of 150 patients, as quantified by number of postoperative complications up to 30 days after surgery and length of hospital stay, both of which were designated as secondary outcome measures in the study protocol.

We hypothesized that there would be no difference between the groups regarding these parameters.

Methods

Ethical approval was obtained from the Regional Ethical Review Board in Linköping in March 2011 (2011/101–31), as was written informed consent from all included patients. The study was prospectively registered at clinicaltrials.gov (NCT 01458678).

This single-blind randomized study was performed at University Hospital Linköping, a 600-bed tertiary care facility in Sweden. As previously described [9], adult patients, ASA class 1–3, planned for elective open abdominal surgery with an expected duration of at least 2 h were screened for inclusion. Exclusion criteria included hepatic resection, severe forms of cardiac arrhythmia, planned central hemodynamic monitoring for cardiac reasons, enrollment in another interventional study or unavailability of research staff.

General management

Patients were recruited from different departments (gynecology, surgery and urology) and therefore preoperative management with regard to fluids and antibiotics followed departmental routines, which could include an explicit enhanced recovery program. After siting a thoracic epidural catheter (when indicated), general anesthesia was induced using fentanyl and propofol or thiopental and maintained using sevoflurane and iterated doses of fentanyl. Intubation was facilitated with rocuronium or succinylcholine. Epidural analgesia was started before the surgery commenced using a continuous infusion of a mixture of bupivacaine, fentanyl and epinephrine supplemented by bolus doses if indicated. All patients were ventilated using a Volume Control mode with a standardized tidal volume of 7 ml kg^{-1} ideal body weight [11].

A maximum of 500 ml of tetrastarch, either Venofundin (B Braun Medical AB, Danderyd, Sweden) or Volulyte (Fresenius Kabi AB, Uppsala, Sweden), could be infused during the epidural catheter placement and the subsequent induction of anesthesia. Both groups received a baseline infusion of 2 ml kg^{-1} h^{-1} (actual body weight) of a 2.5% buffered dextrose solution containing 70 mmol l^{-1} sodium, 45 mmol l^{-1} chloride, and 25 mmol l^{-1} acetate (Glukos Braun 25 mg ml^{-1} with buffer (B Braun Medical AB, Danderyd, Sweden) during surgery. Correction for additional crystalloid fluids given (e.g. antibiotics) was not made. Up to 1000 ml of Ringer's acetate could be infused during surgery to compensate for preoperative dehydration or increased non-hemorrhagic intraoperative fluid loss. Bleeding was replaced 1:1 with a colloid (tetrastarch, albumin 5%, plasma, packed red blood cells or platelets). Infusions with vasoconstrictors (norepinephrine or phenylephrine) and/or inotropes (dobutamine) were used at the discretion of the responsible anesthetist.

Study groups

Patients were recruited and randomized 1:1 by HB or LN, using opaque envelopes prepared by a research nurse from a computerized randomization procedure [12], to receive intraoperative fluid optimization guided by either the pulse oximetric PVI or esophageal Doppler. The PVI was monitored using a Radical-7 Pulse CO-oximeter (Masimo Corporation, Irvine, California, USA) with PVI software (Version SET V7.8.0.1), a re-usable sensor (R2-25r) and a disposable adhesive (R2-25a). The sensor was placed on the middle or index finger of either hand and was covered to avoid room light interference. The placement of a blood pressure cuff on the same arm was avoided.

The esophageal Doppler measurements were performed using a CardioQ apparatus (Deltex Medical, Chicester, United Kingdom) equipped with a DP12 probe, and the signal was averaged over 20 cardiac cycles. In both groups, fluid optimization was initiated after induction of general anesthesia and undertaken by infusing 3 ml kg^{-1} actual body weight (up to 250 ml) of tetrastarch intravenously during 3–5 min, using a 50 ml syringe. As described previously [9], during the first half of the study (patients 1–75), in which the concordance between the methods was studied, all patients were monitored with both PVI and esophageal Doppler. Only the allocated monitor was visible to the responsible anesthetist. For the second part (patients 76–150) only the allocated monitor was used.

Fluid bolus algorithms

In the PVI group, a fluid bolus was given if PVI ≥ 10%. The cut-off value of 10% was chosen based on a previous report [13]. If the PVI 5 min after the fluid bolus fell below 10%, no more fluid was given. If the PVI 5 min after the fluid bolus was still ≥10% but had decreased, a repeat fluid bolus was given. Fluid boluses were repeated until the PVI fell below 10% or did not decrease at all. During surgery, additional optimizations were undertaken in the same way whenever the PVI increased to ≥10%. In order to have at least one fluid bolus available in each patient for analyzing the performance of PVI compared to Doppler during an optimization and in analogy with the Doppler group [9], a fluid bolus was given to all patients in the PVI group after induction of anesthesia, irrespective of the PVI value.

In the Doppler group, volume optimization was guided by the stroke volume changes in accordance with published protocols [14, 15]. Following an initial Doppler measurement, a fluid bolus was given and a new Doppler measurement was performed 5 min later. Fluid boluses were repeated until the stroke volume no longer increased by 10%. The 10% cut-off value is commonly used in studies involving the esophageal Doppler, and is based on measurement characteristics of the device [16]. During surgery, additional optimizations were undertaken in the same way whenever the stroke volume had decreased by ≥10%.

Clinical outcome

Two blinded observers retrospectively documented complications during the first 30 days after surgery using a pre-specified list of complications adapted from Brandstrup et al. [17] (see Additional file 1). A telephone call from the research nurse after postoperative day 30 supplemented the information from the electronic patient chart. If patients received care at another hospital during the 30 day period, copies of relevant reports were requested. Each observer independently scored complications; differences were resolved by discussion.

Length of hospital stay was defined as the number of calendar days spent in hospital, from the day of primary surgery until the 30th postoperative day. In case of in-hospital death within the observation period, a length of stay of 31 days was assumed.

Statistical analysis

In order to calculate a sample size that would be sufficient also for the secondary endpoint postoperative complications, we used combined data from the intervention arms of five previous studies on GDFT during abdominal surgery [18–22]. An expected total of 55 complications per 100 patients with a standard deviation of 19 was calculated. With a power of 90% and a significance level of 5%, 66 patients would need to be included in each group to be able to demonstrate an absolute difference of 10% in postoperative complications [23]. Allowing for dropouts it was decided to include 150 patients in the study. Analysis was done on an intention to treat basis. Between groups differences were analyzed using Student T-test, Mann-Whitney U-test, Fisher's Exact test and chi-square test as appropriate using Statistica, versions 12 and 13 (Dell Incorporated, Tulsa, Oklahoma, USA). A p-value < 0.05 was considered significant.

Results

Patients were recruited between November 14, 2011 and December 8, 2014, and the follow up of the last patient ended on January 8, 2015. A CONSORT flow diagram is presented in Fig. 1. After exclusion of four patients 146 were available for analysis.

Patient and surgical characteristics are presented in Table 1. Median duration of surgery was 3 h in both groups, with some procedures lasting more than 12 h. Types of surgery are specified in Additional file 2.

In two patients in the PVI group (one with increasing lactic acidosis and one with continuing hemodynamic instability), in which the PVI indicated no need for further fluids, Doppler data were requested by the responsible anesthetist. These data confirmed an adequate fluid status, and the Doppler data were blinded for the rest of the procedure. These patients remained in the PVI group for the intention to treat analysis.

There were no differences between the groups in the amounts of colloids used during the optimizations, or in any other intraoperative fluid parameters (Table 2), with

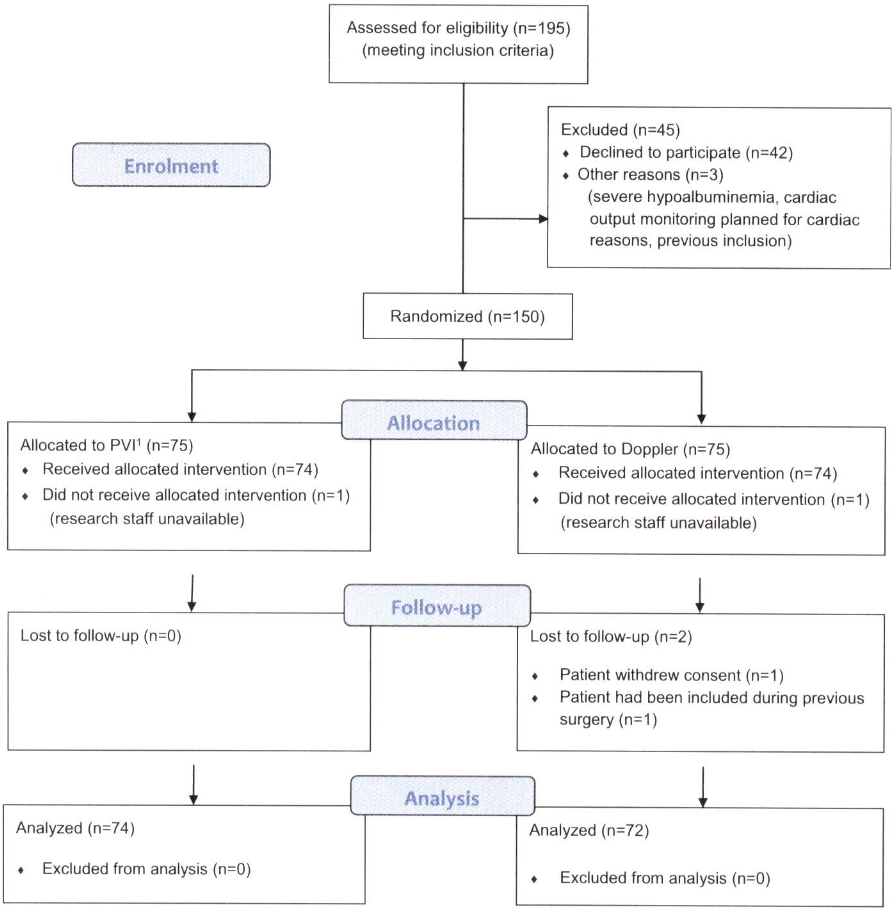

[1] PVI = pleth variability index

Fig. 1 CONSORT 2010 Flow Diagram

the exception of phenylephrine slightly more often being used in the PVI group ($P = 0.04$). Mean increase in body weight 1 day after surgery was 1.3 kg (SD 2.4) in the PVI group and 1.3 kg (SD 1.7) in the Doppler group ($P = 0.97$).

Postoperative complications and length of hospital stay

There was no mortality during the study period. There were in total 64 complications in the PVI group ($n = 74$) and 70 in the Doppler group ($n = 72$) ($P = 0.93$), corresponding to 38 (51%) patients in the PVI group and 35 (49%) patients in the Doppler group ($P = 0.74$) having had at least one complication (Table 3). Eleven complications necessitated surgical intervention requiring general anesthesia (three in the PVI group and eight in the Doppler group ($P = 0.55$)) and in each group two complications required admission to the intensive care unit. Median length of hospital stay was 8.0 days (IQR 8.0) in the PVI group and 8.0 days (IQR 9.5) in the Doppler group ($P = 0.57$).

Discussion

There were no differences in the number of postoperative complications or length of hospital stay when GDFT was guided by PVI instead of esophageal Doppler during major open abdominal surgical procedures.

Previous studies show that both length of stay and incidence of complications were reduced when PVI was used as a part of a colorectal surgery multimodal enhanced recovery protocol in 109 patients, compared to historical controls [24]. The use of PVI also decreased perioperative lactate levels compared to controls [6, 25]. Warnakulasuriya et al. [8] reported no difference in short term outcome when PVI was compared to esophageal Doppler in 40 patients. Based on these reports and our findings, a clinician wishing to pursue GDFT can choose PVI over esophageal Doppler in the large majority of patients undergoing major open abdominal surgery. PVI, in contrast to esophageal Doppler, is not sensitive to interference from diathermy and does not require frequent access to the patient's head for probe

Table 1 Patient characteristics and perioperative data

	PVI ($n = 74$)	Doppler ($n = 72$)
Age, mean (SD), years	63 (12)	61 (14)
Female, n (%)	40 (54)	47 (65)
Body mass index, mean (SD), kg m^{-2}	26.0 (4.1)	26.7 (6.3)
ASA class		
ASA 1, n (%)	22 (30)	27 (38)
ASA 2, n (%)	42 (57)	37 (51)
ASA 3, n (%)	10 (13)	8 (11)
Concomitant morbidity		
Smoker, n (%)	14 (19)	8 (11)
Cardiovascular disease, n (%)	31 (42)	22 (31)
Neurological disease, n (%)	4 (5)	2 (3)
Diabetes, n (%)	11 (15)	8 (11)
Type of surgery		
Gynecology, n (%)	23 (31)	19 (26)
Upper gastrointestinal, n (%)	18 (24)	26 (36)
Lower gastrointestinal, n (%)	22 (30)	21 (29)
Urology, n (%)	11 (15)	6 (9)
Enhanced recovery program, n (%)	7 (9)	8 (11)
Duration of surgery, median {IQR}, h	2.9 {2.2}	3.0 {2.2}
Duration of anesthesia, median {IQR}, h	4.1 {2.3}	3.9 {2.3}
Epidural, n (%)	66 (89)	67 (93)
Lowest temperature during surgery, mean (SD), °C	35.7 (0.5)	35.7 (0.6)
Temperature end of surgery, mean (SD), °C	36.4 (0.6)	36.4 (0.6)

Table 2 Intraoperative fluid data

	PVI ($n = 74$)	Doppler ($n = 72$)	P
Crystalloid fluid, mean (SD), ml	1360 (749)	1240 (662)	0.31
Total colloid fluid, mean (SD), ml	1464 (1000)	1412 (1259)	0.92
Colloid during induction, mean (SD), ml	173 (145)	154 (137)	0.40
Colloid used during optimizations, mean (SD), ml	675 (434)	665 (462)	0.89
Synthetic colloid fluid, mean (SD), ml	1159 (507)	1141 (532)	0.84
Albumin 5%, n (range, ml)	14 (120–1250)	8 (170–500)	0.25
Albumin 20%, n (range, ml)	8 (100–200)	6 (45–100)	0.78
Red blood cells, n (range, ml)	10 (280–1389)	8 (265–2310)	0.80
Plasma, n (range, ml)	6 (776–2734)	5 (265–3300)	1.00
Thrombocytes, n (range, ml)	0	2 (230–250)	0.24
Phenylephrine, n (range, μg)	51 (360–3928)	37 (240–6640)	**0.04**
Norepinephrine, n (range, μg)	29 (52–2180)	30 (11–2726)	0.76
Dobutamine, n (range, mg)	20 (2–110)	20 (1–97)	0.92
Blood loss, median {IQR}, ml	250 {500}	225 {487}	0.41
Urine, median {IQR}, ml	300 {326}	225 {310}	0.22

Statistical differences were analyzed using Student T-test, Mann-Whitney U-test, chi-square test or Fisher's Exact test as appropriate. Significant results in bold

repositioning. Also, PVI can be measured without single-use equipment avoiding the cost for single-use esophageal probes (USD 130 in our setting). However, as illustrated by the request for Doppler data in two PVI patients, the clinician might still want to have access to a reliable method for measuring intraoperative cardiac output to increase the amount of hemodynamic information during unusually complex situations or in cases of known vascular and/or myocardial dysfunction. Data on cardiac output and thus contractility, systemic vascular resistance and oxygen delivery were available in the Doppler group but not incorporated in the treatment protocol, and decisions about inotropic and/or vasoactive support in both groups were left to the clinical judgement of the responsible anesthetist. Despite the more extensive hemodynamic information in the Doppler group, beside more use of the vasopressor phenylephrine in the PVI group, the amount of inotropic support did not differ between the treatment groups.

Other non-invasive methods for dynamic monitoring are available. One meta-analysis reported the offline assessment of respiratory variation in pulse oximetry plethysmographic waveform amplitude (ΔPOP) for predicting fluid responsiveness to be comparable to that of PVI (AUC 0.89 vs 0.95), but this technique is as yet not available in real time [26]. Also, pulse pressure variation and stroke volume variation can now be obtained non-invasively using the Nexfin/Clearsight™ or the CNAP™ systems, but their capacity for predicting fluid responsiveness differs between studies [27–30]. The same applies to measurements of the variability of the diameter of the caval vein or other veins during positive pressure ventilation [31]. Contrary to PVI, the effect on clinical outcome of all these techniques has to the best of our knowledge not been studied.

PVI is a dynamic indicator of fluid responsiveness based on cardiopulmonary interaction while stroke volume optimization is not. As both methods are claimed to be of benefit for fluid management, we argue that these methods, though differing in concept, can be compared with each other in a randomized trial focusing on clinical outcome [3]. Maintaining a patient below a certain PVI value might appear to be less aggressive then aiming for the plateau of the Starling curve, but this depends on the selected cut-off values. Probably, a higher cut off value for PVI with the same settings (such as tidal volume) would have resulted in less fluid administration and vice versa. We have previously shown that a PVI value of 10.5% was optimal in this material [9].

Table 3 Postoperative complications within 30 days after surgery

	PVI ($n = 74$)	Doppler ($n = 72$)	
Major			
Anastomotic insufficiency	3	1	
Lymphatic leakage	0	0	
Bleeding	0	1	
Sepsis	0	1	
Wound dehiscence	0	5	
Intestinal obstruction	0	1	
Stroke	0	0	
Pulmonary embolism	0	0	
Deep vein thrombosis	1	1	
Pulmonary edema/ respiratory insufficiency/ pneumonia	1	2	
Pleural effusion	0	5	
Myocardial infarction	1	0	
Arrhythmia	1	2	
Cardiac arrest	0	0	
Renal dysfunction	13	10	
Liver dysfunction	0	0	
Total	20	29	
Minor			
Superficial wound infection or dehiscence	6	4	
Infection	10	11	
Paralytic ileus	1	0	
Upper GI bleeding	0	1	
Pulmonary congestion	5	0	
Angina pectoris	1	1	
Hypotension	2	6	
Delirium	1	1	
Coagulopathy	4	3	
Severe postoperative nausea and vomiting	8	9	
Urinary retention	6	5	
Total	44	41	
Total number of complications	64	70	($P = 0.93$)
Number (%) of patients with complications	38 (51)	35 (49)	($P = 0.74$)
Mean number of complications in patients with complications	1.7	2.0	($P = 0.28$)

Statistical differences were analyzed using Mann-Whitney U-test or chi-square test as appropriate

Limitations

Limitations of this study include the absence of a control group without either PVI or Doppler to guide volume optimization. Early reports on stroke volume optimization using the esophageal Doppler were favorable [32]. Since then the technique has been questioned, partly because of negative studies on GDFT involving esophageal Doppler [33] and other devices [34, 35], and partly because of questions raised about the Doppler method itself [36]. Based on our results, it is not possible to tell whether PVI and Doppler both result in similar improvements in outcome, or whether neither method improves outcome when compared to treatment without GDFT. Such a control group was reflected upon at the time of designing the study (2011), but deemed unethical since, based on the evidence available at that time, we felt there was no equipoise about the benefits of GDFT. Equipoise about the use of GDFT is supported by our findings previously reported about the limited ability of both PVI and Doppler to predict fluid responsiveness [9]. Also protocol compliance, in terms of time during surgery with achieved PVI and SV goals respectively, was not recorded.

The amount of fluid used during the optimizations represents a part of the total fluid given, because of the per protocol complementary colloid fluid administration during the induction of anesthesia and for bleeding, and crystalloid fluid for maintenance and for the correction of preoperative dehydration. This increased the possibility that both groups would receive similar amounts of fluid; however, we did not find a difference between the groups in the amount of colloids used specifically for the optimizations.

We selected a difference of 10% in number of complications at 30 days to determine required sample size. Therefore the study was not powered to detect smaller albeit still significant differences in postoperative outcome. Also, it could be discussed whether a non-inferiority approach would have been more adequate. This would entail a larger required sample size.

The studies which were used to determine sample size scored complications in different ways and reported incidences of complications which are higher than can be expected in current practice using improved surgical and anesthetic techniques. The findings of this study cannot be applied to laparoscopic surgery. The majority of patients, although undergoing major surgery, were classified as ASA 1 or 2. The potential of GDFT to improve postoperative outcome is more pronounced in patients at higher risk of complications [37], and this could have influenced the possibility to find differences in outcome between the methods. Also, since intraoperative blood pressure is correlated to postoperative outcome, a target MAP should have been specified in the protocol.

Since the reliability of dynamic parameters including PVI increases with increasing tidal volume, a tidal volume of 8 ml kg^{-1} (ideal or actual body weight) or more is often recommended [38]. However, as large tidal volumes are probably detrimental in surgical patients [39] we, in line with earlier reports evaluating PVI, chose a tidal volume of 7 ml kg^{-1} ideal body weight [6, 7, 13]. Whether or not outcome is improved by using larger tidal volumes in surgical patients monitored with dynamic parameters is unknown.

Conclusions

We found no differences regarding number of postoperative complications or length of hospital stay between using PVI or esophageal Doppler for goal directed fluid therapy. PVI appears to be an acceptable alternative to esophageal Doppler for goal directed fluid therapy during major open abdominal surgery.

Abbreviations

ASA: American Society of Anesthesiologists; CONSORT: Consolidated standards of reporting trials; ECG: Electrocardiogram; GDFT: Goal-directed fluid therapy; IQR: Interquartile range; LBBB: Left bundle branch block; MAP: Mean arterial pressure; $PaCO_2$: Partial pressure of carbon dioxide in arterial blood; PaO2/FiO2: Ratio of partial pressure of oxygen in arterial blood divided by fraction of inspired oxygen; PT (INR): Prothrombin time (international normalized ratio); PVI: Pleth variability Index; SD: Standard deviation

Acknowledgements

We are indebted to research nurses Susanne Lind CRNA and Gunilla Gagnö CRNA, Department of Anesthesiology and Intensive Care, University Hospital Linköping, for their assistance with data collection.

Funding

This work was supported by the Department of Anesthesiology and Intensive Care, University Hospital Linköping, Sweden, and Region Östergötland. These organizations did not have any influence on study design, data collection and analysis and the submission process.

Authors' contributions

HB helped conduct the study, collect and analyze data and write the manuscript. RGH helped design the study, analyze data and write the manuscript. LN helped design the study, conduct the study, collect and analyze data and write the manuscript. All the authors read and approved the final manuscript.

Competing interests

RGH has given paid lectures for Baxter Healthcare. HB and LN declare that they have no competing interests.

Author details

[1]Department of Medical and Health Sciences, Linköping University, University Hospital, 58185 Linköping, Sweden. [2]Department of Anesthesiology and Intensive Care, Linköping University, University Hospital, 58185 Linköping, Sweden. [3]Department of Medical and Health Sciences, Linköping University and Research Unit, Södertälje Hospital, 152 86 Södertälje, Sweden.

References

1. Thacker JK, Mountford WK, Ernst FR, Krukas MR, Mythen MM. Perioperative fluid utilization variability and association with outcomes: considerations for enhanced recovery efforts in sample US surgical populations. Ann Surg. 2016;263:502–10.
2. Grocott MP, Dushianthan A, Hamilton MA, Mythen MG, Harrison D, Rowan K. Perioperative increase in global blood flow to explicit defined goals and outcomes after surgery: a Cochrane systematic review. Br J Anaesth. 2013;111:535–48.
3. Benes J, Giglio M, Brienza N, Michard F. The effects of goal-directed fluid therapy based on dynamic parameters on post-surgical outcome: a meta-analysis of randomized controlled trials. Crit Care. 2014;18:e584.
4. Vincent JL, Pelosi P, Pearse R, Payen D, Perel A, Hoeft A, Romagnoli S, Ranieri VM, Ichai C, Forget P, et al. Perioperative cardiovascular monitoring of high-risk patients: a consensus of 12. Crit Care. 2015;19:e224.
5. Sondergaard S. Pavane for a pulse pressure variation defunct. Crit Care. 2013;17:e327.
6. Forget P, Lois F, de Kock M. Goal-directed fluid management based on the pulse oximeter–derived pleth variability index reduces lactate levels and improves fluid management. Anesth Analg. 2010;111:910–4.
7. Forget P, Lois F, Kartheuser A, Leonard D, Remue C, De Kock M. The concept of titration can be transposed to fluid management. But does it change the volumes? Randomised trial on pleth variability index during fast-track colonic surgery. Curr Clin Pharmacol. 2013;8:110–4.
8. Warnakulasuriya SR, Davies SJ, Wilson RJT, Yates DRA. Comparison of esophageal Doppler and plethysmographic variability index to guide intraoperative fluid therapy for low-risk patients undergoing colorectal surgery. J Clin Anesth. 2016;34:600–8.
9. Bahlmann H, Hahn RG, Nilsson L. Agreement between Pleth variability index and oesophageal Doppler to predict fluid responsiveness. Acta Anaesthesiol Scand. 2016;60:183–92.
10. Hahn RG, Bahlmann H, Nilsson L. Dehydration and fluid volume kinetics before major open abdominal surgery. Acta Anaesthesiol Scand. 2014;58:1258–66.
11. Predicted body weight calculator. http://www.ardsnet.org/tools.shtml. Accessed 16 June 2017.
12. Quantitative skills. Random allocator. http://www.quantitativeskills.com/sisa/calculations/randmiz.htm. Accessed 16 June 2017. (Originally accessed at URL: http://home.clara.net/sisa/randmiz.htm).
13. Zimmermann M, Feibicke T, Keyl C, Prasser C, Moritz S, Graf BM, Wiesenack C. Accuracy of stroke volume variation compared with pleth variability index to predict fluid responsiveness in mechanically ventilated patients undergoing major surgery. Eur J Anaesthesiol. 2010;27:555–61.
14. Challand C, Struthers R, Sneyd JR, Erasmus PD, Mellor N, Hosie KB, Minto G. Randomized controlled trial of intraoperative goal-directed fluid therapy in aerobically fit and unfit patients having major colorectal surgery. Br J Anaesth. 2012;108:53–62.
15. Jørgensen CC, Bundgaard-Nielsen M, Skovgaard LT, Secher NH, Kehlet H. Stroke volume averaging for individualized goal-directed fluid therapy with oesophageal Doppler. Acta Anaesthesiol Scand. 2009;53:34–8.
16. Deltex Medical. Accuracy & Precision. http://www.deltexmedical.com/cardioq-odm/accuracy-precision. Accessed 16 June 2017.
17. Brandstrup B, Tønnesen H, Beier-Holgersen R, Beier-Holgersen R, Hjortsø E, Ørding H, Lindorff-Larsen K, Rasmussen MS, Lanng C, Wallin L, et al. Effects of intravenous fluid restriction on postoperative complications: comparison of two perioperative fluid regimens. Ann Surg. 2003;238:641–8.

18. Noblett SE, Snowden CP, Shenton BL, Horgan AF. Randomized clinical trial assessing the effect of Doppler-optimized fluid management on outcome after elective colorectal resection. Br J Surg. 2006;93:1069–76.
19. Wakeling HG, McFall MR, Jenkins CS, Woods WG, Miles WF, Barclay GR, Fleming SC. Intraoperative oesophageal Doppler guided fluid management shortens postoperative hospital stay after major bowel surgery. Br J Anaesth. 2005;95:634–42.
20. Gan TJ, Soppitt A, Maroof M, el-Moalem H, Robertson KM, Moretti E, Dwane P, Glass PS. Goal-directed intraoperative fluid administration reduces length of hospital stay after major surgery. Anesthesiology. 2002;97:820–6.
21. Mayer J, Boldt J, Mengistu AM, Röhm KD, Suttner S. Goal-directed intraoperative therapy based on autocalibrated arterial pressure waveform analysis reduces hospital stay in high-risk surgical patients: a randomized, controlled trial. Crit Care. 2010;14:e18.
22. Benes J, Chytra I, Altmann P, Hluchy M, Kasal E, Svitak R, Pradl R, Stepan M. Intraoperative fluid optimization using stroke volume variation in high risk surgical patients: results of prospective randomized study. Crit Care. 2010;14:e118.
23. Faul F, Erdfelder E, Lang A-G, Buchner A. G*Power 3: a flexible statistical power analysis program for the social, behavioral, and biomedical sciences. Behav Res Methods. 2007;39:175–91.
24. Thiele RH, Rea KM, Turrentine FE, Friel CM, Hassinger TE, McMurry TL, Goudreau BJ, Umapathi BA, Kron IL, Sawyer RG, et al. Standardization of care: impact of an enhanced recovery protocol on length of stay, complications, and direct costs after colorectal surgery. J Am Coll Surg. 2015;220:430–43.
25. Yu Y, Dong J, Xu Z, Shen H, Zheng J. Pleth variability index-directed fluid management in abdominal surgery under combined general and epidural anesthesia. J Clin Monit Comput. 2015;29:47–52.
26. Sandroni C, Cavallaro F, Marano C, Falcone C, De Santis P, Antonelli M. Accuracy of plethysmographic indices as predictors of fluid responsiveness in mechanically ventilated adults: a systematic review and meta-analysis. Intensive Care Med. 2012;38:1429–37.
27. de Wilde RB, de Wit F, Geerts BF, van Vliet AL, Aarts LP, Vuyk J, Jansen JR. Non-invasive continuous arterial pressure and pulse pressure variation measured with Nexfin in patients following major upper abdominal surgery: a comparative study. Anaesthesia. 2016;71:788–97.
28. Stens J, Oeben J, Van Dusseldorp AA, Boer C. Non-invasive measurements of pulse pressure variation and stroke volume variation in anesthetized patients using the Nexfin blood pressure monitor. J Clin Monit Comput. 2016;30:587–94.
29. Monnet X, Dres M, Ferré A, Le Teuff G, Jozwiak M, Bleibtreu A, Le Deley MC, Chemla D, Richard C, Teboul JL. Prediction of fluid responsiveness by a continuous non-invasive assessment of arterial pressure in critically ill patients: comparison with four other dynamic indices. Br J Anaesth. 2012;109:330–8.
30. Biais M, Stecken L, Martin A, Roullet S, Quinart A, Sztark F. Automated, continuous and non-invasive assessment of pulse pressure variations using CNAP® system. J Clin Monit Comput. 2017;31:685–92.
31. de Oliveira OH, Freitas FG, Ladeira RT, Fischer CH, Bafi AT, Azevedo LC, Machado FR. Comparison between respiratory changes in the inferior vena cava diameter and pulse pressure variation to predict fluid responsiveness in postoperative patients. J Crit Care. 2016;34:46–9.
32. Phan TD, Ismail H, Heriot AG, Ho KM. Improving perioperative outcomes: fluid optimization with the esophageal Doppler monitor, a meta-analysis and review. J Am Coll Surg. 2008;207:935–41.
33. Brandstrup B, Svendsen PE, Rasmussen M, Belhage B, Rodt SÅ, Hansen B, Møller DR, Lundbech LB, Andersen N, Berg V, et al. Which goal for fluid therapy during colorectal surgery is followed by the best outcome: near-maximal stroke volume or zero fluid balance? Br J Anaesth. 2012;109:191–9.
34. Pearse RM, Harrison DA, MacDonald N, Gillies MA, Blunt M, Ackland G, Grocott MP, Ahern A, Griggs K, Scott R, et al.; OPTIMISE study group. Effect of a perioperative, cardiac output-guided hemodynamic therapy algorithm on outcomes following major gastrointestinal surgery: a randomized clinical trial and systematic review. JAMA 2014;311:2181–2190.
35. Pestaña D, Espinosa E, Eden A, Nájera D, Collar L, Aldecoa C, Higuera E, Escribano S, Bystritski D, Pascual J, et al. Perioperative goal-directed hemodynamic optimization using noninvasive cardiac output monitoring in major abdominal surgery: a prospective, randomized, multicenter, pragmatic trial: POEMAS study (PeriOperative goal-directed thErapy in major abdominal surgery). Anesth Analg. 2014;119:579–87.
36. Minto G, Struthers R. Stroke volume optimisation: is the fairy tale over? Anaesthesia. 2014;69:291–6.
37. Cecconi M, Corredor C, Arulkumaran N, Abuella G, Ball J, Grounds RM, Hamilton M, Rhodes A. Clinical review: goal-directed therapy-what is the evidence in surgical patients? The effect on different risk groups. Crit Care. 2013;17:209.
38. Desebbe O, Boucau C, Farhat F, Bastien O, Lehot J-J, Cannesson M. The ability of pleth variability index to predict the hemodynamic effects of positive end-expiratory pressure in mechanically ventilated patients under general anesthesia. Anesth Analg. 2010;110:792–8.
39. Serpa Neto A, Hemmes SN, Barbas CS, Serpa Neto A, Hemmes SN, Barbas CS, Beiderlinden M, Biehl M, Binnekade JM, Canet J, et al. PROVE Network Investigators. Protective versus conventional ventilation for surgery: a systematic review and individual patient data meta-analysis. Anesthesiology 2015;123:66–78.

Patient preference survey: are patients willing to delay surgery if obstructive sleep apnea is suspected?

George Ho[1,2], Crispiana Cozowicz[3,4], Jean Wong[1], Mandeep Singh[1,5], Enoch Lam[1], Eva E. Mörwald[3,6], Najia Hasan[1], Stavros G. Memtsoudis[3] and Frances Chung[1*]

Abstract

Background: Screening and optimizing patients for OSA in the perioperative period may reduce postoperative complications. However, sleep studies can be difficult to obtain before surgery. Previous surveys reported that the majority of sleep physicians would delay surgery to diagnose and manage OSA, but most anesthesiologists would not. While disagreements exist, the importance of shared decision making and patient preferences have never been studied on this topic. It is unknown whether patients with suspected OSA, when given information about OSA, would be willing to delay surgery to diagnose and manage their condition preoperatively.

Methods: This study consisted of a self-administered questionnaire that surveyed patients, patient relatives, or any accompanying members. The survey was conducted in the preoperative clinic or in the perioperative patient and family waiting area at two hospitals in Canada and in the United States. A hypothetical scenario was used: participants were given information about OSA, and asked about their preferences regarding preoperative management should they be at risk for OSA in the setting of pending elective surgery. The objective of this study was to determine whether respondents preferred to 1) proceed with surgery as planned, 2) delay surgery to ensure the medical condition of OSA is diagnosed and optimized, or 3) let his/her physician decide.

Results: The final survey contained 19 questions and the survey was conducted from June 2016 to September 2016. Four hundred and seventy-three surveys were collected. Forty-four percent of respondents, when given information about OSA, preferred to delay surgery pending a sleep study and treatment. Forty percent of respondents who preferred to delay surgery would tolerate delaying up to two months.

Conclusion: Increasing emphasis and significant value has been placed on shared-decision making between patients and physicians. Educating patients about the risks of OSA and incorporating patient preferences into the perioperative management of OSA may be warranted.

Keywords: Obstructive sleep apnea, Anesthesiology, Surveys, Decision making

* Correspondence: Frances.Chung@uhn.ca
[1]Department of Anesthesiology and Pain Medicine, Toronto Western Hospital, University Health Network, University of Toronto, Toronto, ON, Canada
Full list of author information is available at the end of the article

Background

Obstructive sleep apnea (OSA) is the most common sleep breathing disorder. The prevalence of OSA in the general population is estimated to be 10–20% [1]. Surgical patients with OSA have an increased risk of postoperative complications, thus identifying OSA patients prior to surgery may ensure optimal perioperative care [2, 3].

There exists significant variation in opinion and practice among anesthesiologists and sleep physicians with respect to the preoperative evaluation and optimization of patients suspected of having OSA. Two surveys conducted amongst anesthesiologists reported that only 25% would delay surgery pending a sleep study to ensure proper diagnosis and treatment if a patient was suspected of having OSA [4, 5]. Another recent questionnaire conducted among four specialties (anesthesiology, primary care, sleep medicine and general surgery), concluded that a mere 4% of anesthesiologists would delay surgery pending a sleep study if a patient was suspected of having OSA, while 22% would simply proceed with surgery [6]. Conversely, among sleep physicians, 54% would prefer to delay surgery and only 5% would proceed with surgery [6].

Since patient preferences have not been studied on this topic, it is unclear whether patients, if suspected to have OSA, would prefer to proceed with or delay surgery pending a sleep study and treatment. Moreover, since 2001 the Institute of Medicine has recognized that adopting patient-centered care is crucial to the improvement of the health care system [7], and the Canadian healthcare system has also placed significant interest and high value on shared decision making that encompasses patient-centered care [8]. Recommendations and treatment should align with patient values and needs, given that it is ultimately the patient who must make informed choices about his or her care [9, 10]. The purpose of this survey was to, for the first time, examine participants' preferences by questioning participants regarding their preferences should they be suspected with having OSA while awaiting elective surgery.

Methods

Study design

This study surveyed patients, patient relatives, or any accompanying members in the preoperative clinic at Toronto Western Hospital (TWH), Toronto, and in the perioperative patient and family waiting area at the Hospital for Special Surgery (HSS), New York, using a self-administered questionnaire. As per the recommendation of the institutional ethics boards, to avoid unnecessary stress before surgery, we did not specifically target patients diagnosed with OSA. Approval from the Research Ethics Board/Institutional Review Board at TWH and HSS was obtained, and written informed consent was waived. Completion of the survey implied consent. The types of surgery performed at TWH include orthopedic, spine, neurosurgery, general surgery, urology, ophthalmology, and hand surgery. The types of surgery performed at HSS include inpatient orthopedic and spine surgery. TWH is a publicly funded healthcare facility, and HSS is a private but not-for-profit healthcare facility.

Primary and secondary objectives

The primary objective of our survey was to determine the preferences of participants when presented with information regarding OSA and a hypothetical scenario in which they are patients scheduled for elective surgery, but are suspected of having OSA. More specifically, which option would participants prefer the most: 1) proceed with surgery as planned, 2) delay surgery to ensure the medical condition of OSA is diagnosed and optimized before surgery, or 3) let his/her physician decide the course of action.

The secondary objectives included: 1) testing the knowledge of participants on OSA (symptoms, risks), 2) inquiry of current treatments amongst participants with OSA, 3) determination of the maximum length of delay that would be tolerated, if respondents preferred to delay surgery, and 4) when making a treatment decision, which domains do participants value the most [e.g. shortest length of stay, lowest risk of intensive care unit (ICU) transfers, etc.].

Survey development

A literature search of PubMed was conducted and no prior surveys investigating the topic of patient preferences presenting for elective surgery with suspected OSA were found. Due to the lack of prior investigations on this topic, content experts were enlisted to develop the survey. Anesthesiologists and sleep physicians were the content experts (FC, SM, CC, NH, MS, and JW) who identified potentially important key categories and themes for evaluation. A list of items was generated from content expert interviews and expanded with input from all of the investigators.

Domains and items reduction

Content experts ranked the importance of each domain and item, and the following domains emerged: knowledge of OSA including OSA diagnosis and current treatment for participants with OSA; when given information regarding OSA and the postoperative risks, do participants understand the information; if given a hypothetical scenario: proceed or delay surgery; participant values ranking: shortest length of hospital stay, risk of complications during surgery, risk of postoperative complications, risk of ICU transfer; and involvement in decision making process with his or her physician.

Survey formatting

The survey consisted of four parts:

1) General socio-demographics of survey participants.
2) General understanding of OSA, OSA diagnosis, and current treatment for participants with OSA.
3a) Presentation of information on OSA and the postoperative risks associated with OSA. The information was presented on one page titled: "Part 3: The following is information about Obstructive Sleep Apnea", and was described in 4 paragraphs. Paragraph 1 explained what OSA is, the symptoms associated with OSA, and the possible consequences of not treating the condition. Paragraph 2 explained what a sleep study is and how it is conducted at a sleep clinic. Paragraph 3 explained possible management modalities (oral appliances, breathing devices, surgery) if a patient has been diagnosed with OSA. Paragraph 4 explained that in the context of OSA patients undergoing surgery, they may be at an increased risk of postoperative complications. Participants were informed: "Compared to surgical patients without sleep apnea, patients with obstructive sleep apnea are:
   - At close to **2.5 times** greater risk of developing breathing problems after surgery
   - At more than **1.5 times greater** risk of developing heart problems after surgery."

Participants were then asked to answer 3 follow-up questions at the bottom of the page so that we could assess participant understanding of the presented information.

3b) Presentation of a hypothetical scenario to evaluate whether participants prefer to delay surgery, proceed with surgery, or let his or her physician decide. Also, for the participants who prefer to delay surgery, the maximum length of delay that would be tolerated. The lengths of delay (2 weeks, 1 month and 2 months) were determined based on a survey of family physicians, ear, nose and throat physicians, and respirologists in Ontario, Canada which reported that the most common response for wait time to undergo a sleep study was 1 to 3 months [11].
4) Five questions were asked to evaluate characteristics participants value the most during the decision making process (e.g. length of hospital stay, risk of intraoperative complications, risk of postoperative complications, risk of ICU transfer, and involvement in the decision making process with his or her physician.

Survey pre/pilot testing

The draft survey was distributed to the investigators who revised the study instrument focusing on clarity and interpretation of the questions. We pilot-tested the survey on ten volunteers from a variety of educational backgrounds. Revisions were made to improve language, and overall clarity of the survey (Additional file 1).

Implementation of the study

Study posters and information were posted in the preoperative clinic at TWH, and in the perioperative waiting area at HSS, while surveys were placed on tables in the respective areas for completion. A response box was set up beside the surveys allowing the study participants to anonymously deposit their completed surveys. Potential participants could pick up the survey, read through the instructions provided on the cover sheet, and complete the survey voluntarily.

The cover sheet indicated that completion of the survey and submission of the survey into the provided response box implied that he or she had consented to participate in the study. Furthermore, the cover sheet instructed respondents to complete the survey in the order that the questions were given, and respondents were asked to answer all questions to the best of their knowledge. Research assistants and other hospital staff informed individuals waiting in the respective clinic areas about the opportunity to complete a survey. As well, the research assistants were available at both sites to answer any questions.

Study participants completed the survey either on the day of the preoperative clinic appointment at TWH, or on the day of the operation at HSS. Both institutions screen patients for OSA, but the surveys were completed when patients were in the waiting room before his/her appointment with nurses and anesthesiologists. Each survey was assigned a coded study identification number. The respondents had the option to skip any question(s) they did not wish to answer. The Table 1 indicates the total number of respondents at both sites, as well as, the total number of responses obtained for each survey question.

Statistical analysis

No estimation of sample size was done, as this was the first study to determine participants' preferences on sleep disorders and treatment before surgery. The target was 500 completed surveys with 250 at each study site. We described the participants' responses using percentages. Statistical analysis was performed between the following subgroups: site (TWH vs. HSS), sex (M vs. F), age (< 65 years old vs. ≥ 65 years old), education level (secondary school education or less vs. college/university education), and respondents indicating they have

Table 1 Summary of the response rates and responses to the survey questions by site

Survey Question	Total *n* (% of total responses)	HSS *n* (% of total responses)	TWH n (% of total responses)	*P*-value
Gender, male/female[a] (T:473, HSS:244, TWH:229)				0.22
Male	187 (40)	103 (42)	84 (37)	
Female	286 (60)	141 (58)	145 (63)	
Age, years[b] (T:405, HSS:181, TWH:224)	55 ± 16	53 ± 17	56 ± 16	0.07
Highest educational attainment[a] (T:473, HSS:244, TWH:229)				< 0.001‡
Less than high school/secondary school	15 (3)	1 (0)	14 (6)	
High school (or equivalent)	88 (19)	33 (14)	55 (24)	
College/University (diploma and/or degree)	365 (77)	208 (85)	157 (69)	
Prefer not to provide this information	5 (1)	2 (1)	3 (1)	
Familiar with sleep apnoea?[a] (T:472, HSS:244, TWH:228)				0.03‡
Yes	421 (89)	225 (92)	196 (86)	
No	51 (11)	19 (8)	32 (14)	
Diagnosed with OSA?[a] (T:430, HSS:224, TWH:206)				0.44
Yes	55 (13)	26 (12)	29 (14)	
No	375 (87)	198 (88)	177 (86)	
If diagnosed with OSA, the current treatment being used[a] (T:55, HSS:26, TWH:29)				1.00
Use CPAP nightly	30 (55)	14 (54)	16 (55)	
Use CPAP sometimes	2 (4)	1 (4)	1 (3)	
Does not use CPAP	4 (7)	2 (8)	2 (7)	
Other treatment (Oral appliances, surgery)	4 (7)	2 (8)	2 (7)	
No treatment	15 (27)	7 (27)	8 (28)	
Participants' knowledge of OSA symptoms[a] (T:469, HSS:242, TWH:227)				
Short episodes where you stop breathing whilst asleep	386 (82)	207 (85)	179 (79)	< 0.001‡
Feeling very tired during the daytime	312 (67)	164 (68)	148 (65)	0.56
Sudden awakening during sleep with choking or gasping	311 (66)	164 (68)	147 (65)	0.49
Loud persistent snoring	306 (65)	167 (69)	139 (61)	0.08
Checked off all four of the above symptoms	208 (44)	112 (46)	96 (42)	0.38
OSA may affect your long-term health[a] (T:470, HSS:243, TWH:227)				0.16
True	430 (91)	227 (93)	203 (89)	
False	11 (2)	6 (2)	5 (2)	
Cannot decide	29 (6)	10 (4)	22 (8)	
OSA is treatable by different therapies[a] (T:469, HSS:243,TWH:226)				0.02‡
True	426 (91)	222 (91)	204 (90)	
False	6 (1)	6 (2)	0	
Cannot decide	37 (8)	15 (6)	22 (10)	
Hypothetical Scenario – Comprehension Questions[a] (T:467, HSS:241, TWH:226)				< 0.001‡
All 3 questions correct	344 (74)	188 (78)	156 (69)	

Table 1 Summary of the response rates and responses to the survey questions by site *(Continued)*

2/3 questions correct	92 (19)	46 (19)	46 (20)	
1 question correct	19 (4)	7 (3)	12 (5)	
0 questions correct	3 (1)	0	3 (1)	
"Cannot Decide" for all 3 questions	9 (2)	0	9 (4)	
Hypothetical Scenario – Proceed/Delay/Physician Decides[a] (T:453, HSS:237, TWH:216)				< 0.001‡
Proceed with surgery	111 (25)	47 (19)	64 (29)	
Delay surgery	201 (44)	126 (53)	75 (35)	
Let my physician decide	141 (31)	64 (27)	77 (36)	
If "Yes" to Delaying Surgery: length of delay tolerated[a] (T:192, HSS:122, TWH:70)				0.41
Up to 2 weeks	49 (26)	34 (28)	15 (21)	
Up to 1 month	66 (34)	38 (31)	28 (40)	
Up to 2 months	77 (40)	50 (41)	27 (39)	
When making a decision as to which method of treatment you most prefer, how do you rate the importance of the following?[b] *(1 = least important, 5 = most important)* (T:448, HSS: 235, TWH: 212)	Mean Rating (Total)	Mean Rating (HSS)	Mean Rating (TWH)	*P*-value
Lowest risk of complications during surgery	4.74 ± 0.7	4.82 ± 0.6	4.67 ± 0.7	0.02‡
Lowest risk of postoperative complications	4.70 ± 0.7	4.82 ± 0.6	4.57 ± 0.8	< 0.001‡
Lowest risk of being transferred to ICU	4.61 ± 0.9	4.65 ± 0.8	4.57 ± 0.9	0.33
Being involved in decision making process	4.46 ± 0.9	4.48 ± 0.9	4.44 ± 0.9	0.67
Shortest length of stay at the hospital	3.64 ± 1.3	3.69 ± 1.2	3.57 ± 1.3	0.33

CPAP = Continuous Positive Airway Pressure; HSS = Hospital for Special Surgery; ICU = Intensive Care Unit; OSA = Obstructive Sleep Apnea; T = total number of responses; TWH = Toronto Western Hospital
[a]Data presented as frequency (%)
[b]Data presented as mean ± SD and the Student Independent 2-sample t-test was used to check the statistical significance
‡Statistical significance ($P < 0.05$)

OSA vs. respondents without OSA (OSA vs. non-OSA). Student's t-tests for continuous variables and chi-square tests for categorical variables were used. P value < 0.05 was considered significant.

Results

The final survey contained 19 questions and the survey was conducted at TWH and HSS from June 2016 to September 2016. Of the 500 distributed surveys, 473 completed surveys were collected. The socio-demographics and response rates of the survey respondents are shown in the Table 1.

Eighty-nine percent (421/472) of respondents were familiar with "Sleep Apnea" and 13% (55/430) of respondents indicated having been diagnosed with OSA. Among the 55 respondents with OSA, 55% (30/55) reported using continuous positive airway pressure (CPAP) nightly, and 27% (15/55) disclosed that they were currently not on any treatment.

For questions 1–3 in Part 3, when given information about OSA, 74% (344/467) of respondents answered all 3 follow-up questions correctly. Nineteen percent (92/467) of respondents answered 2 out of the 3 questions correctly. When given the hypothetical scenario, 44% (201/453) of respondents indicated that he or she would delay surgery to ensure his/her OSA condition was treated and optimized prior to the surgery. Twenty-five percent (111/453) indicated that they would prefer to proceed with the surgery as planned, and 31% (141/453) indicated that they would prefer to let his/her physician make a decision regarding the plan of action. Of those who preferred to delay surgery, 40% (77/192) agreed to delay up to 2 months, pending a sleep study and treatment. If a participant checked yes to all three lengths of delay (2 weeks, 1 month or 2 months delay), it was inferred that the participant would agree to delay surgery for up to two months.

The difference in education levels between the two study sites was significant. Most notably, a higher proportion of respondents at HSS had a College/University education (TWH vs. HSS: 69% vs. 85%). Furthermore, there was a significant difference in the percentage of respondents who would delay surgery between both study sites ($P < 0.001$). Fifty-three percent of respondents at HSS indicated they would prefer to delay surgery. In contrast, only 35% of respondents at TWH indicated they would prefer to delay surgery. A higher percentage of respondents at TWH would prefer to simply proceed with surgery as planned (TWH vs. HSS: 29% vs. 19%).

There was a significant difference in respondents who had secondary school education or less vs. respondents who had college/university education ($p = 0.004$). The same proportion of respondents in both groups would prefer to delay surgery (22%). A lower proportion of respondents with secondary school education or less would prefer to proceed with surgery (secondary school education or less vs. college/university education: 34% vs. 51%). A higher proportion of respondents with secondary school education or less would prefer to let his/her physician decide (secondary school education or less vs. college/university education: 44% vs. 28%).

There was a significant difference between respondents indicating they have OSA vs. respondents without OSA ($p = 0.025$). A higher proportion of respondents with OSA would prefer to proceed with surgery (OSA vs. non-OSA: 37% vs. 21%). A lower proportion of respondents with OSA would prefer to delay surgery (OSA vs. non-OSA: 31% vs. 48%). The same proportion of respondents in both groups would like his/her physician to decide (31%). There was no significant difference between sex (Male vs. Female), and age (< 65 years old vs. ≥ 65 years old) regarding the delay of surgery.

For part 2 question 4 ("What do you believe are the likely symptoms of OSA"), 44% of respondents checked off all 4 symptoms as likely the result of OSA. There was no difference between the two study sites. For questions 5 and 6 (True/False), 91% of respondents believed OSA may affect long-term health, and is treatable by different therapies. There was no difference between the two sites on whether OSA may affect long-term health (question 5), but there was a significant difference on treatment by different therapies (question 6). For question 6, a higher proportion of respondents at TWH indicated they "Cannot decide" (TWH vs. HSS: 10% vs. 6%) and none of the respondents at TWH responded with "False" for this statement ($p = 0.02$).

Discussion

The majority of respondents (89%) were already familiar with OSA as a medical condition. When given information on OSA, 93% were able to answer at least 2 out of the 3 follow-up questions correctly, demonstrating that respondents had a high level of understanding regarding OSA, i.e. how it is diagnosed, types of available treatment, and the associated postoperative risks. When presented with the hypothetical scenario of high risk for OSA and pending surgery, 44% indicated a preference that involved the delay of surgery to ensure that the medical condition of OSA was optimized prior to surgery. In this context, 40% of respondents were willing to tolerate a delay of up to 2 months.

Multiple guidelines have been published on the perioperative management of OSA patients [12–16]. For example, a recently published guideline by the American Society of Anesthesiologists recommends preoperative screening as well as initiation of pre-operative continuous positive airway pressure (CPAP) to optimize the OSA condition [14, 15]. However, access to diagnosis and treatment of OSA is limited, which means that a patient's surgery may be delayed significantly if OSA is suspected and is postponed for further investigation [17]. In fact, the most recent Guideline by the Society of Anesthesia and Sleep Medicine notes that there is limited evidence to guide recommendations with respect to the preoperative decision-making process for patients and clinicians on whether to proceed or delay surgery if a patient is suspected of having OSA [16]. While disagreement exists between sleep physicians and anesthesiologists on whether a delay of surgery is warranted in patients suspected to have OSA [6], a paucity of data exists regarding patient preferences on this issue. At present, physicians have relied on their clinical experience and guidelines have not taken into account patient perspectives in the perioperative management of OSA.

Implementing shared decision making involves understanding patient preferences, while having an open and honest discussion with patients to ensure they are well informed [18]. A recently published article on the implementation of shared decision making in the National Health Service (NHS) recognizes that a change in attitude amongst physicians is key to improving the shared decision making process [18]. It reported that many physicians presume that they already involve their patients in care-related decisions, or physicians may fail to recognize how the values and preferences of patients may differ from their own. These findings have been recognized in Canada and the US, and are not unique to the NHS [10, 19]. In order to improve shared decision making, a true shift in attitude and culture is required [20]. However, none of this can be accomplished if clinicians do not investigate patient preferences or are not aware that patient perspectives may differ from their own perspectives.

OSA is a highly prevalent comorbid condition in the elective surgical population and preoperative identification and treatment of OSA may reduce perioperative complications. It is important for physicians to educate their patients about the potential risks and to involve patients in the decision making process and so it was necessary to investigate the preferences of patients. This study represents the first attempt to examine the preferences of participants using a hypothetical scenario, and demonstrates that a significant proportion of respondents would be willing to delay surgery pending a sleep study and treatment for OSA. Further investigations are warranted on more specific patient populations and the different types of surgical procedures. While an argument could be made that sleep studies and treatments may amount to greater short-term costs, the identification and treatment of OSA will result in reductions in overall healthcare costs in the long term [21, 22]. Anesthesiologists have the opportunity to become major contributors in shared decision making while diagnosing and treating OSA to improve perioperative safety in the healthcare system [17]. Recognition of patient preferences may assist decision making and supplement the formulation and/or modifications of guidelines or institutional policy for the perioperative management of patients with OSA.

There were limitations to this study with regards to the development, distribution and implementation of the survey. Validity testing was not conducted during development. We may have been able to obtain more fully completed surveys and illicit more accurate responses from participants if research assistants were available to guide each respondent through the survey in a one-on-one setting. Due to the nature of the survey, the type (patients and non-patients) and total number of participants attending the clinic or preoperative areas were not collected. The generalizability of the results to individuals with lower educational status may be limited, as most participants in this survey had completed a college/university education. Furthermore, individuals with previous knowledge on OSA may have been more likely to participate in the survey. Only a small portion of participants had OSA, which may have made the scenario more "real" and the data most reliable amongst this group. However, over half of such patients were already on treatment, so the question on delaying surgery would be of little relevance. We presented information on OSA and associated risks to ensure all respondents were informed of OSA, but the presentation of the risks may have biased respondents towards delaying surgery. We acknowledge that the hypothetical nature of the scenario removes respondents from real-life decision-making, and the type of procedure was not specified. The results may differ if respondents were asked to make a real-life decision on their upcoming surgery. The type of procedure may also significantly impact decision-making because elective surgery encompasses a wide range of procedures from cosmetic to cancer surgery. Moreover, when respondents were asked to rate the importance of several factors at the end of the survey, the inclusion of procedure types as a factor may have been of interest.

Conclusions

Despite the limitations of this study, it was the first attempt to understand patient preferences within the preoperative management of suspected OSA. Our study demonstrates that patients do have clear preferences on this topic. Educating patients and incorporating shared decision making when facing a complex condition such as suspected OSA in the surgical setting may help physicians to make decisions about preoperative management of these patients.

Abbreviations

CPAP: continuous positive airway pressure; HSS: Hospital for Special Surgery; ICU: intensive care unit; NHS: National Health Service; OSA: obstructive sleep apnea; TWH: Toronto Western Hospital

Acknowledgements

The authors would like to thank Jacqueline Vlahos, RN, BScN, Patient Care Coordinator, Day Surgery and Preadmission, Toronto Western Hospital, University Health Network, Toronto, Ontario, Canada and the staff of the Preadmission Clinic for the assistance they provided to conduct the survey. The authors would like to thank Sandra Bossi, Associate Director, Innovation and Business Development, Hospital for Special Surgery, New York, New York, USA and the staff of the perioperative waiting area, for their assistance in conducting the survey.

Funding

This research was funded by the Departments of Anesthesia at TWH and HSS, and did not receive any specific grant from funding agencies in the public, commercial, or not-for-profit sectors.

Authors' contributions

GH helped design and conduct the study, analyze the data, and write the manuscript. CC helped design and conduct the study and write the manuscript. JW helped design the study, write and edit the manuscript. MS helped design the study and write the manuscript. EL helped conduct the study, and reviewed the manuscript. EEM helped conduct the study, and reviewed the manuscript. NH helped design the study, and reviewed the manuscript. SGM helped design and conduct the study and write the manuscript. FC helped design and conduct the study and write the manuscript. All authors read and approved the final manuscript.

Competing interests

GH has no conflicts of interest. CC has no conflicts of interest. JW received research grants from Ontario Ministry of Health and Long-Term Care Innovation Fund, Anesthesia Patient Safety Foundation, and Acacia Pharma Ltd. MS received research support from Society of Anesthesia and Sleep Medicine. EL has no conflicts of interest. EEM has no conflicts of interest. NH has no conflicts of interest. SGM is a non-paid consultant for B.Braun, and is funded by the Anna Maria and Stephen Kellen Career Development Award, New York. FC received research grants from Ontario Ministry of Health and Long-Term Care Innovation Fund, University Health Network Foundation, ResMed Foundation, Acacia Pharma Ltd. and Medtronics Inc.

Author details

[1]Department of Anesthesiology and Pain Medicine, Toronto Western Hospital, University Health Network, University of Toronto, Toronto, ON, Canada. [2]Faculty of Medicine, University of Toronto, Toronto, ON, Canada. [3]Department of Anesthesiology, Hospital for Special Surgery, Weill Cornell Medical College, New York, NY, USA. [4]Perioperative Medicine and Intensive Care Medicine, Paracelsus Medical University, Salzburg, Austria. [5]Toronto Sleep and Pulmonary Centre, Toronto, ON, Canada. [6]Perioperative Medicine and Intensive Care Medicine, Paracelsus Medical University, Salzburg, Austria.

References

1. Peppard PE, Young T, Barnet JH, Palta M, Hagen EW, Hla KM. Increased prevalence of sleep-disordered breathing in adults. Am J Epidemiol. 2013; 177(9):1006–14.
2. Opperer M, Cozowicz C, Bugada D, Mokhlesi B, Kaw R, Auckley D, Chung F, Memtsoudis SG. Does obstructive sleep apnea influence perioperative outcome? A qualitative systematic review for the Society of Anesthesia and Sleep Medicine Task Force on preoperative preparation of patients with sleep-disordered breathing. Anesth Analg. 2016;122(5):1321–34.
3. Kaw R, Chung F, Pasupuleti V, Mehta J, Gay PC, Hernandez AV. Meta-analysis of the association between obstructive sleep apnoea and postoperative outcome. Br J Anaesth. 2012;109(6):897–906.
4. Cordovani L, Chung F, Germain G, Turner K, Turgeon AF, Hall R, Gay PC, Bryson GL, Choi PT. Canadian perioperative anesthesia clinical trials G: perioperative management of patients with obstructive sleep apnea: a survey of Canadian anesthesiologists. Can J Anaesth. 2016;63(1):16–23.
5. Turner K, VanDenkerkhof E, Lam M, Mackillop W. Perioperative care of patients with obstructive sleep apnea - a survey of Canadian anesthesiologists. Can J Anaesth. 2006;53(3):299–304.
6. Auckley D, Cox R, Bolden N, Thornton JD. Attitudes regarding perioperative care of patients with OSA: a survey study of four specialties in the United States. Sleep Breath. 2015;19(1):315–25.
7. Crossing the Quality Chasm: A New Health System for the 21st Century. In., EDN Washington (DC): National Academies Press (US); 2001.
8. Legare F, Stacey D, Forest PG. Shared decision-making in Canada: update, challenges and where next! Z Arztl Fortbild Qualitatssich. 2007;101(4):213–21.
9. Canadian Medical Association (CMA). Achieving patient-centered collaborative care. In: CMA POLICY; 2008.
10. Legare F, Witteman HO. Shared decision making: examining key elements and barriers to adoption into routine clinical practice. Health Aff (Millwood). 2013;32(2):276–84.
11. Rotenberg B, George C, Sullivan K, Wong E. Wait times for sleep apnea care in Ontario: a multidisciplinary assessment. Can Respir J. 2010;17(4):170–4.
12. Meoli AL, Rosen CL, Kristo D, Kohrman M, Gooneratne N, Aguillard RN, Fayle R, Troell R, Kramer R, Casey KR, et al. Upper airway management of the adult patient with obstructive sleep apnea in the perioperative period--avoiding complications. Sleep. 2003;26(8):1060–5.
13. Joshi GP, Ankichetty SP, Gan TJ, Chung F. Society for Ambulatory Anesthesia consensus statement on preoperative selection of adult patients with obstructive sleep apnea scheduled for ambulatory surgery. Anesth Analg. 2012;115(5):1060–8.
14. Gross JB, Bachenberg KL, Benumof JL, Caplan RA, Connis RT, Cote CJ, Nickinovich DG, Prachand V, Ward DS, Weaver EM, et al. Practice guidelines for the perioperative management of patients with obstructive sleep apnea: a report by the American Society of Anesthesiologists Task Force on perioperative management of patients with obstructive sleep apnea. Anesthesiology. 2006;104(5):1081–93. quiz 1117-1088
15. American Society of Anesthesiologists Task Force on Perioperative Management of patients with obstructive sleep. A: practice guidelines for the perioperative management of patients with obstructive sleep apnea: an updated report by the American Society of Anesthesiologists Task Force on perioperative management of patients with obstructive sleep apnea. Anesthesiology. 2014;120(2):268–86.
16. Chung F, Memtsoudis SG, Ramachandran SK, Nagappa M, Opperer M, Cozowicz C, Patrawala S, Lam D, Kumar A, Joshi GP, et al. Society of Anesthesia and Sleep Medicine Guidelines on preoperative screening and assessment of adult patients with obstructive sleep apnea. Anesth Analg. 2016;123(2):452–73.
17. Dawson D, Singh M, Chung F. The importance of obstructive sleep apnoea management in peri-operative medicine. Anaesthesia. 2016;71(3):251–6.
18. Joseph-Williams N, Lloyd A, Edwards A, Stobbart L, Tomson D, Macphail S, Dodd C, Brain K, Elwyn G, Thomson R. Implementing shared decision making in the NHS: lessons from the MAGIC programme. BMJ. 2017;357:j1744.
19. Elwyn G, Edwards A, Thompson R: Shared decision making in health care: achieving evidence-based patient choice, 3 edn: Oxford Universiy press; 2016.
20. Rapley T. Distributed decision making: the anatomy of decisions-in-action. Sociol Health Illn. 2008;30(3):429–44.
21. Potts KJ, Butterfield DT, Sims P, Henderson M, Shames CB. Cost savings associated with an education campaign on the diagnosis and management of sleep-disordered breathing: a retrospective, claims-based US study. Popul Health Manag. 2013;16(1):7–13.
22. Skaer TL, Sclar DA. Economic implications of sleep disorders. Pharmacoeconomics. 2010;28(11):1015–23.

10

Analgesic effect of Ropivacaine combined with Dexmedetomidine on brachial plexus block

Zhenqing Liu*, Menglu Jiang, Tongsheng Xu and Hao Hua

Abstract

Background: This randomized controlled study investigated the analgesic effect of ropivacaine in combination with dexmedetomidine versus ropivacaine alone on brachial plexus block to provide alternative anesthetic means for upper limb trauma surgery.

Methods: Totally 114 patients who received upper limb surgeries under brachial plexus block anesthesia in our hospital from February 2013 to July 2015 were enrolled. The patients were randomized to ropivacaine alone (the control group) or ropivacaine combined with dexmedetomidine (the combination group). The blocking effect on sensory and motor neurons, visual analog scale (VAS) score, heart rate (HR), mean arterial pressure (MAP), peripheral capillary oxygen saturation (SPO_2) and adverse reactions were compared between the two groups.

Results: The time to onset of sensory and motor nerve blockade was significantly shorter in the combination group than in the control group (8.9 min vs. 12.4 min for sensation blockade; 7.5 min vs. 12.8 min for motor blockade, $P < 0.05$ for both comparisons), and the duration of the blockade was significantly longer in the combination group (590.2 min vs. 532.1 min, $P < 0.05$). There was no significant difference in VAS scores between the two groups immediately and 4 h after surgery; however, 8, 12 and 24 h after surgery, the VAS scores were all significantly lower in the combination group than the control group (2.4 vs. 3.0 for 8 h; 2.2 vs. 4.2 for 12 h, and 2.1 vs. 5.4 for 24 h, respectively, $P < 0.05$ for all comparisons). There was no statistical difference in HR, MAP and SPO_2 between the two groups before anesthesia, but after anesthesia, the MAP and HR were significantly lower, and the SPO_2 was significantly higher in the combination group than the control group (78 vs. 84 for MAP; 72 vs. 79 for HR; and 95.1 vs. 88.2 for SPO_2, $P < 0.05$ for all comparisons). The rates of adverse reaction was significantly lower in the combination group than the control group (3.6 vs. 7.2, $P < 0.05$).

Conclusion: The brachial plexus blocking effect of ropivacaine combined with dexmedetomidine was superior to that of ropivacaine alone, mainly intra-operatively and postoperatively.

Keywords: Dexmedetomidine, Ropivacaine, Nerve block, Analgesia, Visual analog scale

* Correspondence: Liuzhenqi1208@163.com
Department of Anesthesiology, The Ninth People's Hospital of Wuxi, No.999 Liangxi Road, Wuxi 214062, China

Background

With the dramatic increase in the number of automatic vehicles on the road, the incidence of various types of traffic traumas has been on the rise throughout China. Upper limb fracture is one of them. In order to alleviate severe pain in patients with upper limb fracture, analgesia by brachial plexus blockade is usually applied before surgery. However, due to a myriad of reasons, patients with upper limb fracture are usually very nervous and anxious before and during the operation, leading to heart rate (HR) decrease, blood pressure increase and even shock [1, 2].

Compared with general anesthesia, brachial plexus regional anesthesia is the preferred approach of anesthesia for upper limb surgery because it is easy to perform, and patients can undergo the procedure in the waking state during the operation [3]. However, administration of appropriate analgesics is critical [4]. Traditional analgesics such as fentanyl have strong analgesic effect; however, they were found to be prone to over-anesthesia; thus, they virtually increase perioperative risks and are not conducive to postoperative recovery [5]. At present, a technique of continuous brachial plexus blockade under the guidance of ultrasonography has been developed, where local anesthetics can be intermittently or continuously injected into the location to be blocked through a connection tube installed by visualization technique. This technique is very simple to use, and allows the adjustment of dose of the anesthetic according to operative time; it also meets postoperative analgesic requirement of patients [6].

In addition to the route of anesthesia, the choice of analgesics is also very important. An ideal analgesic is one that can achieve a good anesthetic effect without incurring serious adverse reactions. Ropivacaine is a new local anesthetic that inhibits neuronal excitement and conduction by inhibiting neuronal sodium channels [7]. It has a very strong analgesic effect as it can produce nerve blocking effect at low concentrations; its effect is long lasting, and its central nerve inhibitory activity is low, which makes it a commonly used anesthetic in nerve block anesthesia [8]. In addition, ropivacaine also has vasoconstrictive effect, thereby reducing absorption of drugs into the plasma and leading to a long lasting effect. The drug is also one of the ideal anesthetics to relieve a variety of postoperative pain. Dexmedetomidine is a highly selective $\alpha 2$ adrenergic receptor agonist. It shows a high affinity for its receptor that is 7 to 8 times stronger than clonidine, which belongs to the same category. It also shows a fast onset time and long lasting effect. Clinically, dexmedetomidine is used as an analgesic, sedative and anxiolytic medication [9]. Studies have shown that dexmedetomidine also has a neuroprotective effect, possibly by increasing intravascular calcium levels and reducing the concentration of catecholamines [10, 11]. Thus, dexmedetomidine has been as an anesthesia adjuvant.

In this study, we evaluated the efficacy and safety of ropivacaine in combination with dexmedetomidine versus ropivacaine alone in 114 patients requiring upper limb surgery with the primary outcome being changes in postoperative visual analog scale (VAS) scores versus baseline.

Methods

Patients

This randomized controlled study enrolled patients who were scheduled to undergo elective upper limb surgery, including tendon repair, fracture internal fixation, and flap transfer, at our hospital between February 2013 and July 2015. Patients were included 1) if they had an American Society of Anesthesiologists (ASA) physical status classification I or II; 2) if they were aged between 20 and 50 years; 3) if they had no known allergy to anesthetics; 4) if they had no history of heart, kidney and brain diseases. Patients were excluded 1) if they had chronic heart and lung diseases; 2) if they were obese (body mass index, BMI ≥ 30 kg/m^2); 3) if they refused to provide consent to the study.

This study was approved by the local Institute Ethic Committee at the authors' affiliated institution and all patients signed informed consent to voluntarily participate in the study.

Randomization

Sample size calculation was based on the primary outcome of changes in postoperative VAS scores versus baseline. We calculated the sample size using the SAS Proc Power, and 48 patients for each group were required, assuming a two-sided type I error (α) of 0.05 and a power of 80%. Allowing for approximately 20% incomplete follow-up or dropout, a total of 120 patients were enrolled in this study.The patients were randomly assigned either to the control group or the combination treatment group in a 1:1 ratio using a computer-generated randomization number sequence performed by a clinician who was not involved in the study. Group assignment was sealed in sequentially numbered opaque envelopes. The patients, attending anaesthesiologists, surgeons, and data collectors were all blinded to patient group assignment.

Brachial plexus block

Phenobarbital sodium (0.1 g) was administered intramuscularly 30 min before surgery. Immediately before the operation, oxygen was provided conventionally, an intravenous route was established and the vital signs including heart rate (HR), mean arterial pressure (MAP) and oxygen saturation (SpO2) were monitored conventionally. Brachial plexus block anesthesia was then started. Briefly, the patient was placed in a supine position, and the upper limbs were placed on the corresponding side of the body. The needle was inserted into the muscle layer at the circular cartilage level, and moved towards the posterolateral and lower direction of the grove. The needle was then turned slightly towards C6 cervical transverse process. When the stimulating electric current reached 0.5 mA, if the distal muscle of the deltoid muscle group contracted concurrently, the puncture was deemed successful. After the successful puncture, anesthetics were injected. The control group received 20 mL 0.375% ropivacaine within 30 s; the combination treatment group received 20 mL 0.375% ropivacaine in combination with 100 μg dexmedetomidine within 30 s.

Study outcomes

During the whole procedure, vital signs of the patients were recorded. Pain was evaluated using the VAS, with 0 for no pain, and 10 for the worst possible pain. VAS scores at baseline (0 h), and 4, 8, 12 and 24 h after surgery were recorded. The primary outcome was changes in postoperative VAS scores versus baseline. The secondary outcomes included time to onset of blockade, time to recovery of sensation and movement and the total analgesic maintenance time, changes in HR, MAP and SPO_2 and safety. Time to onset of blockade was defined as the time between injection of the anesthetics and loss of sensation to needle prick, and the time between injection of the anesthetics and loss of thumb movement. Time to onset of blockade of the radial nerve, median nerve, ulnar nerve and musculocutaneous nerve was recorded. In addition, time to recovery of sensation and movement and the total analgesic maintenance time were also recorded. Adverse reactions during the perioperative period were recorded.

Statistical analysis

Data was expressed as mean ± SD and analyzed using the SPSS 13.0 software (SPSS Inc., Chicago, IL, USA). Comparison between the two groups was performed using Student's t test. Count data were analyzed with χ^2 test. $P < 0.05$ was considered statistically significant.

Results

Patient demographic and baseline data

The study flowchart is shown in Fig. 1. Totally 150 patients were screened for enrollment, 25 patients did not meet the eligibility requirements and were excluded, and 5 did not provide consent to the study and were not included. One hundred twenty patients were eligible; 6 patients were excluded because they were not cooperative during the study. Finally, 114 patients were included in the study. They included 37 (64.9%) male patients and 20 (35.1%) female patients in the combination treatment group and 36 (63.2%) male patients and 21 (36.8%) female patients in the control group. The age of patients in the combination treatment group (30.4 ± 10.1 years; range 20 to 55 years) was comparable with that of the control group (30.8 ± 11.2 years; range 21 to 55 years). The two groups were comparable in demographic variables ($P > 0.05$).

Ropivacaine in combination with dexmedetomidine is more effective than ropivacaine in alleviating postoperative pain

The VAS scores of the two groups before and at different time points after surgery are summarized in Table 1. As shown in Table 1, there was no statistically significant difference between the VAS scores of the two groups at baseline and 4 h after the surgery. At 8, 12 and 24 h after surgery, the VAS scores of the combination treatment group were significantly lower than those of the

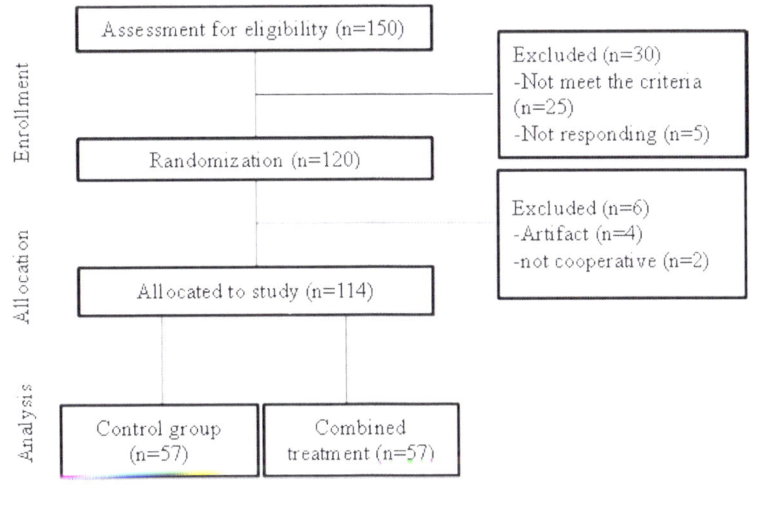

Fig. 1 The study flowchart

Table 1 Comparison of VAS score between the two groups

Group	Cases	Preoperative	4 h postoperative	8 h postoperative	12 h postoperative	24 h postoperative
Combination	57	1.7 ± 0.4	1.8 ± 0.9	2.4 ± 0.6[a]	2.2 ± 0.9[a]	2.1 ± 0.4[a]
Control	57	1.8 ± 0.5	1.9 ± 0.7	3.0 ± 1.5	4.2 ± 1.1	5.4 ± 0.8

Note: [a]t test, $P < 0.05$ compared with the control group

control group (8 h: 2.4 vs. 3.0; 12 h: 2.2 vs. 4.2, and 24 h: 2.1 vs. 5.4, respectively, $P < 0.05$ for all comparisons).

Ropivacaine in combination with dexmedetomidine exerts significantly longer blocking effects on sensory and motor nerves than ropivacaine alone

The sensory and motor nerve blocking effects in both groups are shown in Table 2. Compared with that of the control group, the time to onset of nerve blockade of both sensory nerves and motor nerves in the combination treatment group was significantly shorter (8.9 min vs. 12.4 min for sensation blockade; 7.5 min vs. 12.8 min for motor blockade, $P < 0.05$ for both comparisons). Furthermore, the blockade maintenance time for both sensory nerve and motor nerve was significantly longer in the combination treatment group than the control group (482.1 min vs. 380.2 min for sensation blockade; 430.1 min vs. 350.1 min for motor blockade, $P < 0.05$ for both comparisons), and the analgesic maintenance time was also significantly longer in the combination treatment group (590.2 min vs.532.1 min, $P < 0.05$).

Ropivacaine in combination with dexmedetomidine leads to greater improvement in HR, MAP and SPO_2 than ropivacaine

The vital signs of the study patients at different time points are shown in Table 3. HR, MAP and SPO_2 exhibited no statistically significant changes after surgery versus baseline in both groups. However, a statistically significant difference was found in HR, MAP and SPO_2 between the two groups during the surgery: HR and MAP of the combination treatment group were significantly lower than those of the control group (MAP: 78 vs. 84; HR: 72 vs. 79; $P < 0.05$ for both comparisons), and SPO_2 of the combination treatment group was significant higher than that of the control group (95.1 vs. 88.2; $P < 0.05$), indicating that the combination treatment was more beneficial to the patients.

Ropivacaine in combination with dexmedetomidine has significantly fewer adverse reactions than ropivacaine alone

The adverse reactions of the two groups are summarized in Table 4. The major adverse reactions in both groups were lethargy and nausea; however, the incidence rate of adverse reaction in the combination treatment group was significantly lower than that of the control group (3.6 vs. 7.2; $P < 0.05$). However, the cases of the adverse reaction were too few to reach a final conclusion yet, and more studies are needed to verify this.

Discussion

This study evaluated the efficacy and safety of ropivacaine in combination with dexmedetomidine versus ropivacaine alone in 114 patients requiring upper limb surgery. The findings showed that ropivacaine in combination with dexmedetomidine was associated with a significantly greater reduction of VAS scores at 8 to 24 h postoperatively compared with ropivacaine alone, suggesting that the combination regimen is more effective than ropivacaine alone in alleviating postoperative pain. We further demonstrated that this improvement in pain reduction was at least partially due to significantly longer blocking effects by the combination therapy on sensory and motor nerves than ropivacaine alone. The study indicates that along with its more benign safety profile, ropivacaine in combination with dexmedetomidine offers a more effective and safer alternative to ropivacaine alone in analgesia for patients undergoing upper limb surgery.

Theoretically, the combined use of two kinds of anesthetics would yield a synergistic effect, leading to a low dosage use of each drug. Several studies have evaluated the dosages and efficacy of the combination of the two anesthetics in different race cohorts [12, 13]. However, few studies on the ropivacaine-dexmedetomidine combination have been reported in Chinese cohorts [14]. In this study, we investigated the analgesic effect of ropivacaine in combination with dexmedetomidine in brachial plexus block and compared its effect with that of

Table 2 Comparison of sensory and motor nerve blocking effects between the two groups

Group	No. of cases	Onset of blockage time (min)		Blockage maintenance time (min)		Analgesia maintenance time (min)
		Motor	Sensation	Motor	Sensation	
Combination	57	7.5 ± 2.3[a]	8.9 ± 2.5[a]	430.1 ± 35.7[a]	482.1 ± 39.4[a]	590.2 ± 40.5[a]
Control	57	12.8 ± 3.7	12.4 ± 2.4	350.1 ± 32.4	380.2 ± 37.2	532.1 ± 36.7

Note: [a]t test, $P < 0.05$ compared with control group

Table 3 Comparison of HR, MAP and SPO2 at different time points between the two groups

Group	Timing	HR	MAP	SPO_2
Combination	Preoperative	81.0 ± 5.8	84.2 ± 6.5	97.2 ± 3.2
	Intraoperative	72.2 ± 7.4[a]	78.0 ± 5.4[a]	95.1 ± 3.9[a]
	Postoperative	80.2 ± 6.4	84.1 ± 6.2	97.1 ± 3.7
Control	Preoperative	81.5 ± 7.3	84.7 ± 7.1	97.0 ± 4.0
	Intraoperative	79.4 ± 6.8	84.0 ± 5.9	88.2 ± 2.0
	Postoperative	80.0 ± 5.7	84.3 ± 6.8	97.3 ± 4.0

Note: [a]t test; $P < 0.05$ compared with the control group

ropivacaine alone. The results showed that compared with the control group, nerve blockade onset time in the combination treatment group was significantly shorter, and the blockade maintenance time was markedly longer; the VAS scores of the combination treatment group were significantly lower than that of control group at 8, 12 and 24 h after the operation; furthermore, MAP and HR in combined treatment were significantly lower than those of the control group, and SPO_2 was significantly higher than that of the control group; the major adverse reactions in both groups were lethargy and nausea, while the incidence rate of adverse reaction in combined treatment group was significantly lower than that of the control group.

Compared with similar studies performed by other investigators [12–14], our results are consistent with their conclusions. Moreover, our study is superior to those already published in several aspects: 1) we had a larger sample size (114 patients in our study compared with 80 patients in the study published). 2) Our study parameters were broader, i.e., VAS score for assessing the effect of analgesia was also included in our study. 3) Detailed study of the adverse reactions was also included in our study.

We found that the major adverse reactions in both groups were lethargy and nausea, and the incidence rate of adverse reaction in the combined treatment group was significantly lower than that of the control group, which is somewhat surprising, as per common sense, one would assume that the combination of two anesthetics would cause more adverse reactions than single anesthetic. For example, Das reported a higher incidence of somnolence in the combination group than the control group [13]. One explanation for the discrepancy is that we used a lower dose of the anesthetics in our study so that they might not cause somnolence in our patient.

Table 4 Comparison of adverse reactions between the two groups {case (%)}

Group	Cases	Lethargy	Nausea	Incidence rate (%)
Combination	57	1(1.8)	1(1.8)	3.6[a]
Control	57	2(3.6)	2(3.6)	7.2

Note: [a]χ^2 test; $P < 0.05$ compared with the control group

In the meantime, it is worthy of pointing out that the cases of the adverse reaction in our study were too few (one case vs. two cases) to reach a final conclusion yet, more studies are needed to verify this.

The study also has limitations. The study was undertaken in a tertiary care setting and the findings may not be applicable to primary or secondary care settings. Second, we only evaluated the effect on pain reduction up to 24 h postoperatively. In addition, we only limited the study patients to those undergoing upper limb surgery and the study findings may not be applicable to other types of surgery. Moreover, ultrasonography was not used in the current study as it was not available in our surgical ward.

Conclusions

To summarize, from this study, it can be concluded that combination use of dexmedetomidine and ropivacaine in the brachial plexus block has a good analgesic effect. Compared with use of ropivacaine alone, the combination regimen has faster nerve blockade onset, longer nerve blocking effect and lower VAS score, it can significantly improve vital signs such as HR, blood pressure and SPO_2, and can also reduce the incidence of adverse reactions; thus, its application is worth promoting widely.

Abbreviations

ASA: American Society of Anesthesiologists; HR: heart rate; MAP: mean arterial pressure; SPO_2: peripheral capillary oxygen saturation; VAS: visual analog scale

Authors' contributions

ZQL: conceived and designed the study, reviewed and edited the manuscript. MLJ: Collecting and Organizing Data, TSX: Data Analysis, HH: wrote the paper, All authors read and approved the manuscript.

Competing interests

All the authors declare that they have no conflict of interest.

References

1. She Y. Clinical effect of Dexmedetomidine combined with bupivacaine and lidocaine in brachial plexus block. Chin J Clin Rational Drug Use. 2015;21:113–4.
2. Qu B, Yu Y, Guan R, Zheng Y, Chen X. Application of Dexmedetomidine combined with Ropivacaine in brachial plexus block. Chin J Surg of Integrated Traditional and West Med. 2015;05:515–7.

3. Kang H, Cao S. The sedation effect of Dexmedetomidine in assisting brachial plexus block. Jiangsu Pharm. 2015;14:1674–6.
4. Zhou L, Cao X, Liao X. Effects of different doses of Dexmedetomidine combined with Ropivacaine on brachial plexus block. Chin Pharm. 2015;30:4210–2.
5. Zhan L, Chen Z. Application of Tozoxin combined with Ropivacaine hydrochloride in brachial plexus block. World Latest Med. 2015;50:76.
6. Hu G, Song X, Tao J. The effect of Ropivacaine combined with Dexmedetomidine on brachial plexus block. J Clin Anesth. 2014;06:546–9.
7. Ma M, Han Y. Clinical observation of lidocaine combined with Ropivacaine or bupivacaine in brachial plexus block. Qinghai Med J. 2015;11:16–7.
8. Huang J, Hu H, An X, Zhang Q, Zhu F, Wang X. The effect of application of same dose and different volume of Ropivacaine to block brachial plexus under ultrasound guidance on the movement of diaphragm. J Clin Anesth. 2015;31(12):1176–9.
9. Yang H, Zhou J, Sun J, Chen H. Clinical application of Dexmedetomidine combined with Ropivacaine in pediatric axillary brachial plexus block. Hainan Med J. 2015;26(23):3481–3.
10. Chen M, Wan Z, Xu P, Cai L, Liu J, Hu N. Preventive effect of intravenous administration of Dexmedetomidine under brachial plexus block anesthesia on pain caused by tourniquet. Shanghai Med. 2015;38(10):767–70.
11. Jin Y, Zhao X. Effect of Ropivacaine combined Dexmedetomidine on ultrasound-guided axillary brachial plexus block anesthesia. Shanghai Med. 2015;02:110–4.
12. Bangera A, Manasa M, Krishna P. Supraclavicular brachial plexus block using ropivacaine alone or combined with dexmedetomidine for upper limb surgery: a prospective, randomized, double-blinded, comparative study. Saudi J Anaesth. 2016;10(1):38–44.
13. Das B, Lakshmegowda M, Sharma M, Mitra S, Chauhan R. Dexmedetomidine as an adjuvant to ropivacaine in supraclavicular brachial plexus block. Rev Esp Anestesiol Reanim. 2016;63(3):135–40.
14. Zhang Y, Wang CS, Shi JH, Sun B, Liu SJ, Li P, Li EY. Perineural administration of Dexmedetomidine in combination with Ropivacaine prolongs axillary brachial plexus block. Int J Clin Exp Med. 2014;7(3):680–5.

Survey of postoperative pain control in different types of hospitals: a multicenter observational study

Michał Borys[1*], Klaudia Zyzak[1], Agata Hanych[2], Michał Domagała[3], Piotr Gałkin[4], Katarzyna Gałaszkiewicz[1], Agata Kłaput[1], Kai Wróblewski[1], Justyna Miękina[1], Dariusz Onichimowski[5] and Mirosław Czuczwar[1]

Abstract

Background: Current pain assessment and treatment does not address every patient's requirements. Although the Polish national guidelines for post-operative pain management have been published, many patients experience severe pain in the postoperative period. The main goal of our study was to assess pain severity among patients from different types of hospitals (primary, secondary, and tertiary centers) after similar types of surgeries. We also aimed to determine if there were any differences in pain severity associated with anesthesia technique, type of surgery, and the patient's age and sex.

Methods: This was a prospective, observational study. A questionnaire form was used to collect demographic data, type of hospital, surgery, anesthesia, and patient satisfaction of pain control in the postoperative period. The visual analogue scale (VAS) was used to measure pain severity at four time points after surgery (4, 8, 12, and 24 h).

Results: The study was conducted from November 2015 to June 2016 in seven hospitals in Eastern Poland, and 269 women and 293 men participated. At the 4-h measurement, 39.32% of patients assessed the pain as moderate and 19.75% as severe. A difference was found in pain intensity between patients treated in primary and secondary hospitals. Vascular surgery patients had the lowest pain intensity (19 (13–26)), especially in comparison to those undergoing thoracic surgery (30 (27–33)). A sudden elevation in pain severity among patients anesthetized with single-shot spinal technique was observed. Only 4.9% of participants received strong opioids during the first 24 h after surgery

Conclusions: Postoperative pain control seems to be unexpectedly poor after single-shot subarachnoid anesthesia. Despite concerns, the use of analgesics may be insufficient in some groups of patients. Our study indicates new variables that influence the severity of pain, such as operated region, anesthetic technique, and type of surgical department. The results obtained in our study are in discrepancy with recommendations presented by the national guidelines for post-operative pain management.

Keywords: Postoperative pain management, Analgesia, Analgesics, Multimodal analgesia

* Correspondence: michalborys1@gmail.com
[1]The Second Department of Anaesthesiology and Intensive Therapy, Medical University of Lublin, ul. Staszica 16, 20-081 Lublin, Poland
Full list of author information is available at the end of the article

Background

Over 200 million major surgeries are performed worldwide annually [1]. Even though the World Health Organization proclaimed pain relief and management as a fundamental human right, many patients experience moderate or severe pain in the postoperative period [2]. According to different variables, such as type of surgery, pain-measurement tool, time of assessment, and patient's sex and age, pain may be classified as moderate and severe in approximately 60 to 80% of cases [3–6].

Surprisingly, the introduction of new analgesic techniques and drugs, as well as the implementation of national guidelines for acute pain management, did not significantly influence inadequately-treated postoperative pain. The guidelines endorsed by the Polish Society of Anesthesiology and Intensive Therapy in 2014 comprise many analgesic approaches that are relevant in most clinical scenarios [7]. However, most data included in these guidelines were not acquired in the population of patients treated in Polish hospitals. The data presented in the recent paper by Tomaszek and Debska indicated that postoperative pain treatment is still unsatisfactory in Polish hospitals [8]. A similar conclusion was found in the study by Mędrzycka-Dabrowska and co-workers [9], which emphasizes the lack of a separate team for acute pain management and administration of insufficient quantities of medication for pain alleviation. Although pain monitoring is mandatory during the first postoperative day in all hospitals in Poland, there is no registry like that of other countries, such as Germany [10, 11]. Furthermore, it is likely that nurses, who are obliged to monitor the NRS (numerical rating scale) in the postoperative period across all surgical wards in Poland, do not have a significant impact on the prescription of analgesics or implementation of more sophisticated methods of pain control [8, 9]. According to recent papers, there are several barriers to postoperative pain management mentioned by Polish nurses [8, 9]. However, the most important factors are, in their opinion, their lack of independence in decisions concerning pharmacological treatment, as well as poor cooperation from physicians.

The first step to assess the current pain control policies in the Polish healthcare system is to acquire data from a variety of hospitals across the country. Therefore, the main goal of our study was to assess the current postoperative pain management practices after publication of the guidelines endorsed by the Polish Society of Anesthesiology and Intensive Therapy in 2014.

Materials and methods

Study design

Ethical approval for this study (permit number KE-0254/282/2015) was provided by the Medical University of Lublin Ethics Committee. This was a prospective, observational, multi-center study, that involved postoperative patients who underwent scheduled surgeries in seven hospitals across eastern Poland. The data were collected by medical students, after obtaining written consent from eligible patients.

Patients and data collection

The questionnaire form contained seven sections as follows: (1) patient demographics; (2) type of anesthesia; (3) type of operated region; (4) pain evaluation with visual-analogue scale (VAS); (5) drugs, routes of their administration, and techniques used to relieve pain; (6) patient satisfaction, apprehension, and complications associated with the perioperative period; and (7) type of department and hospital. The entire form is shown in Additional file 1. The medical students helped patients to complete the questionnaire form if needed.

Patients over 18 years of age, who were able to sign the consent form and fill out the questionnaire and VAS scale form, were included in the study. Furthermore, only participants who underwent major surgical procedures that required hospitalization were asked to participate.

The following patients were excluded from the study: (1) minors under 18 years of age, (2) patients admitted to the ICU (intensive care unit) after surgery, (3) patients who did not sign the written consent, (4) patients who were unable to fill out the form or mark pain severity on the VAS scale, (5) patients who received local anesthesia, and (6) patients who were not able to fill out the questionnaire form or the VAS form within 4 h after surgery.

The main variable measured in the study was the VAS value (given in mm) obtained at 4, 8, 12, and 24 h following the end of the surgery. We also analyzed the relationship between the pain intensity scores and the following parameters obtained during data collection: patient demographics, type of surgery, type of anesthesia, hospital type, kind of surgical ward, and operated region.

Statistics

The analysis of variances (ANOVA), t-test, and multivariate regression were used for statistical analysis. Tukey's HSD (honest significant difference) was used for post-hoc analysis. VAS results were presented as means and confidence intervals (CI). All measurements were performed using Statistica 12.5 software (StatSoft Inc., Tulsa, OK, USA).

Results

Hospitals and patients

The study was conducted from November 2015 to June 2016 in seven hospitals in eastern Poland, which were comprised of two university (284 patients), two secondary

Table 1 Patient demographics

	Number	Percent	Mean age	Height [cm]	Weight [kg]
Women	269	47.8	52.78	162.42 (161.10–163.74)	71.82 (69.93–73.73)
Men	293	52.2	50.78	174.10 (173.06–175.14)	82.68 (80.54–84.82)
Overall	562	100	51.74	168.51 (167.55–169.47)	77.49 (75.98–78.99)

Type of ward	Thoracic surgery	Gynecology	Orthopeady	Laryngology	Neurosurgery	Urology	Obstetrics	General surgery	Vascular surgery
Number of patients	113	82	112	75	22	42	16	70	25
Patients' sex W/M (n)	35/78	82/0	50/62	23/52	10/12	13/29	16/0	33/37	4/21
Patients mean age	58.73	49.88	50.94	39.16	47.86	46.80	31.23	54.56	59.20

Patient demographics are presented as means and confidence intervals (CI).The second part of the table shows the number of patients (total and divided into sex) in every type of surgical department. *W* women, *M* men

(154 patients), and three primary (local) (124 patients) hospitals. Each hospital was granted two weeks during the study period for data gathering. The VAS forms were collected from a total of 565 patients. Three patients were excluded from further analysis because of a local anesthesia procedure. The data regarding patient demographics and type of surgical ward are presented in Table 1.

Total pain intensity

Pain severity is summarized in Table 2. The pain was described as moderate (40–59)) or severe (≥60).

Postoperative analgesics

The prevalence of analgesics used in the study is presented in Table 3. Approximately 91.3% (512/562) of patients received analgesics after surgery. Twenty-eight patients received strong opioids (morphine and nalbuphine), and tramadol was used in 150 cases (26.69%). Metamizole and ketoprofen were, by far, the most frequently administered analgesics for post-surgical pain. Of the patients, 8.7% (49/561) did not receive any drugs postoperatively.

Pain severity according to the type of hospital

There was no difference in the overall pain intensity (measured with VAS) according to the reference type of hospital. However, significant difference was found between primary and secondary hospitals at the 4- and 12-h assessments ($F = 10.77$; $p = 0.00001$) (Fig. 1). The mean VAS at 4 h was 40 (36–45) for primary and 28 (24–32) for secondary hospitals ($p = 0.0026$). On the other hand, at 12 h after surgery, the mean VAS result was 20 (16–24) for primary and 31 (27–34) for secondary hospitals ($p = 0.026$).

Table 2 Patient pain intensity expressed by VAS at the 4, 8, 12 and 24 h after surgery

VAS	Mean (CI)	Moderate pain N (%)	Severe pain N (%)
4-h	34 (32–36)	221 (39.32)	111 (19.75)
8-h	32 (30–34)	187 (33.27)	81 (14.41)
12-h	27 (25–29)	135 (24.02)	67 (11.92)
24-h	25 (23–27)	116 (20.64)	48 (8.54)

VAS visual-analogue scale, *CI* confidence interval. Moderate and severe data are given as N and (%)

Pain severity according to the type of operated region

On data from the four VAS measurements, the highest level of pain was associated with surgery on the upper abdomen (36 (30–41)), while the lowest pain scores were found in patients undergoing surgical procedures in the head/neck region (26 (23–30) However, the difference was not significant ($F = 2.09$; $p = 0.065$).

At the 4-h measurement, the highest VAS results were obtained in patients undergoing thoracic (41 (37–46)) and upper abdomen procedures (43 (34–51)). These results were significantly higher than the lower limb VAS measurements (24 (18–29)) in our study ($p = 0.00012$ and 0.02).

A statistical difference was not found at the 8-h measurement, yet similar to previous assessments, the most painful procedures seemed to be associated with the upper abdomen (39 (31–46)) and, surprisingly, the lower limb (36 (31–41)).

At the 12-h measurement, there was a significant difference in VAS ($p = 0.039$) between surgeries of the chest (21 (17–25)) and lower limb (31 (27–36)).

Furthermore, this tendency was maintained at the 24-h measurement, and lower limb procedures were associated with the highest pain intensity scores (32 (28–36)). A significant difference was demonstrated between lower limb surgeries and head/neck (19 (16–23) $p = 0.00064$) and hypogastrium operations (22 (19–25) $p = 0.011$). The results are presented in Fig. 2.

Pain severity according to the type of surgical ward

The total difference in VAS values (mean of the four measurements) between patients treated in vascular surgery (19 (13–26)) and thoracic surgery (30 (27–33)) were significant ($F = 2.49$, $p = 0.012$).

Table 3 Analgesics used after surgery

Postoperative analgesics	number
no analgesics	49
acetylsalicylic acid	1
bupivacaine + fentanyl (epidural)	33
diclofenac	37
gabapentin	1
ibuprofen	1
ketoprofen	202
lidocaine	2
mefenamic acid	1
metamizol	384
morphine	27
nalbuphine	1
paracetamol	169
tramadol	150

Drugs are presented in alphabetical order

At the 4-h measurement, a difference was found between orthopedic (29 (24–34)) and thoracic surgeries (42 (37–47); $p = 0.0058$). VAS results at the 8-h measurement demonstrated no statistical significance between studied wards. At the 12-h assessment, there was a significant difference in VAS scores between the thoracic (20 (16–24)) and the orthopedic (34 (30–38); $p = 0.0001$) and urology procedures (37 (31–44); $p = 0.0093$). Furthermore, at the 24-h VAS assessment, orthopedic procedures (33 (30–37)) seemed to be the most painful, especially in comparison to gynecology (20 (16–24); $p = 0.0005$), laryngology (19 (14–24); $p = 0.00037$)), and general surgery procedures (21 (16–26); $p = 0.0085$). The results are presented in Fig. 3.

Type of anesthesia and pain severity

The types of anesthesia that were performed in our study are presented in Table 4.

For statistical analysis, in order to avoid bias associated with the small number of cases in some groups, patients were assigned to four groups as follows: general anesthesia (335), subarachnoid (111), epidural (43), and regional peripheral (73) (Fig. 4).

At the 4-h VAS measurement, a difference was found between the general anesthesia group (39 (37–42)) and the subarachnoid (26 (21–30); $p = 0.00033$) and peripheral regional groups (26 (20–32); $p = 0.0077$). No difference was found at the 8-h measurement; however, the most severe pain was noted in the subarachnoid group (36 (31–40)). Furthermore, statistical significance was detected at the 12-h VAS measurement between the subarachnoid (33 (29–37) and general anesthesia groups (24 (23–28); $p = 0.017$). No difference was found between groups at the 24-h VAS measurement.

Pain severity according to the patient's sex

There was a significant difference in overall pain intensity according to the patient's sex (Fig. 5). Women experienced more intense pain than men, with VAS values of 31 (29–33) and 28 (26–30), respectively; $p = 0.044$. However, that difference was only significant during the two first measurements (at 4 and 8 h). At the 4-h measurement, the mean VAS results for women and men subsequently reached 37 (34–40) and 31 (28–34), respectively;

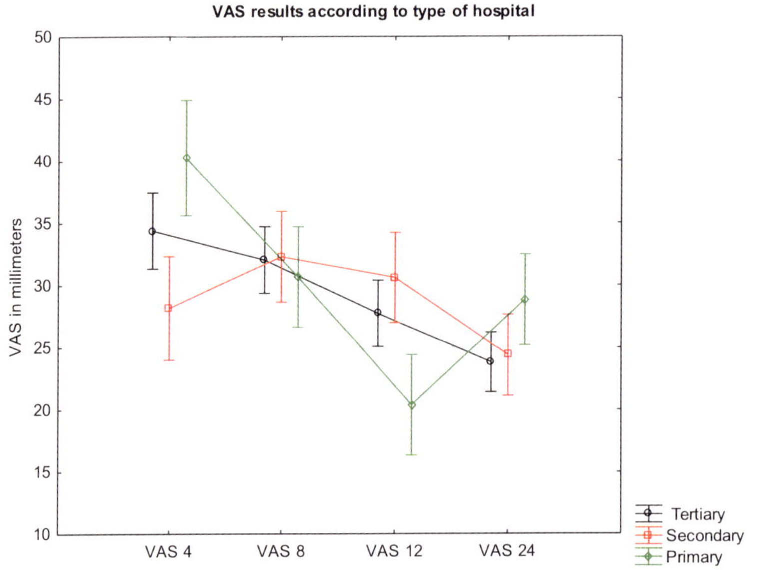

Fig. 1 Legend: VAS results in millimeters during the first day after surgery in different types of hospitals. VAS are presented as means and confidence intervals

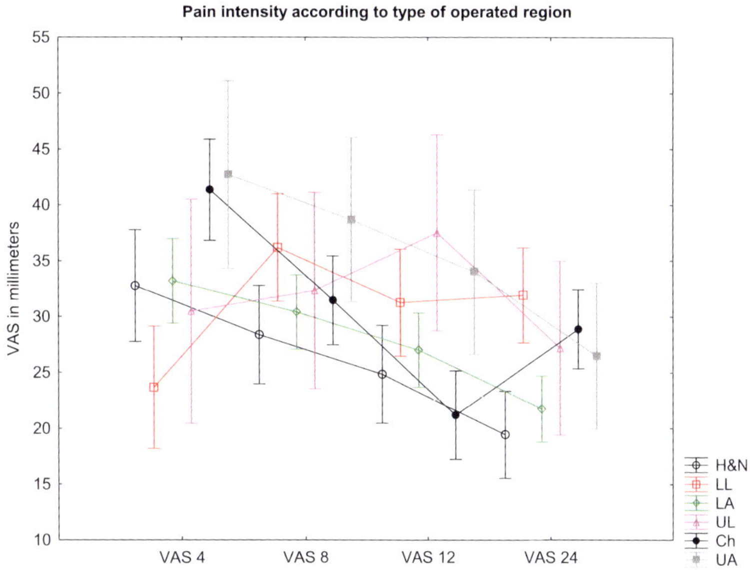

Fig. 2 Legend: Pain intensity measured by VAS in millimeters during the first day after surgery according to operated region. VAS are presented as means and confidence intervals. H&N – head&neck; LL – lower limb; LA – lower abdomen; UL – upper limb; Ch – chest; upper abdomen

$p = 0.012$. At the 8-h measurement, the VAS values were 34 (32–37) for women and 30 (27–32) for men ($p = 0.012$).

Correlation between patient's age and VAS value

A statistical correlation was found at the 12-h measurement on the linear regression model between the patient's age and VAS value. Although the p-value was 0.0027, the calculated r^2 value was 0.0159. However, after dividing the participants of our study into three groups, younger (up to 45 years), middle-aged (45–60 years), and older patients (over 60 years), a significant difference was found between the older patients (21 (18–24), $n = 180$) and the younger (29 (26–33), $n = 176$; $p = 0.0031$) and middle-aged patients (30 (26–33), $n = 205$; $p = 0.0022$).

Patient satisfaction with pain control

Of the 562 patients, 526 (93.6%) were satisfied with the quality of postoperative pain control (good or very good

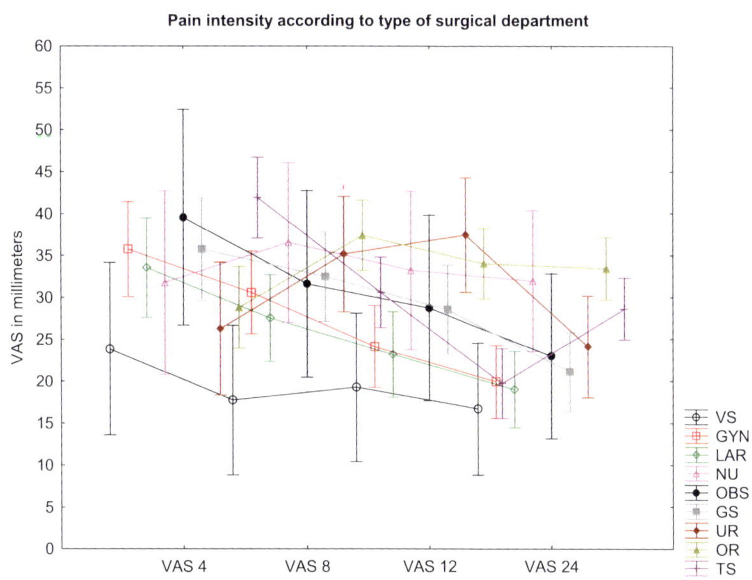

Fig. 3 Legend: Pain intensity measured by VAS in millimeters during the first day after surgery according to surgical ward. VAS are presented as means and confidence intervals. VS – vascular surgery, GYN – gynecology; LAR – laryngology; NU – neurosurgery; OBS – obstetrics; GS – general surgery; UR – urology; OR – orthopedic surgery; TS – Thoracic surgery

Table 4 Number and percent of anesthesia types performed in the study

Type	Number (n)	Percent
General	335	59.61
Subarachnoid	111	19.75
Epidural	31	5.52
Peripheral regional	32	5.69
Combined spinal&epidural	4	0.71
General + epidural	8	1.42
General + peripheral regional	33	5.87
Subarachnoid + peripheral regional	8	1.42

marks in the questionnaire). In contrast, 33 patients were not satisfied with the quality of postoperative pain control (poor marks), and five ranked the postoperative analgesia as not satisfactory. Overall VAS values (given as a mean of the four measurements) reached 51 (45–57) among the patients with poor pain control and was significantly higher than in the patients with satisfactory pain control (28 (27–30)).

Impact of patient's preoperative concerns on postoperative pain control

Patients who were afraid of poor postoperative pain control had slightly higher overall VAS values (32 (29–35)) in comparison to participants with no preoperative concerns (26 (22–30)), but these results were not significant.

However, when comparing VAS values at the specific time measurements, statistically significant differences were found. At the 4-h VAS measurement, there was a significant difference in pain intensity between patients who were afraid of either awareness or intraoperative pain (22 (13–32)) and those whose main concern was death (40 (34–45); $p = 0.038$) or postoperative pain (39 (34–45); $p = 0.032$). The same difference was observed at the 8-h measurement, but it was not significant. At the 12-h measurement, patients whose main concern was awareness indicated pain severity on the VAS score as the most intense (contrary to the previous observations), but this result was not significant. Furthermore, at the 24-h measurement, no difference in VAS scores was found, but slightly reduced pain was noted among the patients who were afraid of perioperative death (22.1 (17.8–26.3)).

Discussion

Our results highlighted new aspects of postoperative pain control, such as unsatisfactory analgesia of patients with single-shot subarachnoid anesthesia at 8 and 12 h after the surgery and a low number of strong opioids administered in the hospitals studied.

The prevalence of moderate and severe pain was high among the study population, especially during the first hours after the surgery (39 for the 4-h VAS). However, at the same time, 93.6% of patients recognized pain control as good or very good.

Of the patients, 50.5% were anesthetized in two university hospitals. Lower numbers of surgeries in low-volume units might have been more vulnerable to random deviations during statistical analysis. However, the impact of the patient distribution in our study is difficult to predict. The difference in pain intensity between

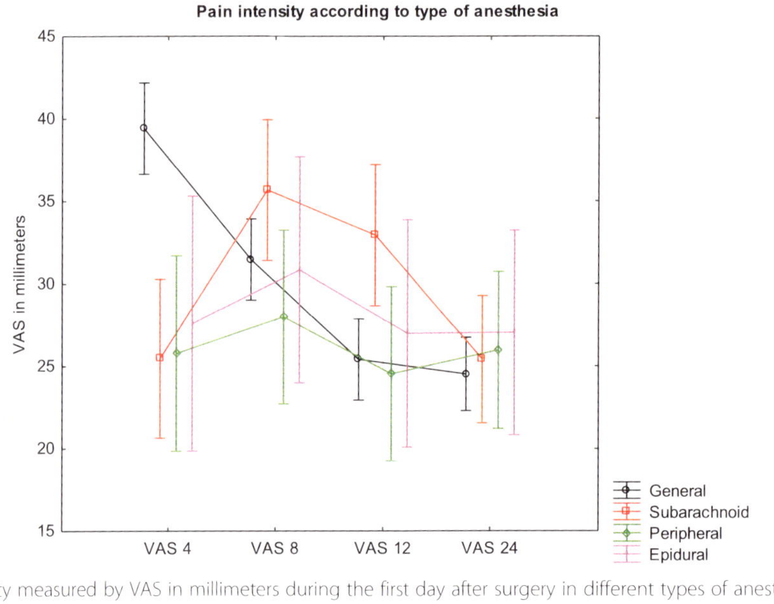

Fig. 4 Legend: Pain intensity measured by VAS in millimeters during the first day after surgery in different types of anesthesia. VAS are presented as means and confidence intervals

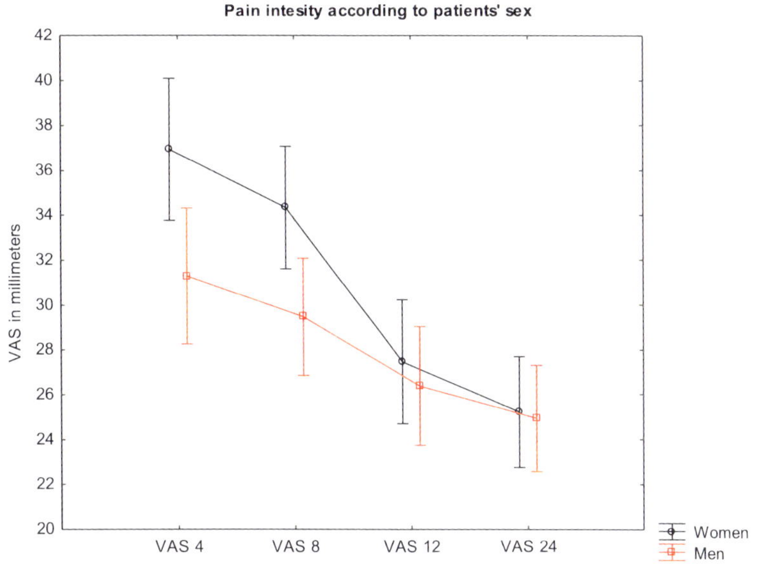

Fig. 5 Legend: Pain intensity measured by VAS in millimeters during the first day after surgery according to sex. VAS are presented as means and confidence intervals

primary and secondary hospitals at 4- and 12- h after surgery became evident after further analysis and is likely due to the presence of orthopedic wards and the quantity of these surgeries performed in secondary hospitals. Furthermore, the probable cause of the 12-h peak in VAS values in orthopedic patients, with the high prevalence of lower limb operations, was the use of subarachnoid anesthesia. Although spinal, single-shot anesthesia is a standard approach for hip and knee surgeries, and more intense pain at the 12-h measurement was a result of insufficient supplementary analgesic techniques. Currently, the early mobilization of patients after hip or knee replacements is one of the main goals and possesses beneficial effects [11, 12].

The combined spinal-epidural technique or systemic opioid administration may postpone the rehabilitation process and delay the patient's discharge. The femoral nerve, lumbar plexus, or adductor canal blocks are well-established alternatives [13, 14]. However, in our study, such analgesic techniques were only implemented in 11 cases.

Younger age of patients seems to be an independent risk factor for higher postoperative pain in our investigation. Nevertheless, such a difference was not presented in the study of Gagliese and Katz if non-verbal scales, such as VAS or NRS were utilized [15]. Conversely, in the study of Sommer et al., as well as two more recent studies from Germany, a difference was found between younger and older patients (younger perceived more intense pain) [10, 16, 17].

Moreover, the authors of these articles identified women as more vulnerable to postoperative pain. These results are consistent with those found by our study.

Although opioid-related side effects are common, omitting these drugs in the postoperative period can lead to augmentation of pain. In the very recent study of Thiels et al., 93.9% of surgical patients received opioid prescriptions at discharge [18]. In contrast, only 4.9% of participants in our study obtained strong opioids (morphine and nalbuphine) during the first 24 h after surgery. Even though the results presented by Breivik et al. regarding chronic pain in Europe showed that Polish patients used the lowest number of opioids and the highest number of non-opioid drugs in comparison to other European patients, the low amount of parenteral opioids used in our study was unexpected [19].

The Polish national guidelines for post-operative pain management present multiple analgesic methods and regimens [6]. The guidelines emphasize the role of multimodal analgesia, as well as the broader implementation of loco-regional techniques. This statement is consistent with recommendations of the American Pain Society [20]. The other aspect presented in the Polish guidelines is preemptive analgesia and regular administration of painkillers, not only on the patient's demand. However, there is a discrepancy between our results and the guidelines. The majority of our patients did not receive preemptive or multimodal analgesia. Moreover, in many cases, drugs were not administered at regular intervals. Only 13% of our study participants received peripheral regional anesthesia/analgesia methods. We suppose that the main reason for this fact is insufficient time spent with patients due to the lack of staff in most hospitals. Moreover, drugs are not administered according to VAS or NRS results, but by medical staff habits [9]. The improvement of communication and cooperation between nurses and physicians could be the solution in many clinical scenarios, and the majority of problems could be solved by the organization of specialized teams for acute pain management and continuous training of healthcare providers.

Conclusions

Results presented in our study show that many patients still experience moderate or severe pain in the postoperative period, even though there are guidelines and methods to treat pain after surgical procedures. Moreover, postoperative pain control seems to be unexpectedly poor after single-shot subarachnoid anesthesia. Despite concerns, the use of analgesics may be insufficient in some groups of patients. Our study also indicates new variables that influence the severity of pain, such as operated region, anesthetic technique, and the type of surgical department. The results obtained in our study are in discrepancy with recommendations presented by the national guidelines for post-operative pain management.

Abbreviations

ANOVA: The analysis of variances; CI: confidence interval; N: number; NRS: numerical rating scale; VAS: visual-analogue scale

Acknowledgements

Assistance with the study: students from Medical University of Lublin.

Authors' contributions

MB and KZ made substantial contributions to the study design. These authors conducted the study, collected and analyzed data, and prepared the manuscript. JM and MC helped to analyze and prepare the manuscript. AH, MD, PG, KG, AK, KW, DO helped in collection and data interpretation. All authors read and approved the final manuscript.

Competing interests

The authors declare that they have no competing interests.

Author details

[1]The Second Department of Anaesthesiology and Intensive Therapy, Medical University of Lublin, ul. Staszica 16, 20-081 Lublin, Poland. [2]The Department of Anaesthesia and Intensive Therapy, The Podkarpackie Center of Lung Disease, Rzeszów, Poland. [3]The Department of Anaesthesia and Intensive Therapy, Saint Lukash Hospital, Końskie, Poland. [4]The Department of Anaesthesia and Intensive Therapy, Jedrzej Sniadecki Hospital, Białystok, Poland. [5]The Department of Anaesthesia and Intensive Therapy, University of Warmia and Mazury, Olsztyn, Poland.

References

1. Weiser TG, Regenbogen SE, Thompson KD, et al. An estimation of the global volume of surgery: a modelling strategy based on available data. Lancet. 2008;372:139–44.
2. Brennan F, Carr DB, Cousins M. Pain management: a fundamental human right. Anesth Analg. 2007;105:205–21.
3. Apfelbaum JL, Chen C, Mehta SS, Gan TJ. Postoperative pain experience: results from a national survey suggestpostoperative pain continues to be undermanaged. AnesthAnalg. 2003;97:534–40.
4. Sauaia A, Min SJ, Leber C, Erbacher K, Abrams F, Fink R. Postoperative pain management in elderly patients: correlation between adherence to treatment guidelines and patient satisfaction. J Am Geriatr Soc. 2005;53: 274–82.
5. Gan T, Habib A, Miller T, White W, Apfelbaum J. Incidence, patientsatisfaction, and perceptions of post-surgical pain: results from a US nationalsurvey. Curr Med Res Opin. 2014;30:149–60.
6. Misiołek H, Cettler M, Woroń J, et al. The 2014 guidelines for post-operative pain management. Anaesthesiol Intensive Ther. 2014;46: 221–44.
7. Erlenwein J, Stamer U, Koschwitz R, et al. Inpatient acute pain management in German hospitals: results from the national survey "Akutschmerzzensus 2012". Schmerz. 2014;28:147–56.
8. Tomaszek L, Dębska G. Knowledge, compliance with good clinical practices and barriers to effective control of postoperative pain among nurses from hospitals with and without a "hospital without pain" certificate. J Clin Nurs. 2017 Dec 8; https://doi.org/10.1111/jocn.14215.
9. Mędrzycka-Dąbrowska WA, Dąbrowski S, Basiński A, Pilch D. Perception of barriers to postoperative pain management in elderly patients in polish hospitals with and without a "hospital without pain" certificate – a multi-center study. Archives of Medical Science : AMS. 2016;12(4):808–18. https://doi.org/10.5114/aoms.2015.54768.
10. Meißner W, Komann M, Erlenwein J, et al. The quality of postoperative pain therapy in German hospitals. —the effect of structural and procedural variables Dtsch Arztebl Int. 2017;114:161–7.
11. Chandrasekaran S, Ariaretnam SK, Tsung J, et al. Early mobilization after total knee replacement reduces the incidence of deep venous thrombosis. ANZ J Surg. 2009;79:526–9.
12. Guerra ML, Singh PJ, Taylor NF. Early mobilization of patients who have had a hip or knee joint replacement reduces length of stay in hospital: a systematic review. Clin Rehabil. 2015;29:844–54.
13. Chan EY, Fransen M, Parker DA, et al. Femoral nerve blocks for acute postoperative pain after knee replacement surgery. Cochrane Database Syst Rev. 2014;13(5):CD009941.
14. Amiri HR, Zamani MM, Safari S. Lumbar plexus block for Management of hip Surgeries. Anesth Pain Med2014;4(3):e19407.
15. Gagliese L, Katz J. Age differences in postoperative pain are scale dependent: a comparison of measures of pain intensity and quality in younger and older surgical patients. Pain. 2003;103:11–20.
16. Sommer M, de Rijke JM, van Kleef M, et al. The prevalence of postoperative pain in a sample of 1490 surgical inpatients. EurJ Anaesthesiol. 2008;25:267–74.
17. Gerbershagen HJ, Pogatzki-Zahn E, Aduckathil S, et al. Procedure specific risk factor analysis for the development of severe postoperative pain. Anesthesiology. 2014;120:1237–45.
18. Thiels CA, Anderson SS, Ubl DS, et al. Wide variation and over prescription of opioids after elective surgery. Ann Surg. 2017;266:564–73.
19. Breivik H, Collett B, Ventafridda V, et al. Survey of chronic pain in Europe: prevalence, impact on daily life, and treatment. EurJ Pain. 2006; 10:287–333.
20. Chou R, Gordon DB, de Leon-Casasola OA, Rosenberg JM, Bickler S, et al. Management of Postoperative Pain: a clinical practice guideline from the American pain society, the American Society of Regional Anesthesia and Pain Medicine, and the American Society of Anesthesiologists' committee on regional anesthesia, executive committee, and administrative council. J Pain. 2016;17:131–57. https://doi.org/10.1016/j.jpain.2015.12.008.

12

Risk prediction tool for use and predictors of duration of postoperative oxygen therapy in children undergoing non-cardiac surgery: a case-control study

Maliwan Oofuvong*, Siriwimol Ratprasert and Thavat Chanchayanon

Abstract

Background: We aimed to construct a prediction tool for postoperative oxygen therapy and determine predictors of duration of use among children undergoing non-cardiac surgery.

Methods: Data from this case-control study was obtained from a database of 9820 children aged < 15 years who underwent general anesthesia between January 2010 and December 2013 at a tertiary care hospital in southern Thailand. The primary outcomes were the use and duration (hours) of postoperative oxygen therapy (cases). Cases were matched with controls on age group and year of surgery in a ratio of 1:4. A negative binomial hurdle model was used to obtain significant predictors of any use and number of hours of oxygen therapy. A risk score was derived from the coefficients of the significant predictors. The risk score, adjusted odds ratio (OR) for any use and count ratio (CR) for duration of postoperative oxygen therapy and 95% confidence interval (CI) were determined.

Results: A total of 288 cases and 1152 controls were included. The median (inter-quartile range) duration of oxygen therapy delivered was 17 (9–22) hours. An optimal risk score for predictors of oxygen use was 12 (0–32) giving an area under the receiver operating characteristic curve of 0.93. Predictors of high risk need for oxygen therapy (score ≥ 12) were thoracic surgery (OR = 278, 95% CI = 44.6–1733) and having desaturation perioperatively (OR = 459.8, 95% CI = 169.7–1246). Intermediate risk factors (score 8–11) were having bronchospasm (OR = 92.4, 95% CI = 29.7–287.5) and upper airway obstruction/laryngospasm (OR = 61.5, 95% CI = 14.4–262.4) perioperatively. Significant predictors of duration of oxygen therapy were probably difficult airway (CR = 2.2, 95% CI = 1.4–3.5), history of delayed development (CR = 2.3, 95% CI = 1.5–3.6), airway (CR = 3.0, 95% CI = 1.6–5.8), orthopedic (CR = 2.1, 95% CI = 1.1–4.3), thoracic (CR = 4.9, 95% CI = 2.3–10.1) and abdominal surgery (CR = 4.2, 95% CI = 2.1–8.1), compared to eye surgery.

Conclusions: Our risk prediction tool for the use of postoperative oxygen therapy provided a high predictive ability. Children who have thoracic surgery, desaturation, bronchospasm, upper airway obstruction or laryngospasm will most likely need postoperative oxygen therapy, regardless of other factors, while those with a probably difficult airway, history of delayed development, or thoracic/abdominal surgery will most likely need longer duration of oxygen therapy.

Keywords: Predictors, Duration of use, Postoperative oxygen therapy, Pediatric anesthesia

* Correspondence: oomaliwa@gmail.com
Department of Anesthesiology, Faculty of Medicine, Prince of Songkla University, 15 Kanjanavanich Road, Songkhla 90112, Thailand

Background

At the post-anesthetic care unit (PACU), postoperative oxygen therapy is often given to patients, particularly children, after finishing general anesthesia. Studies have shown that general anesthesia, which induces airway closure, ventilation, and perfusion mismatch, can decrease the functional residual capacity causing hypoxemia and necessitates supplemental oxygen during the first postoperative hour that continues into the postoperative period [1–5]. Since the prevalence of hypoxemia at the PACU in children can be as high as 21% [5], supplemental oxygen therapy during transfer to the PACU [6] and throughout the PACU stay is recommended [7].

Despite the usefulness of oxygen therapy, longer use of postoperative oxygen therapy can be harmful to children [8]. In addition, surgery-related or anesthesia-related factors may also be important. However, a risk prediction tool for the need of postoperative oxygen therapy in children has never been developed and predictors of the duration and use of postoperative oxygen therapy in children have not been determined. Therefore, the objectives of this study were to develop a risk prediction tool for postoperative oxygen therapy and to determine predictors of duration of use in children undergoing non-cardiac surgery with general anesthesia. The results of this study may help guide anesthesia personnel determine which patient groups are more likely to require postoperative oxygen therapy as well as those who may require longer use.

Methods

This was a matched case-control study among children who underwent non-cardiac surgery at Songklanagarind Hospital which is an 853-bed tertiary care university hospital in southern Thailand. The study was approved by the Institutional Ethics Committee of the Faculty of Medicine, Prince of Songkla University, Songkhla, Thailand (Chairperson Assoc. Prof. Boonsin Tangtrakulwanich) on October 8, 2014 [EC57294081].

Participants

The surveillance anesthetic database under quality assurance conference by nurse anesthetists performed every 2 months was used to identify children aged less than 15 years who received postoperative oxygen therapy after undergoing non-cardiac surgical procedures as well as digital imaging or other interventions under general anesthesia with or without regional anesthesia or peripheral nerve block between January 2010 and December 2013. All identified children were confirmed eligible by chart review of electronic anesthetic records by two investigators (MO, SR). Patients were excluded if they were classified as American Society of Anesthesiologists (ASA) physical status 4 or 5, had preoperative oxygen saturation by pulse oximetry (SpO_2) < 95% at room air, received preoperative oxygen therapy, were endotracheally intubated, or their lungs were mechanically ventilated or both before or after surgery, had congenital cyanotic heart disease, or had cardiac surgery. These criteria were used to exclude pre-existing active respiratory problems before surgery or cardiopulmonary problems after surgery. The children who needed postoperative mechanical ventilation have more severe respiratory insufficiency and may have different risk factors compared to children who need only postoperative oxygen and were therefore excluded from the study.

Anesthetic practice and standard operating procedure [9]

The choice of anesthesia, anesthetic agents, and type of airway devices were made by a certified anesthesiologist. The decision to give general anesthesia combined with epidural analgesia, caudal block, or peripheral nerve block was made by a certified anesthesiologist with at least 1 year experience. There were on average 18 certified anesthesiologists per year during the four-year study period. The anesthetic resident and anesthetic nurse observed children from induction until discharge from the recovery room under supervision of staff anesthesiologists. At the end of the operation, children were transferred either to the PACU or pediatric intensive care unit. Children who had SpO_2 < 95% would receive 100% oxygen via facemask during transfer to the PACU. Children who received massive transfusion, or had potential cardiovascular or respiratory problems were transferred to the pediatric intensive care unit to continue intubation with mechanical ventilation.

At the PACU, anesthetic nurses gave an oxygen facemask (aerosol mask) via high flow air/oxygen blender with a dial setting at fractional inspired oxygen 0.4 up to 0.6. The flow rate was adjusted depending on the patient's respiratory pattern to achieve fractional inspired oxygen at the set point. If a patient refused to wear an oxygen facemask, oxygen insufflation was performed by blowing into the patient's nostrils and mouth. Low flow oxygen via nasal cannula is rarely used because it causes nasal discomfort and more humidity is needed. Oxygen therapy via oxygen facemask was continued at the pediatric ward depending on the discretion of the anesthesiologist based on three conditions. First, in some high-risk patients, such as those with obstructive sleep apnea syndrome or prolonged operation, oxygen therapy was not discontinued. Second, after oxygen therapy was discontinued, oxygen therapy was reinstituted in case of dyspnea, having respiratory events, or if SpO_2 fell below 95%. Third, in case of suspected upper airway edema, the patient was endotracheally intubated with spontaneous breathing via oxygen T-piece.

Outcome of interest

Postoperative oxygen therapy

Postoperative oxygen therapy was defined when patients were given postoperatively an oxygen facemask, oxygen insufflation, or oxygen T-piece at the PACU and pediatric ward. Children who did not immediately receive postoperative oxygen but required oxygen at or after postoperative day 1 or needed postoperative mechanical ventilation were excluded at the beginning of the study process and were not included in the analysis. Use of postoperative oxygen therapy was retrieved from the validated anesthetic records by two investigators (MO, SR) and confirmed by the nurses' notes from the hospital information system. Children who were given postoperative oxygen therapy were defined as cases and each case was randomly matched with four patients who were not given postoperative oxygen therapy (controls). The four controls increased the power of the study due to the low number of cases.

Duration of postoperative oxygen therapy

Oxygen saturation by pulse oximetry was continuously monitored during oxygen therapy. Weaning off oxygen therapy was attempted at the pediatric ward when the patient had no signs or symptoms of respiratory disturbance, or the SpO_2 reached 95% while the patient was breathing room air. The duration of postoperative oxygen therapy in hours was defined from the time of starting oxygen therapy at the PACU until terminating oxygen therapy and the patient could breathe spontaneously. This information was retrieved from the nurses' notes from the electronic hospital information system. The start and stopping dates of oxygen therapy were recorded by agreement of the two investigators (MO, SR).

Matching procedure

All cases were identified from the anesthetic records and the hospital information system according to the above-mentioned criteria. To avoid selection bias and imbalance between cases and controls, a matching algorithm was constructed. The list of controls was selected from the pool of patients kept in the department of pediatrics database. Data management with application of the exclusion criteria was managed by MO to accomplish the qualified controls. Each case was randomly matched with four qualified controls based on age group (< 1, 1–6, > 6 years) and year of operation.

Potential predictors and confounding variables

Covariates were categorized into 11 patient-related factors, two surgery-related factors (elective/emergency and site of procedure), seven anesthesia-related factors, and occurrence of respiratory events during anesthesia. Patient-related factors included sex, body mass index (kg/m^2), history of upper respiratory tract infection (URI) (defined as any sign or symptom of rhinitis, cough, pharyngitis, or an active or recent URI within 2 weeks), history of hyper-reactive airway (defined as a history of allergic rhinitis or asthma), history of pulmonary disease (defined as a history of pneumonia, atelectasis, or bronchiectasis within 2 weeks), history of snoring, history of non-cyanotic heart disease, history of delayed development (defined as a history of cerebral palsy or mental retardation), preoperative anemia (males and females having a hemoglobin below 13 g/dl and 12 g/dl, respectively), having a probable difficult airway, and having a risk of aspiration (defined as inadequate nothing-by-mouth time, full stomach, or history of gastroesophageal reflux) (Table 1). Anesthesia-related factors included ASA physical status, choice of anesthesia, airway device, neuromuscular blocking agent used, volatile anesthetic agent used, narcotic used, and anesthetic time (Table 2). A respiratory event during anesthesia was defined as having an event such as laryngospasm (defined as a partial or complete upper airway obstruction from a spasm of the vocal cords), upper airway obstruction (defined as soft tissue obstruction or secretion obstruction after the airway device was removed), bronchospasm (defined as a lower airway obstruction from a spasm of bronchial smooth muscle) or wheezing, or desaturation < 95% for at least 10 s [10] during the intraoperative period or at the PACU.

Statistical analysis

All variables are presented descriptively with mean and standard deviation or median and interquartile range as appropriate for continuous variables, and frequency and percent for categorical variables. Unpaired Student's t-tests or Wilcoxon's rank sum tests were used to compare normally or non-normally distributed variables, respectively, between the two outcome groups. The chi-square test or Fisher's exact test was used to compare categorical variables. Predictors of the use and duration of postoperative oxygen therapy were determined using a hurdle model with adjustment for potential confounders [11, 12]. The hurdle model had two sets of predictors. The first set predicted whether the patient used any oxygen therapy postoperatively. The second set predicted the duration of oxygen therapy among the cases. The model was refined by sequential backward elimination of non-significant variables performed by the likelihood ratio test that provided coefficients and their 95% confidence intervals. The exponential of these coefficients gave adjusted odds ratios to assess the effects of various factors on any oxygen therapy and adjusted count ratios to assess the multiplying effects of various factors on duration (hours) of oxygen therapy. Factors were considered significant if the likelihood ratio test p values were < 0.05.

Table 1 Demographic data among children who received postoperative oxygen therapy compared with those who did not

Factor	No oxygen therapy (n = 1152)	Oxygen therapy (n = 288)	p value
Age (years)			0.99
<1	216 (18.8)	54 (18.8)	
1–6	552 (47.9)	138 (47.9)	
>6	384 (33.3)	96 (33.3)	
Male	684 (59.4)	182 (63.2)	0.26
Weight, median (IQR) (kg)	16.0 (9.8-25.0)	14.3 (8.4-33.4)	0.41
Height, median (IQR) (cm)	104.0 (80-128.0)	98.5 (75.0-130.0)	0.19
Body mass index (kg/m^2)			<0.001*
5–14.9	479 (41.6)	130 (45.1)	
15–24.9	629 (54.6)	128 (44.4)	
25-60	44 (3.8)	30 (10.4)	
URI (Y/N)	72 (6.2)/1080 (93.8)	23 (8)/265 (92.0)	0.35
Pulmonary disease (Y/N)	8 (0.7)/1144 (99.3)	16 (5.6)/272 (94.4)	<0.001*
Hyper-reactive airway (Y/N)	65 (5.6)/1087 (94.4)	24 (8.3)/264 (91.7)	0.12
Anemia (Y/N)	526 (45.7)/626 (54.3)	127 (44.1)/161 (55.9)	0.68
Snoring (Y/N)	14 (1.2)/1138 (98.8)	4 (1.4)/284 (98.6)	0.95
Non-cyanotic heart (Y/N)	41 (3.6)/1111 (96.4)	30 (10.4)/258 (89.6)	<0.001*
Probable difficult airway (Y/N)	12 (1.0)/1140 (99.0)	21 (7.3)/267 (92.7)	<0.001*
Risk of aspiration (Y/N)	24 (2.1)/1128 (97.9)	11 (3.8)/277 (96.2)	0.13
Delayed development (Y/N)	34 (3.0)/1118 (97.0)	22 (7.6)/266 (92.4)	<0.001*

Data are presented as frequency (percentage) unless otherwise stated
*<0.05 by chi-squared test
IQR inter-quartile range, *URI* Upper respiratory tract infection

Hurdle model

Hurdle models are one type of regression model for count data that can handle zero inflated outcomes, i.e., many zero observations. There are two-components in the modeling process: a truncated count component which is often modeled using a Poisson or negative binomial distribution for non-zero counts (in this study the number of hours of postoperative oxygen therapy), and a hurdle component which models the probability of a zero count, i.e., no oxygen therapy, versus non-zero count, i.e., use of oxygen. The zero count process is modeled using logistic regression. Due to over-dispersion, i.e., a situation where the variance is much larger than the mean, in the number of hours of oxygen therapy and the fact that many children in our study did not receive oxygen therapy, a negative binomial hurdle model was chosen for this analysis. This distribution also fit our data better than the Poisson model.

The hurdle model is given by the following equation:

$$f_{hurdle}(y; x, z, \beta, \gamma) = \begin{cases} f_{zero}(0; z, \gamma), & \text{if } y = 0 \\ (1 - f_{zero}(0; z, \gamma)) \times \dfrac{f_{count}(y; x, \beta)}{1 - f_{count}(0; x, \beta)}, & \text{if } y > 0 \end{cases}$$

y = outcome (number of hours of postoperative oxygen therapy)

x = potential predictors of the truncated count data model

z = potential predictors of the zero hurdle model

β = vector of regression coefficients of f_{count}

γ = vector of regression coefficients of f_{zero}

The regression coefficients are estimated using maximum likelihood. The corresponding mean regression relationship is given by:

$$\text{Log}\,(\mu_i) = x_i{}^T\beta + \log\{1 - f_{zero}(0; z_i, \gamma)\} - \log\{1 - f_{count}(0; x_i, \beta)\}$$

where μ_i = mean number of hours using oxygen.

Risk prediction tool

The risk prediction tool was developed using the first set of predictors from the hurdle model. A test for discrimination was used to attain the predictive accuracy of the tool. The risk score of postoperative oxygen therapy was calculated from the coefficients of the significant covariates in the final model [13]. Scores were obtained by multiplying each coefficient by 2 and then rounding the result to the nearest integer for simple interpretation. Model discrimination performance was examined using

Table 2 Anesthesia- and surgical-related risk among children who received postoperative oxygen therapy compared with those who did not

Factor	No oxygen therapy (n = 1152)	Oxygen therapy (n = 288)	p value
ASA physical status			<0.001*
1	242 (21.0)	21 (7.3)	
2	742 (64.4)	136 (47.2)	
3	168 (14.6)	131 (45.5)	
Type of case			<0.001*
Elective	984 (85.4)	212 (73.6)	
Emergency	168 (14.6)	76 (26.4)	
Site/ type of procedure			<0.001*
Eye	226 (19.6)	11 (3.8)	
Urologic	212 (18.4)	33 (11.5)	
Airway	187 (16.2)	66 (22.9)	
Ear-nose-face	93 (8.1)	19 (6.6)	
Thoracic	2 (0.2)	23 (8.0)	
Intra-abdomen	84 (7.3)	49 (17.0)	
Orthopedic	238 (20.7)	50 (17.4)	
Intra-cranial	14 (1.2)	9 (3.1)	
Gastrointestinal scope	53 (4.6)	13 (4.5)	
Cardiac catheterization	43 (3.7)	15 (5.2)	
Choice of anesthesia			0.04*
GA only	948 (82.3)	252 (87.5)	
GA with epidural/caudal	151 (13.1)	31 (10.8)	
GA with peripheral nerve block	53 (4.6)	5 (1.7)	
Airway device			<0.001*
Facemask/laryngeal mask airway	411 (35.7)	31 (10.8)	
Spontaneous breathing with non-rebreathing mask	28 (2.4)	4 (1.4)	
Endotracheal tube intubation	713 (61.9)	253 (87.8)	
Neuromuscular blocking agent			<0.001
Succinylcholine	84 (7.3)	45 (15.6)	
Aminosteroid derivatives	39 (3.4)	29 (10.1)	
Benzylisoquinolines	456 (39.6)	141 (49.0)	
None	573 (49.7)	73 (25.3)	
Inhalation agent			0.99
Sevoflurane	945 (82.0)	236 (81.9)	
Desflurane	24 (2.1)	6 (2.1)	
None	183 (15.9)	46 (16.0)	
Narcotic			0.006*
Fentanyl	841 (73.0)	204 (70.8)	
Morphine	100 (8.7)	42 (14.6)	
None	211 (18.3)	42 (14.6)	
Anesthetic time (hour)			<0.001*
<1	281 (24.4)	27 (9.4)	
1–<3	737 (64.0)	201 (69.8)	
≥3	134 (11.6)	60 (20.8)	

Table 2 Anesthesia- and surgical-related risk among children who received postoperative oxygen therapy compared with those who did not *(Continued)*

Factor	No oxygen therapy (n = 1152)	Oxygen therapy (n = 288)	p value
PRAE			<0.001*
None	1,130 (98.1)	129 (44.8)	
Upper airway obstruction	0 (0)	9 (3.1)	
Laryngospasm	9 (0.8)	3 (1.0)	
Desaturation	7 (0.6)	126 (43.8)	
Bronchospasm/wheezing	6 (0.5)	21 (7.3)	

Data are presented as frequency (percentage) unless otherwise stated
*<0.05 by chi-squared test
ASA American Society of Anesthesiologists, *GA* General anesthesia, *PRAE* Perioperative respiratory adverse events

the area under the receiver operating characteristic (ROC) curve providing sensitivity and specificity based on the optimal cut-point of the risk score.

Sample size determination

We estimated the lowest prevalence of exposure (potential predictor) among the controls to be 5% with a ratio of controls to cases of 4:1 to detect an odds ratio of at least 2.0 using a significance level of 0.05 and a power of 80% that resulted in a required sample size of 250 cases and 1000 controls. The mean prevalence of postoperative oxygen therapy among non-cyanotic children in our hospital between 2010 and 2013 was 3%. Therefore, 4 years of retrospective data were required to obtain this sample size.

Results

From the database, 9614 children received general anesthesia during the four-year study period. After applying the exclusion criteria, 8044 children were eligible for the study. Figure 1 shows the flow diagram of the study which contained 288 cases and 1152 matched controls. Five percent of height data were missing and replaced by the mean height of children of the same age and sex. The reasons for giving postoperative oxygen therapy were prophylaxis in high risk patients or high risk operations (43.8%), perioperative desaturation (44.4%), perioperative wheezing/rhonchi (4.5%), spontaneous breathing via T-piece (3.8%), perioperative upper airway obstruction (2.4%), and shivering (1%). Some children (< 50%) who had either a probable difficult airway or airway surgery were endotracheally intubated and received oxygen via the T-piece connector. Table 1 compares the demographic data of children who received postoperative oxygen therapy to those who did not. High body mass index, history of pulmonary disease, history of non-cyanotic heart disease, having a probable difficult airway, and history of delayed development were significantly different between the two groups. Table 2 shows a similar comparison of anesthesia-related and surgery-related risk factors. There were significant differences between the two groups in terms of ASA physical status, elective/emergency case, site and type of surgery, choice of anesthesia, airway device, neuromuscular blocking agents used, narcotic used, anesthetic time, and having a respiratory event during anesthesia.

Analysis of postoperative oxygen therapy

Seven variables having a p value ≤ 0.2 from the univariate analysis were included in the initial multivariate hurdle model but were not significant: history of pulmonary disease, history of non-cyanotic heart disease, history of delayed development, having risk of aspiration, elective/emergency, choice of anesthesia, and narcotic used. Table 3 shows the results of the final hurdle model predicting postoperative oxygen therapy.

Development of risk prediction tool

Risk scores from the model are shown in Table 3. We selected the reference group based on the subgroup which had a lowest risk. The scores were summed to obtain an individual risk score which ranged from 0 to 32. Figure 2 shows the ROC curve of the individual risk scores predicting oxygen therapy. The area under the curve was 0.93 and the optimal cut-point based on the highest summation of sensitivity (85%) and specificity (86%) of the model was 12. The risk scores were then classified into three groups: high (≥ 12), intermediate (8–11), and low (≤ 7) that indicated the level of need for postoperative oxygen therapy.

Duration of postoperative oxygen therapy

The median (inter-quartile range) duration of oxygen therapy among the cases was 17 h (range 9–22 h). The distribution of the number of hours of oxygen use was over-dispersed, thus using a negative binomial hurdle model fit the data much better than the Poisson hurdle model (Additional file 1). Nine variables that had a p value ≤ 0.2 in the univariate analysis were included in the initial multivariate hurdle model but were not significant: body mass index, history of URI, history of pulmonary disease, history of snoring, anemia, choice of anesthesia, airway

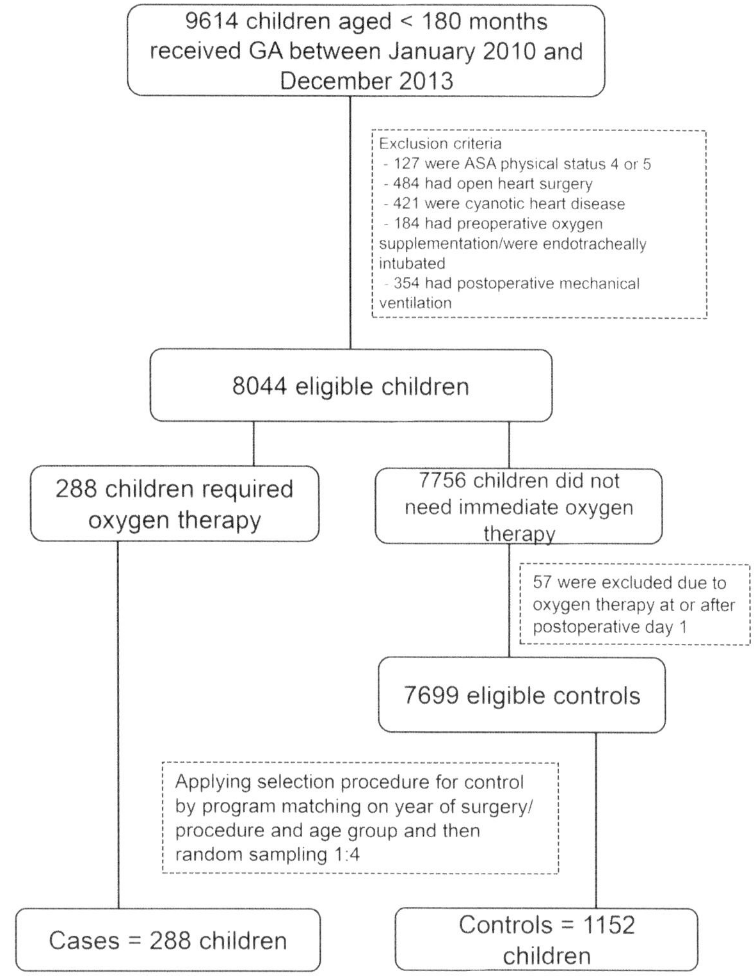

Fig. 1 Flow diagram of the study. *GA* General anesthesia, *ASA* American Society of Anesthesiologists

device, neuromuscular blocking agent used, and having a respiratory event during anesthesia (Additional file 2). Table 4 shows the results of the final hurdle model predicting duration of postoperative oxygen therapy.

Discussion

This matched case-control study determined predictors of the use and duration of postoperative oxygen therapy using a hurdle model to present two sets of predictors. A risk prediction tool for postoperative oxygen therapy was developed giving an area under the ROC curve of 0.93. Using the risk scores obtained from the model coefficients, children were classified into high (score ≥ 12), intermediate (8–11), or low (≤7) risk groups. These risk scores can be used to determine the level of need for postoperative oxygen therapy among children with similar risk factors.

Risk prediction tool for postoperative oxygen therapy

The optimal cut-point from the ROC curve was 12; therefore, we classified children with a score of ≥12 as high risk. A score of 8 showed high sensitivity (98.6%) which was consistent with a very low false negative rate (1.4%) (Fig. 2). Therefore, we considered a risk score < 8 to be a low risk (negative test) with a chance to require postoperative oxygen therapy < 1.4%. Thus, an individual risk score between 8 and 11 was classified as intermediate risk.

High risk group

The high risk group (score ≥ 12) included those who had thoracic surgery or had desaturation perioperatively. Children undergoing thoracic surgery (score of 11) usually need to be intubated with an endotracheal tube (score of 4) and are at high risk for postoperative oxygen therapy because they have a decrease of pulmonary functional residual capacity and high disturbance of cardiopulmonary function [14–16]. Provision of oxygen supplementation at the PACU and at a ward is necessary to prevent pulmonary complications. Children who had perioperative desaturation were also classified as high

Table 3 Multivariate hurdle model of factors predicting postoperative oxygen therapy use and risk scores in children undergoing non-cardiac surgery

Factor	Coefficient	Adjusted OR (95% CI)	*p* value	Risk score
Body mass index (Ref: 15-24.9)				
5–14.9	0.51	1.66 (1.07, 2.58)	0.024	1
25-60	1.04	2.82 (1.30, 6.11)	0.009	2
Hyper-reactive airway (Ref: No)				
Yes	0.92	2.50 (1.12, 5.59)	0.025	2
Probable difficult airway (Ref: No)				
Yes	1.61	4.99 (1.74, 14.32)	0.003	3
ASA physical status (Ref: 1)				
2	0.31	1.36 (0.73, 2.53)	0.327	0
3	1.55	4.73 (2.43, 9.18)	<0.001	3
Site/ type of procedure (Ref: Eye)				
Urologic	1.46	4.32 (1.39, 13.41)	0.01	3
Airway	2.04	7.72 (2.62, 22.70)	0.0002	4
Ear-nose-face	0.82	2.27 (0.60, 8.52)	0.22	0
Thoracic	5.63	277.9 (44.56, 1733)	<0.0001	11
Intra-abdomen	1.96	7.12 (2.30, 22.04)	0.0007	4
Orthopedic	1.95	7.00 (2.30, 21.33)	0.0006	4
Intra-cranial	2.01	7.45 (1.62, 34.20)	0.01	4
Gastrointestinal scope	1.23	3.42 (0.88, 13.37)	0.07	0
Cardiac catheterization	1.98	7.28 (2.04, 25.96)	0.002	4
Airway device (Ref: Facemask/LMA)				
Spontaneous breathing with non- rebreathing mask	1.38	3.98 (0.64, 24.88)	0.14	0
Endotracheal tube intubation	1.89	6.64 (2.54, 17.32)	0.0001	4
Neuromuscular blocking agent (Ref: None)				
Succinylcholine	0.67	1.95 (0.92, 4.13)	0.080	0
Aminosteroid derivatives	1.06	2.89 (1.18, 7.05)	0.02	2
Benzylisoquinolines	0.07	1.07 (0.58, 1.96)	0.83	0
Anesthetic time (hours) (Ref: <1)				
1–2.9	1.09	2.99 (1.38, 6.44)	0.005	2
≥3	1.57	4.79 (1.99, 11.6)	0.0005	3
PRAE (Ref: None)				
UAO and laryngospasm	4.12	61.5 (14.4, 262)	<0.0001	8
Desaturation	6.18	481.2 (177.9, 1302)	<0.0001	12
Bronchospasm/wheezing	4.53	92.4 (29.7, 288)	<0.0001	9

Ref Reference group; *OR* Odds ratio, *CI* Confidence interval, *ASA* American Society of Anesthesiologists, *LMA* Laryngeal mask airway, *UAO* Upper airway obstruction, *PRAE* Perioperative respiratory adverse events

risk. Strategies to identify risk or develop a risk prediction tool to predict the occurrence of perioperative respiratory events would help to reduce the need for postoperative oxygen therapy [9, 13, 17, 18].

Intermediate risk group

The intermediate risk group (score of 8–11) included those who had bronchospasm, upper airway obstruction or laryngospasm perioperatively, or from a combination of patient risk factors, such as high body mass index (score of 2), history of hyper-reactive airway (score of 2), having probable difficult airway (score of 3), other types of operations (score of 0–4), and anesthesia risk factors, such as ASA physical status 3 (score of 3), endotracheal tube intubation (score of 4), and anesthetic time ≥ 1 h (score of 2–3).

Obesity was found to be associated with the limitation of functional residual capacity and cardiovascular comorbidities

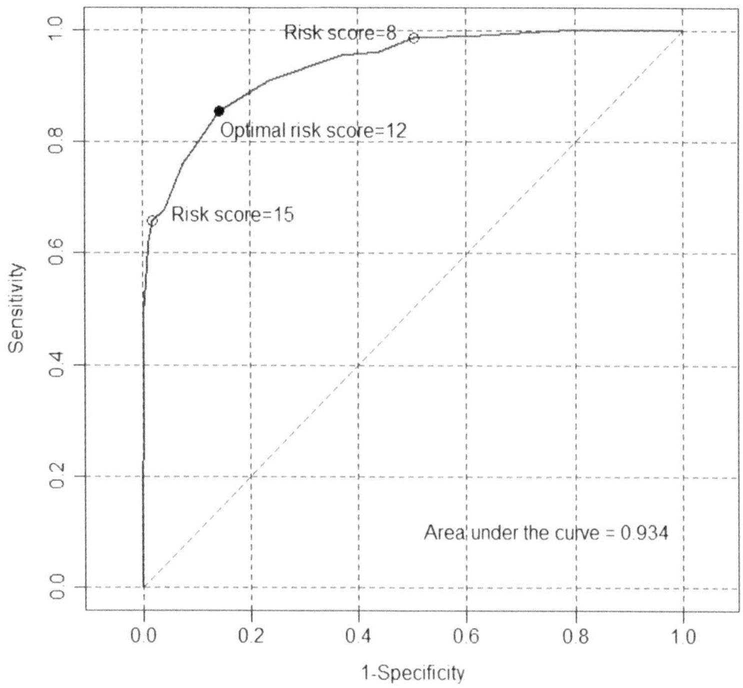

Fig. 2 Receiver operating characteristic curve of the risk score predicting postoperative oxygen therapy

that caused desaturation [13, 19–21] which may necessitate postoperative oxygen therapy. A child with a hyper-reactive airway (due to asthma) is prone to develop bronchospasm or desaturation due to airway hypersensitivity to stimuli during anesthesia. Having a probable difficult airway [22, 23] and prolonged anesthetic time [19, 24] may lead to the need for postoperative oxygen therapy due to upper airway obstruction, desaturation, and perioperative reintubation. The ability to quickly and easily calculate a risk score for children undergoing non-cardiac surgery might help anesthesia personnel make decisions concerning the child's management both at the preoperative and intraoperative periods. For example, if a child has an individual risk score of 6 or 7, the health personnel may try to reduce this score by preventing desaturation in difficult airway cases or by avoiding both endotracheal tube intubation and long or intermediate use of neuromuscular blocking agents intraoperatively, if feasible.

Predictors for duration of postoperative oxygen therapy

The median duration of postoperative oxygen therapy in our study was 17 h which is a duration that is quite safe from the harmful effects of oxygen therapy in children. The significant predictors for longer use of oxygen therapy included: history of delayed development, having probable difficult airway, thoracic, abdominal, airway and orthopedic surgery, and ASA physical status 3.

Having a probable difficult airway and airway surgery were predictors for both postoperative oxygen therapy and duration of use. Most of the children who were given oxygen via the T-piece connector ($n = 11$) had a probably difficult airway and airway surgery, thus they had a longer duration of oxygen therapy since duration (in hours) included the timing from receiving oxygen T-piece, removing endotracheal tube to weaning oxygen therapy via facemask. Children with cerebral palsy and mental retardation, defined as having delayed development, was another strong predictor for longer use of oxygen therapy (count ratio = 2.3). Most children with delayed development have several comorbidities, including cognitive disability, and have a higher risk of respiratory problems such as lower airway infection, airway secretion, or aspiration which may require longer use of postoperative oxygen therapy [25].

Compared with eye surgery, which had the lowest risk for postoperative oxygen therapy, ear-nose-face surgery and gastrointestinal endoscopy were also predictors for longer use of oxygen therapy. Ear-nose-face surgery cases included fractures of the face bones which necessitated postoperative endotracheal intubation and oxygen therapy via the T-piece connector, while children who had gastrointestinal endoscopy were more likely to have a history of delayed development. Use of morphine decreased the duration of postoperative oxygen therapy by a factor of about two-thirds compared to fentanyl. In this study, morphine was usually given (> 80%) in both older children (> 10 years) and those with ASA physical status 1 or 2 which may result in earlier discontinuation of postoperative oxygen therapy compared to those who received

Table 4 Multivariate hurdle model of factors predicting duration of postoperative oxygen therapy use in children undergoing non-cardiac surgery

Factor	Adjusted count ratio (95% CI)	*p* value
Probable difficult airway	2.19 (1.39, 3.48)	0.0008
History of delayed development	2.31 (1.49, 3.57)	0.0002
ASA physical status (Ref: 1)		0.03[a]
2	0.75 (0.43, 1.32)	
3	1.07 (0.61, 1.88)	
Site/type of procedure (Ref: Eye)		<0.0001
Urologic	1.98 (0.99, 3.96)	
Airway	3.01 (1.55, 5.83)	
Ear-nose-face	2.27 (1.06, 4.82)	
Thoracic	4.86 (2.34, 10.1)	
Intra-abdomen	4.15 (2.13, 8.11)	
Orthopedic	2.14 (1.08, 4.25)	
Intra-cranial	1.26 (0.52, 3.02)	
Gastrointestinal scope	2.73 (1.23, 6.04)	
Cardiac catheterization	1.18 (0.53, 2.60)	
Narcotic used (Ref: None)		0.049[b]
Morphine	0.69 (0.40, 1.20)	
Fentanyl	1.10 (0.72, 1.68)	

Ref Reference group, *ASA* American Society of Anesthesiologists
[a]The contrast of ASA physical status 3 vs ASA physical status 2 gave a significant count ratio of 1.42 and 95% CI of 1.10 and 1.84.
[b]The contrast of morphine vs fentanyl gave a significant count ratio of 0.63 and 95% CI of 0.44 and 0.90.

fentanyl. However, since age group was matched between cases and controls and ASA physical status was adjusted in the final model (Table 4), an explanation of this result is inconclusive as no other study has reported a similar result. Further studies focusing on opioids for postoperative oxygen therapy may help to explain this result.

Since 80% of respiratory events during anesthesia were mild desaturation (SpO_2 90–94%) and brief in duration (< 60 s), which required oxygen therapy for a short duration (< 17 h), it was not a predictor for duration of oxygen therapy. Thus, low flow oxygen or a lower oxygen concentration should be considered for those at high risk to reduce the risk of oxygen toxicity [26, 27]. Therefore, we attempted to limit the fraction of inspired oxygen between 0.4 and 0.6. We also provided continuous oxygen saturation monitoring and weaned off the oxygen therapy as soon as possible in almost 25% of the children who received oxygen therapy for more than 24 h.

Important issues and implications for clinical management

Our risk prediction tools have implications for aiding physicians in their clinical decision making peri-operatively. These can be divided into four strategic steps.

First, pre-operatively, physicians can utilize the risk prediction tool to quickly calculate a risk score indicating the degree of need for post-operative oxygen therapy. For example, an obese child (score + 2), or one with hyperactive airway (+ 2), history of difficult airway (+ 3), or with an ASA physical status 3 (+ 3), would have an increased risk of requiring post-operative oxygen therapy. Having multiple risk factors would also increase the requirement substantially.

Second, combining pre-operative with intra-operative risk factors can help physicians determine which children have an increased need for post-operative oxygen therapy, for example, children who undergo thoracic surgery or cardiac catheterization. In addition, children with a history of delayed development or those requiring a gastrointestinal scope may not only require post-operative oxygen therapy but may require prolonged use.

Third, children who score highly (≥ 12) on pre- and intra-operative risk factors can be targeted for receiving extra attention by anesthetic personnel. On the other hand, children who have low scores (≤ 7) may be given short-acting neuromuscular blocking agents, or given an anesthetic device that has a low risk of oxygen therapy postoperatively such as a laryngeal mask airway or face-mask, or given shorter anesthetic time (if feasible), or tried to minimize the incidence of respiratory events during anesthesia.

Fourth, minimizing the risk of prolonged oxygen therapy, by minimizing the risk score, should also result in a reduced duration of postoperative oxygen therapy. If oxygen therapy is absolutely necessary, for example when given as a prophylaxis in high risk children or when a respiratory event occurs during anesthesia, weaning children off oxygen therapy should be considered in those who have a low (≤ 7) or intermediate (8–11) risk score as soon as possible when signs and symptoms of hypoxia have improved in order to minimize the consequences of excessive use of postoperative oxygen therapy [28, 29]. It has been suggested that an audit of the criteria used for prescribing oxygen such as target saturations, oxygen device used, and indication for use, would help wean children off postoperative oxygen therapy [30]. However, if the prolonged need for postoperative oxygen therapy cannot be avoided, the lowest fraction of inspired oxygen concentration (< 0.5) should be considered to prevent long term complications and enhance patient safety.

Strengths and limitations

This study has some strengths. Matching cases to controls was done using age groups and year of surgery to reduce selection bias and to balance the two groups in terms of age. The multivariate hurdle model to predict both outcomes (any use and duration of postoperative oxygen therapy) was performed to adjust for potential confounding variables. The sample size was adequate which resulted in a high area under the ROC curve (0.93).

Even though we attempted to minimize the selection bias, some information bias from the database could have occurred. The incidence of a respiratory event during anesthesia in our study as well as some patient-related factors such as snoring and URI were quite low compared to a previous prospective study [24]. Finally, the child's age, which might affect the need for postoperative oxygen therapy, could not be evaluated since it was used for matching.

Even though this was a retrospective study, the reliability and accuracy of our results are quite high because the outcomes were determined from records confirmed by two experienced anesthesiologists, the study was matched on age and year of operation, and the sample size was large. The external validity to other children in the same setting should be convincing although the subjects were recruited from a single university hospital.

Conclusions

Our risk prediction tool for postoperative oxygen therapy provided a high predictive ability and severity of risk prediction score. For both outcomes, the common risk factors were: probable difficult airway, ASA physical status 3, and operations involving the airway, thorax, and abdomen. Anesthesia-related and surgery-related factors played an important role in the longer use of postoperative oxygen therapy. Some patient-related and surgery-related risks may not be preventable but the adjustment of oxygen therapy can be made under patient safety issues.

Abbreviations

ASA: American Society of Anesthesiologist; PACU: Post-anesthetic care unit; ROC: Receiver operating characteristic; URI: Upper respiratory tract infection; SpO_2: Oxygen saturation by pulse oximetry

Acknowledgements

We would like to thank Assistant Professor Edward McNeil for editing the manuscript and Glenn Shingledecker for correcting some grammatical errors in the manuscript.

Funding

This work was funded by the Faculty of Medicine, Prince of Songkla University, Hat Yai, Songkhla, Thailand.

Authors' contributions

All those listed as authors contributed to the preparation of the manuscript. Each listed author participated in the work that they can defend its content. MO coordinated the study, participated in the study design, undertook the statistical analysis and wrote the draft manuscript. SR participated in its design, collected the data and revised the draft manuscript. TC participated in its design and coordinated the drafting of the manuscript. All authors have read and approved the final version.

Competing interests

The authors declare that they have no competing interests.

References

1. Singh V, Gupta P, Khatana S, Bhagol A. Supplemental oxygen therapy: important considerations in oral and maxillofacial surgery. Natl J of Maxillofac Surg. 2011;2:10–4.
2. Lerman J. Perioperative respiratory complications in children. Lancet. 2010; 376:745–6.
3. von Ungern-Sternberg BS. Respiratory complications in the pediatric postanesthesia care unit. Anesthesiol Clin. 2014;32:45–61.
4. Baijal RG, Bidani SA, Minard CG, Watcha MF. Perioperative respiratory complications following awake and deep extubation in children undergoing adenotonsillectomy. Paediatr Anaesth. 2015;25:392–9.
5. Xue FS, Tong SY, Liao X, Liu JH, Zhang RJ, An G, Luo LK. Observation of the correlation of postanesthesia recovery scores with early postoperative hypoxaemia in children. Paediatr Anaesth. 1999;9:145–51.
6. Siddiqui N, Arzola C, Teresi J, Fox G, Guerina L, Friedman Z. Predictors of desaturation in the postoperative anesthesia care unit: an observational study. J Clin Anesth. 2013;25:612–7.
7. Hintong T, Klanarong S, Suksompong S, Chua-in W, Chatmongkolchat S, Werawatganon T. The Thai Anesthesia Incident Monitoring Study (Thai AIMS) of oxygen desaturation in the post-anesthetic care unit. J Med Assoc Thail. 2008;91:1531–8.
8. Kallstrom TJ. American Association for Respiratory Care (AARC).AARC clinical practice guideline: oxygen therapy for adults in the acute care facility--2002 revision & update. Respir Care. 2002;47:717–20.
9. Oofuvong M, Geater AF, Chongsuvivatwong V, Pattaravit N, Nuanjun K. Risk over time and risk factors of intraoperative respiratory events: a historical cohort study of 14,153 children. BMC Anesthesiol. 2014;14:13. https://doi.org/10.1186/1471-2253-14-13.
10. Xue FS, Luo LK, Tong SY, Liao X, Deng XM, An G. Study of the safe threshold of apneic period in children during anesthesia induction. J Clin Anesth. 1996;8:568–74.
11. Hu MC, Pavlicova M, Nunes EV. Zero-inflated and hurdle models of count data with extra zeros: examples from an HIV-risk reduction intervention trial. Am J Drug Alcohol Abuse. 2011;37:367–75. https://doi.org/10.3109/00952990.2011.597280.
12. Neelon B, Chang HH, Ling Q, Hastings NS. Spatiotemporal hurdle models for zeroinflated count data: exploring trends in emergency department visits. Stat Methods Med Res. 2016;25:2558–76.
13. Subramanyam R, Yeramaneni S, Hossain MM, Anneken AM, Varughese AM. Perioperative respiratory adverse events in pediatric ambulatory anesthesia: development and validation of a risk prediction tool. Anesth Analg. 2016; 122:1578–85. https://doi.org/10.1213/ANE.0000000000001216.
14. Nomori H, Kobayashi R. Postoperative pulmonary complications in patients undergoing thoracic surgery with special reference to preoperative respiratory muscle strength and nutrition. Nihon KyobuGeka Gakkai Zasshi. 1994;42:1272–5.

15. Katz LE. Postoperative complications of thoracic surgery: their recognition and treatment. AANA J. 1980;48:222–9.
16. Saito H, Minamiya Y, Kawai H, Motoyama S, Katayose Y, Kimura K, Saito R, Ogawa JI. Estimation of pulmonary oxygen consumption in the early postoperative period after thoracic surgery. Anesthesia. 2007;62:648–53.
17. Tait AR, Voepel-Lewis T, Christensen R, O'Brien LM. The STBUR questionnaire for predicting perioperative respiratory adverse events in children at risk for sleep-disordered breathing. Paediatr Anaesth. 2013;23:510–6.
18. von Ungern-Sternberg BS, Boda K, Chambers NA, Rebmann C, Johnson C, Sly PD, Habre W. Risk assessment for respiratory complications in pediatric anesthesia: a prospective cohort study. Lancet. 2010;376:773–83.
19. Oofuvong M, Geater AF, Chongsuvivatwong V, Pattaravit N, Nuanjun K. Association between intraoperative and post-anesthetic care unit respiratory events among 12,641 children in southern Thailand. BJMMR. 2015;6:1101–12.
20. Uakritdathikarn T, Chongsuvivatwong V, Geater AF, Vasinanukorn M, Thinchana S, Klayna S. Perioperative desaturation and risk factors in general anesthesia. J Med Assoc Thail. 2008;91:1020–9.
21. Tait AR, Voepel-Lewis T, Burke C, Kostrzewa A, Lewis I. Incidence and risk factors for perioperative adverse respiratory events in children who are obese. Anesthesiology. 2008;108:375–80.
22. Oofuvong M, Valois T, Withington DE. Laryngeal mask airway and difficult airway management in adolescent: a case report. Paediatr Anaesth. 2008;18:1228–9. https://doi.org/10.1111/j.1460-9592.2008.02724.x.
23. Chanchayanon T, Suraseranivongse S, Chau-in W. The Thai Anesthesia Incidents Study (THAI Study) of difficult intubation: a qualitative analysis. J Med Assoc Thail. 2005;88(Suppl 7):S62–8.
24. Oofuvong M, Geater AF, Chongsuvivatwong V, Chanchayanon T, Sriyanaluk B, Saefung B, Nuanjun K. Excess costs and length of hospital stay attributable to perioperative respiratory events in children. Anesth Analg. 2015;120:411–9.
25. Proesmans M, Vreys M, Huenaerts E, Haest E, Coremans S, Vermeulen F, Feys H. Respiratory morbidity in children with profound intellectual and multiple disability. Pediatr Pulmonol. 2015;50:1033–8.
26. Milési C, Boubal M, Jacquot A, Baleine J, Durand S, Odena MP, Cambonie G. Highflow nasal cannula: recommendations for daily practice in pediatrics. Ann Intensive Care. 2014;4:29. https://doi.org/10.1186/s13613-014-0029-5 eCollection 2014.
27. AARC. AARC clinical practice guideline. Oxygen therapy in the home or alternate site health care facility--2007 revision & update. Respir Care. 2007;52:1063–8.
28. Yeh J, McGrath-Morrow SA, Collaco JM. Oxygen weaning after hospital discharge in children with bronchopulmonary dysplasia. Pediatr Pulmonol. 2016;51:1206–11. https://doi.org/10.1002/ppul.23442.
29. Jindal SK. Oxygen therapy: important considerations. Indian J Chest Dis Allied Sci. 2008;50:97–107.
30. Wheeler L, James J, Byrne S, Forton J. Audit of oxygen prescribing in a children's hospital. Arch Dis Child. 2016;101:e2. https://doi.org/10.1136/archdischild-2016-311535.36.

13

Deferoxamine preconditioning ameliorates mechanical ventilation-induced lung injury in rat model via ROS in alveolar macrophages: a randomized controlled study

Weilin Zhu*, Yuansi Huang, Yuqiong Ye and Yafeng Wang

Abstract

Background: Mechanical ventilation (MV) can provide effective breathing support; however, ventilatior-induced lung injury (VILI) has also been widely recognized in clinical practice, including in the healthy lung. Unfortunately, the morbidity and mortality of VILI remain unacceptably high, and no satisfactory therapeutic effect can be achieved. The current study aimed to examine the effects of iron chelator preconditioning on the mitochondrial reactive oxygen species (ROS) in alveolar macrophages and pathological lung injury in VILI.

Methods: Twenty four healthy male Sprague–Dawley (SD) rats (250–300 g in weight) were randomly divided into 3 groups, including the control group (NC group, $n = 8$), the high-volume mechanical ventilation group (HV group, $n = 8$), and the deferoxamine treatment group (HV + DFO group, n = 8). Rats in the HV and HV + DFO groups were subjected to high-volume MV at a dose of 40 ml/kg. DFO was administered at a dose of 200 mg/kg 15 min prior to over-ventilation. Spontaneously breathing anesthetized rats were used as the controls. The animals were sacrificed after 4 h of high-volume ventilation or under control conditions, the animals were sacrificed. Purified alveolar macrophages from bronchoalveolar lavage fluid (BALF) and lung tissue were collected for further analysis through light microscopy and flow cytometry.

Results: Compared with the controls, the high-volume-ventilated rats had exhibited typical lung edema and histological lung injury, and ROS were markedly increased in alveolar macrophages and mitochondria. Moreover, all indices of VILI were remarkably different in rats treated with DFO preconditioning. DFO could ameliorate lung injury in the mechanically ventilated SD rat model.

Conclusions: DFO preconditioning contributes to mitigating the histological lung damage while reducing ROS levels in alveolar macrophages and mitochondria, suggesting that iron metabolism in alveolar macrophages may participate in VILI.

Keywords: Ventilator-induced lung injury, Deferoxamine, Reactive oxygen species, Mitochondria, Alveolar macrophages

* Correspondence: zhuwl2002@sina.com
Department of Anesthesia, People's Hospital of Guangxi Zhuang Autonomous Region, Nanning 530021, China

Mechanical ventilation (MV) is necessary for patients under anesthesia during surgery, which can provide respiratory support for the whole body. It is also used to treat patients with acute lung injury (ALI), acute respiratory distress syndrome (ARDS) and other diseases. MV can provide effective breathing support; nonetheless, VILI has also been widely recognized in clinical practice [1, 2].

At present, biological lung injury is known to be associated with the release of inflammatory factors, apoptosis, endothelial injury, and activation of the coagulation system [3, 4]. However, the existing therapeutic effect is limited targeting the above mechanisms. Consequently, it is important to explore new treatment ideas and mechanisms. Alveolar macrophages, which reside in the alveolar space, have accounted for 90% of all leukocytes, and the remainders are mainly dendritic cells and T cells. Alveolar macrophages (AMs) play a crucial role in maintaining immunological homeostasis and host defense, which are also the primary producers of pro-inflammatory cytokines in lung following exposure to noxious stimuli [5, 6]. Oxidative stress in mitochondria can promote the pathology of degenerative diseases and tumorigenesis [7]. Mitochondrion is the main organelle involved in the action of AMs, and also the key initiating factor of the pulmonary inflammatory reaction in early ALI [8]. Previous data reveal that AMs exposed to asbestos fibers can produce H_2O_2. In addition, the production of reactive oxygen species (ROS) can be reduced by knocking down the iron-sulfur protein of complex III in the mitochondrial electron transport chain (ETC), a major site responsible for ROS production [9]. Lung diseases can be treated through targeting oxidative stress with antioxidant agents, such as thiol molecules, polyphenols and superoxide dismutase (SOD) [10]. Moreover, the introduction of low tidal volume ventilation has improved the clinical outcome [11].

However, the morbidity and mortality of VILI remain unacceptably high at present; besides, the therapeutic effect is limited for the previously discovered mechanisms. Unfortunately, no preventive therapeutic agent is available currently. Iron chelators are the important antioxidant drugs [12, 13]. There is currently no more effective method to change the ROS levels in the mitochondria of AMs in VILI, and whether an iron chelator is effective in lung MV remains to be further studied.

The current study aimed to explore whether the iron chelator deferoxamine (DFO) had a lung protective effect against VILI in rats and to preliminarily extract a potential new mechanism of MV-induced lung injury.

Materials and methods

Animals

The Sprague-Dawley (SD) rat model of VILI was established as previously described [14]. Healthy male adult SD rats weighing 250-300 g were provided by the Laboratory Animal Center of Guangxi Medical University (Nanning, China, License number: SCXK GUI 2009–0002), and raised in an environmentally controlled room at 23 ± 2 °C and 50–70% humidity under a 12/12 h light/dark cycle. All animals were allowed free access to food and water.

The study was performed in accordance with the guidelines for the Care and Use of Laboratory Animals approved by Ethics and Animal Welfare Committee of the People's Hospital of Guangxi Zhuang Autonomous Region (Nanning, China, Permission number 2014–034). All possible efforts were undertaken to avoid animal suffering at each stage of the experiments.

Establishment of the VILI rat model

16 male SD rats were randomly divided into two groups, including the control group (group NC) and lung injury group (group HV) Group NC received an intraperitoneal injection of 10% chloral hydrate (1.5 mL/kg) to induce anesthesia. The rats were intubated with a tracheal cannula after tracheotomy upon the cease of body movement. The animals were fixed in a supine position on the operating table and were performed thoracotomy to remove the lung tissues under aseptic conditions. Group HV underwent an intraperitoneal injection of 10% chloral hydrate (1.5 mL/kg) to induce anesthesia. The animals were also fixed in a supine position on the operating table, intubated with a tracheal cannula after tracheotomy, and fixed with surgical line nodes connected to a small animal ventilator (TOPO, Kent Scientific, Torrington, USA) for MV. The respiratory parameter settings were as follows: a tidal volume of 40 mL/kg, a respiratory frequency of 40–60/min, a respiratory ratio of 1:1, and a positive end-expiratory pressure of 0. All rats were given supplemental oxygen at approximately 40–50%. Blood samples were collected from the anatomical femoral artery indwelling tube for blood gas analysis. The respiratory rate was adjusted using the partial pressure of carbon dioxide in arterial blood ($PaCO_2$) and maintained at 35–45 mmHg. After MV for 4 h, lung tissues were collected under sterile conditions. Animals in both groups were sacrificed by bloodletting.

Hematoxylin and eosin (HE) staining

Tissues from the left lung were cut into 3 blocks 0.1 cm × 0.1 cm × 0.1 cm in size, fixed with 10% formalin, and sent to the Department of Pathology of Guangxi Zhuang Autonomous Region People's Hospital for pathological sectioning and observation under a light microscope (Olympus, Japan). The pathological observation results showed that the lung injury model had been successfully established by MV with a high tidal volume (tidal volume of 40 mL/kg, respiratory frequency of 40–60/min, and ventilation for 4 h).(Fig. 1).

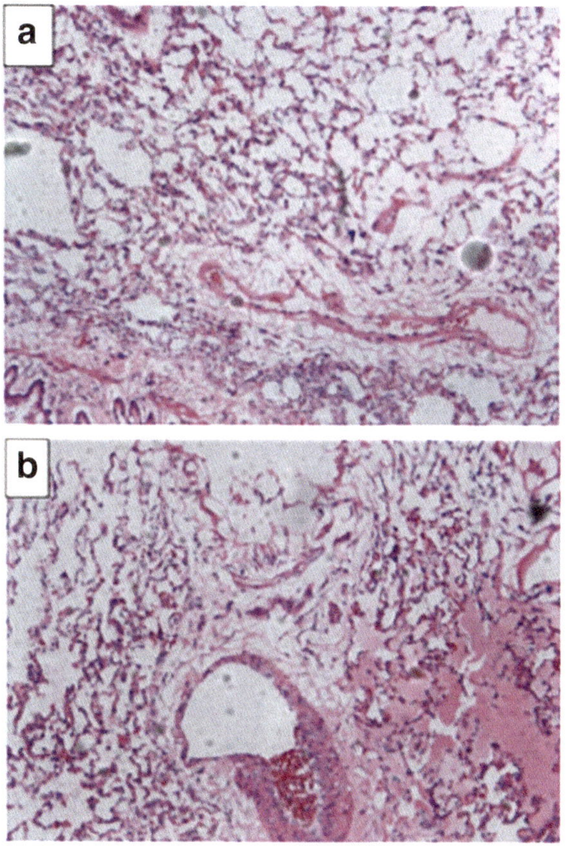

Fig. 1 Estblishment of a VILI rat model. **a** Group NC showed lung alveolar structure and clear alveolar exudate, × 100. **b** In group HV, epithelial shedding in the lung alveoli was visible after 4 h of VILI tidal volume of 40 mL/kg, × 100

Establishment of a MV model with preconditioning

Twenty four healthy adult male SD rats weighing 250–300 g were randomly divided into three groups, with 8 rats in each group. The control group (group NC) underwent intraperitoneal injection of 10% chloral hydrate (1.5 mL/kg) 5 min after tracheal intubation and thoracotomy. The high tidal volume ventilation group (group HV) received intraperitoneal injection of 10% chloral hydrate (1.5 mL/kg). 5 min later, 2 mL saline was injected intraperitoneally. Ventilator-controlled breathing and tracheal intubation were initiated 15 min later based on the following parameters, a tidal volume of 40 mL/kg, a frequency of 40–60/min, a I:E ratio of 1:1, and a positive end-expiratory pressure of 0. All rats were administered supplemental oxygen at approximately 40–50%. Blood samples were collected from the anatomical femoral artery indwelling tube for blood gas analysis. The respiratory rate was adjusted using the partial pressure of carbon dioxide in arterial blood ($PaCO_2$) and maintained at 35–45 mmHg. The group DFO (group HV + DFO) was given an intraperitoneal injection of 10% chloral hydrate (1.5 mL/kg), followed by intraperitoneal injection of DFO (200 mg/kg, Sigma, USA) 5 min later. 15 min later, tracheal intubation with a ventilator was performed to control breathing in the same way as that in the group HV. After MV for 4 h, the left lung was ligated, and the lung blood was flushed through the pulmonary artery with solution 2. Animals in the three groups were sacrificed by rapid bloodletting, the whole trachea, heart and lungs were removed, and the corpses were disposed properly.

Lung wet/dry ratio (W/D)

Part of left lung tissues were collected and weighed on an electronic balance, and the total wet weight was recorded as W. The samples were then incubated at 80 °C in a drying oven for 48 h to obtain the total dry weight, which was recorded as D. Finally, the W/D ratio was calculated to assess pulmonary edema.

Lung tissue pathological injury

Fresh left lung tissue blocks approximately 0.1 cm × 0.1 cm × 0.1 cm in size were fixed with 10% formaldehyde and sent to the Department of Pathology of Guangxi Zhuang Autonomous Region People's Hospital for observation. Paraffin sections were produced, stained with HE, observed under a light microscope (Olympus, Japan), and graded according to both histological and morphometric analysis introduced by Smith [15].

Preparation of the AM suspension solution

The right lung with endotracheal tube was placed into a 50 ml beaker, and washed with 1 x PBS using the transtracheal catheter for 10 times. The lavage fluid was collected and placed into a 50 ml 130 g × 8 min centrifuge tube for centrifugation. The supernatant was collected, and 3 ml red blood cell lysate was added, followed by ice cracking for 10 min. The mixture was sufficiently mixed and centrifuged at 440G for 10 min to collect the supernatant. 2 ml red blood cell lysate was then added to centrifuge at 440G for 10 min, and the supernatant was collected, which was the macrophage suspension. According to related literature, the alveolar lavage fluid mainly consisted of AMs.

Tracheal intubation with lung lavage was performed after washing with 6 mL PBS for 10 times. The lavage fluid was collected and transferred to a 50 mL centrifuge tube for centrifugation (Hettich, Germany) at 4 °C at 130 g for 8 min. The supernatant was discarded, and then 3 ml red blood cell lysate was added, followed by ice cracking for 10 min, centrifugation at 440 g for 10 min, for twice. The precipitate was suspended in PBS, and the cell concentration was adjusted to 2 × 106/mL-3 × 106/mL. The purity was detected by Giemsa staining, the cell activity was detected by the trypan blue exclusion assay and counted using a hemocytometer.

Detection of ROS in macrophages

Cytometric detection of ROS in macrophages was conducted through assay (Beyotime Biotechnology, China) by flow cytometry (BD FacsCalibur, USA). Samples loaded with probes were detected by flow cytometry. The excitation and emission wavelengths were 510 nm and 580 nm, respectively, which were used to detect the stimulated fluorescence intensity in a real-time manner.

Detection of mitochondrial ROS in macrophages

Detection of mitochondrial ROS in macrophages through assay (Life Technologies, USA) by flow cytometry. Alveolar macrophages were suspended in MitoSOXTM liquid by dilution. Samples loaded with probes were detected by flow cytometry. The excitation and emission wavelengths were 510 nm and 580 nm, respectively, which were used to detect the fluorescence intensity in a real-time manner using the Reactive Oxygen Detection Kit (Life Technologies, USA).

Statistical analysis

Animals were required to obtain a power of 0.80 with a $p < 0.05$ and a SD = 1/2 mean.

Some data had to be excluded due to technical problems; as a result, the subsequent lung analyses were done with 8 samples per group as indicated. SPSS 24 statistical software was employed to determine the mean ± SD and perform single factor analysis of variance. Intracellular and mitochondrial ROS were analyzed using the Flowjo 7.6.2 software (BD, USA). Data were compared using the chi-squared test or Fisher's test, and differences with a value of $p < 0.05$ were considered statistically significant.

Results

Lung W/D ratio

The W/D ratio was markedly increased in group HV compared with that in group NC group ($p = 0.02$). In the meantime, the W/D ratio was outstandingly decreased in group HV + DFO relative to that in group HV ($p = 0.015$) (Fig. 2).

Lung tissue pathological damage under a light microscope

In group NC, the lung tissue was clear, the alveoli were intact and free of congestion and edema, and no inflammatory exudation was present. In comparison, the lung tissue in group HV showed inflammatory cell infiltration. Group HV + DFO displayed mild pathological changes, which mainly manifested as capillary congestion, alveolar fibrin with little exudation, slight alveolar septum widening, occasional exfoliated epithelial cells in the lumen, as well as rare alveolar and interval neutrophilic exudation (Fig. 3).

Lung injury score by both histological and morphometric analysis

Compared with group NC, the he lung injury score was markedly increased in group HV ($p = 0.000$). In group HV + DFO, the lung injury score ($p = 0.047$) was increased to

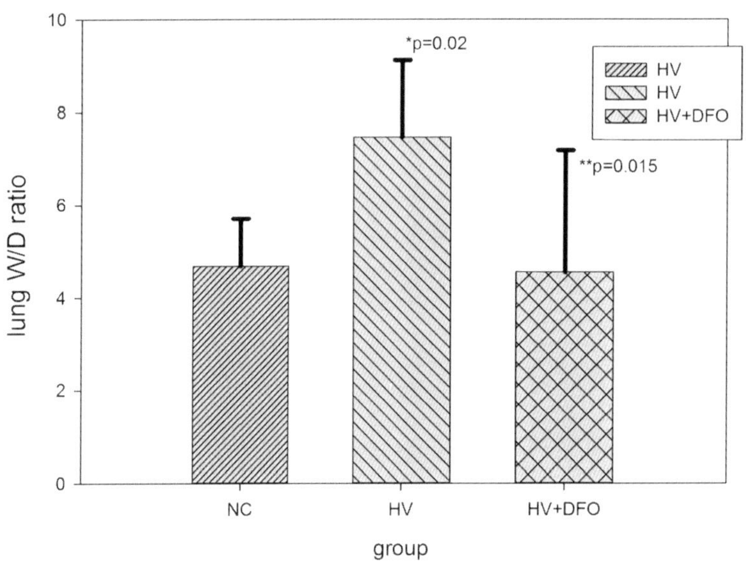

Fig. 2 Comparison of lung W/D ratio among the three groups ((Mean ± SD). Part of the left lung tissues were collected and weighed on an electronic balance, and the total wet weight was recorded as W. The samples were then incubated at 80 °C in a drying oven for 48 h to obtain the total dry weight, which was recorded as D. The value of W/D ratio was calculated to assess pulmonary edema. $p = 0.054$ by Levene statistics; $F = 53.39$ and $p = 0.000$ between groups. *$p = 0.02$ (95%CI 4.01, 5.17), compared with group NC, and **$p = 0.015$(95%CI -5.30,-0.53) compared with group HV by Tukey HSD statistics

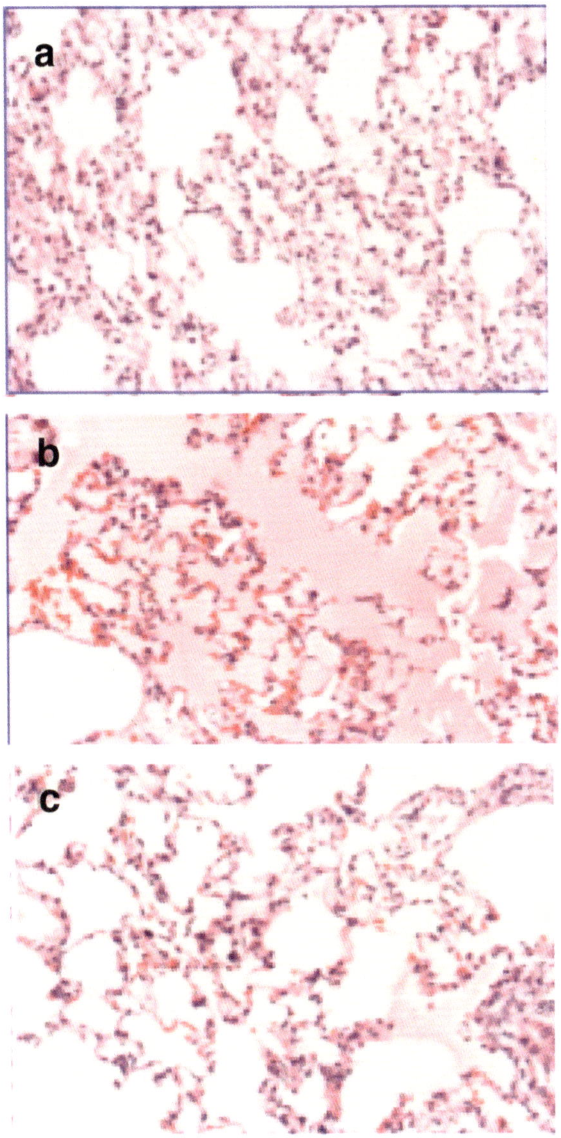

Fig. 3 Pathological sections of lung tissue were observed under a light microscope. **a** Normal lung tissue morphology, with no protein exudation in alveolar cavity and no alveolar epithelium peeling (group NC, × 200). **b** Visible alveoli with fibrin exudation, and the epithelial cavity was visible (group HV, × 200). **c** Small amount of alveolar epithelial shedding, along with normal lung interval (group HV + DFO, × 200)

a certain extent, but was apparently lower than that in group HV ($p = 0.000$) (Fig. 4).

The purity and activity of alveolar macrophages

Macrophage suspensions were prepared and purified using BALF. The purity was detected through Giemsa staining. The cell concentration was adjusted to 2×10^6/mL- 3×10^6/mL. The cell activity was detected by trypan blue exclusion assay and counted using a hemocytometer. According to the trypan blue exclusion assay, the cell survival rate was as follows, group NC: 90.42 ± 3.70%, group HV: 88.37 ± 5.21%, and group HV + DFO:87.00 ± 4.83% ($F = 0.79, p = 0.467$). Results of Giemsa staining and cell suspensions by flow cytometry analysis suggested that the cell liquid purity rates were as follows, group NC: 90.87 ± 4.36%, group HV: 86.50 ± 6.00%, and group HV + DFO: 87.75 ± 8.15% ($F = 1.03, p = 0.384$).

Determination of ROS in cells and macrophage mitochondria

Results of flow cytometry showed that the mean fluorescence intensity (MFI) of ROS in cells and macrophage mitochondria in group HV was dramatically increased compared with that in group NC ($p = 0.03, p = 0.000$). In contrast, the MFI in cells and mitochondria was notably decreased in group HV + DFO compared with that in group HV ($p = 0.017, p = 0.000$) (Figs. 5, 6, 7).

Discussion

The important findings of this study are that VILI in AMs and mitochondrion-released ROS are involved in the injury process, while DFO preconditioning can outstandingly reduce ROS release from AMs and mitochondria, mitigate pulmonary edema, alleviate pathological damage, and show lung protection.

MV, which can provide effective respiratory support, can also lead to severe lung injury known as VILI. An increasing number of studies have been conducted to examine the inflammatory factors and cells involved in lung injury, which suggest that macrophages are important cells involved in the pathogenesis of VILI [5, 6], and the main cells participating in the inflammatory response [16].

Additionally, relevant literature shows that the BALF cells mainly consist of AMs [17], which conforms to our results. Recent studies have found that oxidative stress is involved in mechanical injury [18–20], and ROS production is increased in many cells with increased tensile stress [21–23]. ROS is an important target of VILI, as discovered from ROS generated by antioxidant treatment [24, 25]. However, the origin and possible mechanism of ROS production remain unclear. Mitochondria are the main sites responsible for ROS production [26, 27]. Nonetheless, the role of macrophage mitochondria in MV-induced lung injury remains to be further elaborated. Besides, it has not been reported whether preventive medication can prevent MV-induced lung injury.

Increasing evidence indicates that oxidative stress originating from iron overload plays an important role in various lung diseases, including asthma, chronic obstructive pulmonary disease (COPD), ALI, pulmonary fibrosis and the pathogenesis of lung cancer [28–31]. Chelation of free iron with iron amine has been shown to protect against lung injury caused by oxidative stress in some lung diseases [32, 33].

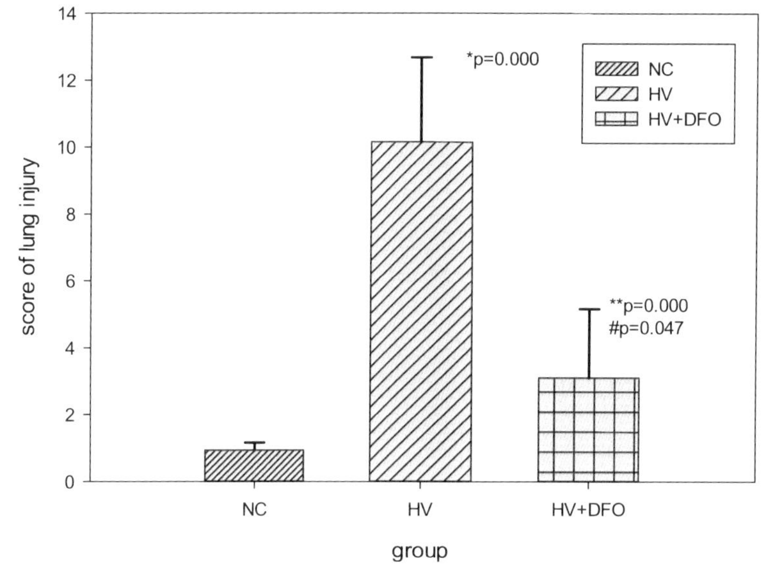

Fig. 4 Both histological and morphometric analysis of lung injury among the three groups ((Mean ± SD). $p = 0.001$ by Levene statistics; Welch statistic F = 53,39, and $p = 0.000$ between groups. *$p = 0.000$ (95%CI 11.85, 6.59), #$p = 0.047$(95% CI 0.37, 4.30) compared with group NC, and **$p = 0.000$ (95% CI -10.07, – 4.03) compared with group HV by Games-Howell statistics

DFO has a specific hydroxylamine group iron chelator and shows a high affinity for Fe^{3+}. Thus, reducing ROS attack generated by iron ions on biofilms is a very effective way to prevent iron ions from being reduced to ferrous ions and participating in oxidative stress. Therefore, iron chelators have gradually become the focus in the tissue protection field. Iron overload will result in increased ROS release in cancer, brain injury and other diseases, giving rise to tissue damage [34–37]. However, it remains unclear whether this reaction is involved in iron overload. Our findings reveal that ROS production in AMs and mitochondria are increased in VILI ($p < 0.05$), and the ROS increasing range in mitochondria is higher than in macrophages. In addition, intracellular or mitochondrial ROS can be reduced by DFO preconditioning ($p < 0.05$). However, DFO is a non-selective mitochondrial antioxidant; consequently, further study is required to determine whether intracellular ROS is derived from mitochondrial deformation. Group HV + DFO has exhibited reduced pathological damage, and the lung W/D ratio is remarkably decreased ($p < 0.05$), which is consistent with the ROS production trend

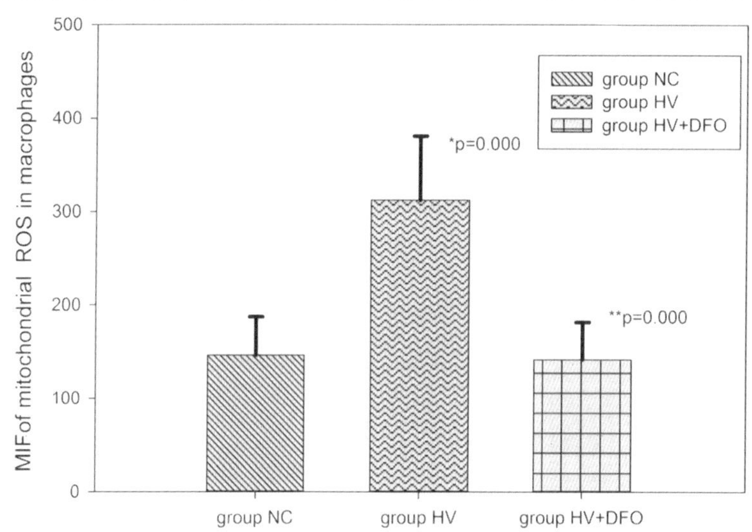

Fig. 5 The mean fluorescence intensity (MFI) of mitochondrial ROS in AMs among the three groups ((Mean ± SD). *$p = 0.03$ compared with group NC, and **$p = 0.017$ compared with group HV

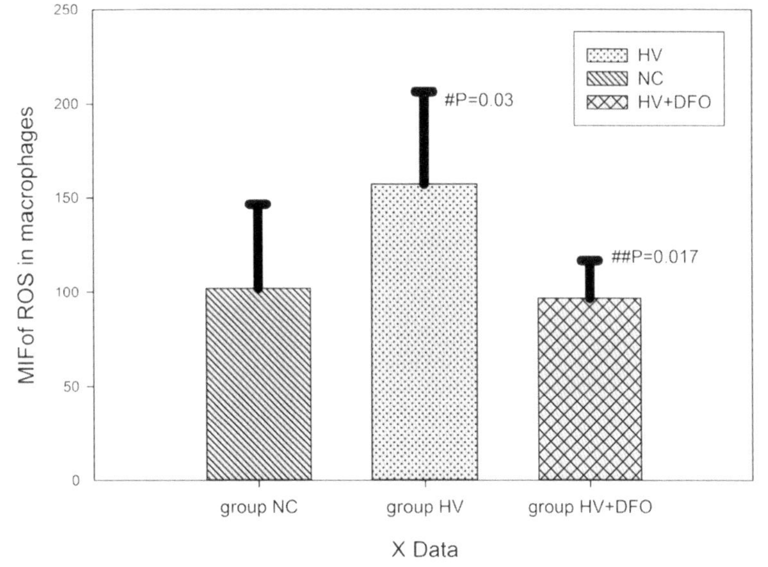

Fig. 6 Comparison of MFI of ROS in AMs among the three groups ((Mean ± SD). # $p = 0.03$ compared with group NC, and ##$p = 0.017$ compared with group HV

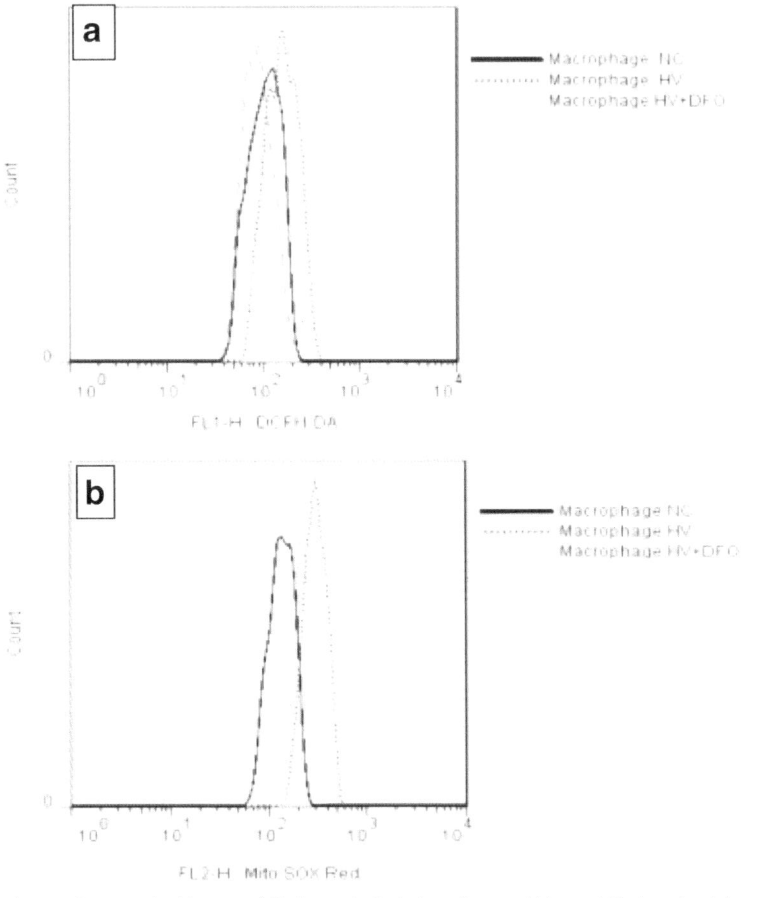

Fig. 7 **a** MFI of ROS in macrophages. Compared with group NC, the peak deviation of group HV was shifted to the right, and the peak left deviation of group HV + DFO was similar to that of group NC. **b** MFI of ROS in macrophage mitochondria by flow cytometry. Compared with group NC, the peak deviation of group HV was shifted to the right, and the peak left deviation of group HV + DFO was similar to that of group NC

observed in macrophages and mitochondria. Such result suggests that prophylactic intraperitoneal injection of the iron chelator DFO can effectively reduce ROS formation in macrophages and mitochondria in SD rats. Additionally, it can also inhibit the oxidative damage to biological membranes, and reduce pulmonary edema as well as lung pathological damage. Such finding indicates that iron overload may be involved in VILI. The current study is inevitably associated with certain limitations. Specifically, DFO displays no specificity in inhibiting mitochondrial ROS production; therefore, it can not be ensured that ROS originate in mitochondria. On this account, our next step will be to further study the effects of the mitochondrion specific iron chelator on MV-induced lung injury, and the role of DFO preconditioning in hyperoxic alveolar damage.

In conclusion, preconditioning with intraperitoneal injection of the iron chelator DFO can effectively reduce the ROS production in macrophages and mitochondria, as shown in the MV-induced lung injury SD rat model, resulting in reduced pathological damage and showing lung protection. It is also suggested that oxidative stress induced by iron overload in macrophages may be involved in VILI, which should be further verified in studies.

Conclusions

DFO preconditioning contributes to mitigating the histological lung damage while reducing ROS levels in alveolar macrophages and mitochondria, suggesting that iron metabolism in alveolar macrophages may participate in VILI.

Acknowledgements

We thank Professor Linghui Pan (Tumor Hospital of Guangxi Medical University, China) and Professor Bingwen He (Guangxi Medical University, China) for their assistance in the establishment of animal model.

Funding

This work was supported by the Guangxi Natural Science Foundation of China [0640060].

Authors' contributions

WZ contributed to the overall study design, data analysis, and co-writing of the paper; YH had carried out experiments, collected and analyzed data, and co-wrote the paper. YY had performed the experiments, collected and analyzed data with YW. All authors had read and approved the final manuscript.

Competing interests

The authors declare that they have no competing interests.

References

1. Cagle LA, Franzi LM, Linderholm AL, Last JA, Adams JY, Harper RW, Kenyon NJ. Lung-Protective Ventilation With Low Tidal Volumes and the Occurrence of Pulmonary Complications in Patients Without Acute Respiratory Distress Syndrome: A Systematic Review and Individual Patient Data Analysis. Crit Care Med. 2015;43:2155–63.
2. Serpa Neto A, Hemmes SN, Barbas CS, Beiderlinden M, Biehl M, Binnekade JM, Canet J, Fernandez-Bustamante A, Futier E, Gajic O, Hedenstierna G, Hollmann MW, Jaber S, Kozian A, Licker M, Lin WQ, Maslow AD, Memtsoudis SG, Reis Miranda D, Moine P, Ng T, Paparella D, Putensen C, Ranieri M, Scavonetto F, Schilling T, Schmid W, Selmo G, Severgnini P, Sprung J, Sundar S, Talmor D, Treschan T, Unzueta C, Weingarten TN, Wolthuis EK, Wrigge H, Gama de Abreu M, Pelosi P, Schultz MJ. Protective versus conventional ventilation for surgery: a systematic review and individual patient data meta-analysis. Anesthesiology. 2015;123:66–78.
3. Li LF, Huang CC, Liu YY, Lin HC, Kao KC, Yang CT, Liao SK. Hydroxyethyl starch reduces high stretch ventilation-augmented lung injury via vascular endothelial growth factor. Transl Res. 2011;157:293–305.
4. Huang LT, Chou HC, Wang LF, Chen CM. Tissue plasminogen activator attenuates ventilator-induced lung injury in rats. Acta Pharmacol Sin. 2012;33:991–7.
5. Dai H, Pan L, Lin F, Ge W, Li W, He S. Mechanical ventilation modulates Toll-like receptors 2, 4, and 9 on alveolar macrophages in a ventilator-induced lung injury model. J Thorac Dis. 2015;7:616–24.
6. Hamanaka K, Ming YJ, Mary I, et al. TRPV4 channels augment macrophage activation and ventilator-induced lung injury. Am J Physiol Lung Cell Mol Physiol. 2010;299:L353–62.
7. Rowlands DJ. Mitochondria dysfunction: a novel therapeutic target in pathological lung remodeling or bystander? Pharmacol Ther. 2016;166:96–105.
8. Murthy S, Adamcakova-Dodd A, Perry SS, Tephly LA, Keller RM, Metwali N, Meyerholz DK, Wang Y, Glogauer M, Thorne PS, Carter AB. Modulation of reactive oxygen species by Rac1 or catalase prevents asbestos-induced pulmonary fibrosis. Am J Physiol Lung Cell Mol Physiol. 2009;297:L846–55.
9. Osborn-Heaford HL, Ryan AJ, Murthy S, Racila AM, He C, Sieren JC, Spitz DR, Carter AB. Mitochondrial Rac1 GTPase import and electron transfer from cytochrome c are required for pulmonary fibrosis. J Biol Chem. 2012;287:3301–12.
10. Liu X, Chen Z. The pathophysiological role of mitochondrial oxidative stress in lung diseases. J Transl Med. 2017;15:207.
11. Xie J, Jin F, Pan C, Liu S, Liu L, Xu J, Yang Y, Qiu H. The effects of low tidal ventilation on lung strain correlate with respiratory system compliance. Crit Care. 2017;21:23.
12. Haskova P, Koubkova L, Vavrova A, et al. Comparison of various iron chelators used in clinical practice asprotecting agents against catecholamine-induced oxidative injury and cardiotoxicity. Toxicology. 2011;289:122–31.
13. Al-Rousan RM, Paturi S, Laurino JP, Kakarla SK, Gutta AK, Walker EM, Blough ER. Deferasirox removes cardiac iron and attenuates oxidative stress in the iron-overloaded gerbil. Am J Hematol. 2009;84:565–70.
14. Matute-Bello G, Downey G, Moore BB, Groshong SD, Matthay MA, Slutsky AS, Kuebler WM. An official American Thoracic Society workshop report: features and measurements of experimental acute lung injury in animals. Am J Respir Cell Mol Biol. 2011;44:725–38.
15. Smith KM, Mrozek JD, Simonton SC, et al. Prolonged partial liquid ventilation using conventional and high-frequency ventilatory techniques: gas exchange and lung pathology in an animal model of respiratory distress syndrome. Crit Care Med. 1997;25:1888–97.
16. Zhang Y, Liu G, Dull RO, Schwartz DE, Hu G. Autophagy in pulmonary macrophages mediates lung inflammatory injury via NLRP3 inflammasome activation during mechanical ventilation. Am J Physiol Lung Cell Mol Physiol. 2014;307:L173–85.
17. Misharin AV, Morales-Nebreda L, Mutlu GM, Budinger GR, Perlman H. Flow cytometric analysis of macrophages and dendritic cell subsets in the mouse lung. Am J Respir Cell Mol Biol. 2013;49:503–10.
18. Li LF, Kao KC, Yang CT, Huang CC, Liu YY. Ethyl pyruvate reduces ventilation-induced neutrophil infiltration and oxidative stress. Exp Biol Med. 2012;237:720–7.
19. Liao CC, Kau YC, Ting PC, Tsai SC, Wang CJ. The Effects of Volume-Controlled and Pressure-Controlled Ventilation on Lung Mechanics, Oxidative Stress, and Recovery in Gynecologic Laparoscopic Surgery. J Minim Invasive Gynecol. 2016;23:410–7.

20. Spassov SG, Faller S, Hummel M, Helo K, Ihle A, Ryter SW, Strosing KM, Hoetzel A. Hydrogen sulfide confers lung protection during mechanical ventilation via cyclooxygenase 2, 15-deoxy Δ12,14-prostaglandin J2, and peroxisome proliferator-activated receptor gamma. Crit Care Med. 2017;45:e849–57.
21. Ali MH, Pearlstein DP, Mathieu CE, Schumacker PT. Mitochondrial requirement for endothelial responses to cyclic strain: implications for mechanotransduction. Am J Physiol Lung Cell Mol Physiol. 2004;287:L486–96.
22. Grote K, Flach I, Luchtefeld M, Akin E, Holland SM, Drexler H, Schieffer B. Mechanical stretch enhances mRNA exp ression and proenzyme release of matrix metalloproteinase-2 (MMP-2) via NAD (P) H oxidase-derived reactive oxygen species. Circ Res. 2003;92:e80–6.
23. Wung BS, Cheng JJ, Shyue SK, Wang DL. NO modulates monocyte chemotactic protein-1 expression in endothelial cells under cyclic strain. Arterioscler Thromb Vasc Biol. 2001;21:1941–7.
24. Spassov SG, Donus R, Ihle PM, Engelstaedter H, Hoetzel A, Faller S. Hydrogen sulfide prevents formation of reactive oxygen species through PI3K/Akt signaling and limits ventilator-induced lung injury. Oxidative Med Cell Longev. 2017;2017:3715037.
25. Faller S, Strosing KM, Ryter SW, et al. The volatile anesthetic isoflurane prevents ventilator-induced lung injury via phosphoinositide 3-kinase/Akt signaling in mice. Anesth Analg. 2012;114:747–56.
26. Osborn-Heaford HL, Ryan AJ, Murthy S, Racila AM, He C, Sieren JC, Spitz DR, Carter AB. Mitochondrial Rac1 GTPase import and electron transfer from cytochrome c are required forpulmonary fibrosis. J Biol Chem. 2012;287: 3301–12.
27. Murthy S, Ryan A, He C, Mallampalli RK, Carter AB. Rac1-mediated mitochondrial H2O2 generation regulates MMP-9 gene expression in macrophages via inhibition of SP-1 and AP-1. J Biol Chem. 2010;285: 25062–73.
28. Henricks PA, Nijkamp FP. Reactive oxygen species as mediators in asthma. Pulm Pharmacol Ther. 2001;14:409–20.
29. MacNee W. Oxidative stress and lung inflammation in airway disease. Eur J Pharmacol. 2001;429:195–207.
30. Repine JE, Bast A, Lankhorst I. Oxidative stress in chronic obstructive pulmonary disease. Am J Respir Crit Care Med. 1997;156:341–57.
31. Halliwell B, Gutteridge JM, Cross CE. Free radicals, antioxidants, and human disease: where are we now? J Lab Clin Med. 1992;119:598–620.
32. Ritter C, da Cunha AA, Echer IC, Andrades M, Reinke A, Lucchiari N, Rocha J, Streck EL, Menna-Barreto S, Moreira JC, Dal-Pizzol F. Effects of N-acetylcysteine plus deferoxamine in lipopolysaccharide-induced acute lung injury in the rat. Crit Care Med. 2006;34:471–7.
33. La londe C, Ikeganik K, Demling R. Aerosolized deferoxamine prevents lung and systemic injury caused by smoke inhalation. J Appl Physiol. 1994;77:2057–64.
34. Paradkar PN, Zumbrennen KB, Paw BH, Ward DM, Kaplan J. Regulation of mitochon- drial iron import through differential turnover of mitoferrin1 and mitoferrin2. Mol Cell Biol. 2009;29:1007–16.
35. Zhang WJ, Wei H, Frei B. The iron chelator, esferrioxamine, reduces inflammation and atherosclerotic lesion development in experimental mice. Exp Biol Med. 2010;235:633–41.
36. Weinreb O, Mandel S, Youdim MB, Amit T. Targeting dysregulation of brain iron homeostasis in Parkinson's disease by iron chelators. Free Radic Biol Med. 2013;62:52–64.
37. Umemura M, Kim JH, Aoyama H, Hoshino Y, Fukumura H, Nakakaji R, Sato I, Ohtake M, Akimoto T, Narikawa M, Tanaka R, Fujita T, Yokoyama U, Taguri M, Okumura S, Sato M, Eguchi H, Ishikawa Y. The iron chelating agent, deferoxamine detoxifies Fe (Salen)-induced cytotoxicity. J Pharmacol Sci. 2017;134:203–10.

14

Gender differences in career development awards in United States' anesthesiology and surgery departments, 2006–2016

Lena M. Mayes[1], Cynthia A. Wong[2], Shanta Zimmer[3], Ana Fernandez-Bustamante[1] and Karsten Bartels[1*]

Abstract

Background: Although the status of women in anesthesiology has advanced by many measures, obtaining career development funding remains challenging. Here, we sought to compare the characteristics of funded career development awards from the National Institutes of Health (NIH) between the specialties of anesthesiology and surgery. We hypothesized that the two groups differ in percentage of faculty with awards, gender distribution among principal investigators, as well as the number of awards promoting diversity.

Methods: The NIH grant-funding database RePORT was queried for career development awards for the years 2006–2016 using the filters "Anesthesiology" and "Surgery." Grants were characterized based on the gender of the principal investigator and whether the funding opportunity announcement indicated promotion of underrepresented minorities (URM). The 2016 Association of American Medical Colleges (AAMC) report on "Distribution of U.S. Medical School Faculty by Sex and Rank" was used to adjust comparisons according to baseline gender distributions in anesthesiology and surgery departments. Cohorts were characterized using descriptive methods and compared using Chi-square or Fisher's exact test.

Results: Based on our AAMC data query, in 2016, the number of women faculty members at the instructor or assistant professor level in U.S. medical schools was 2314 (41%) for anesthesiology and 2281 (30%) for surgery. Between 2006 and 2016, there were 88 career development grants awarded to investigators in anesthesiology departments compared to 261 in surgery departments. Of the grantees in each specialty, 29 (33%) were women in anesthesiology and 72 (28%) in surgery ($P = 0.344$). Awards to promote URM were identified for two grants (2%) in anesthesiology and nine grants (3%) in surgery ($P = 0.737$). Faculty members in surgery were more likely to receive an award than in anesthesiology ($P < 0.0001$), and women were less likely to receive an award than men ($P = 0.026$).

Conclusions: The major difference between US anesthesiology and surgery departments is that the number of faculty career development awards is significantly higher in surgery departments. Future efforts should aim to identify the reasons for such differences in order to inform strategies that can improve the likelihood for junior faculty members to receive career development funding.

Keywords: Grants, Funding, Career development, Gender, Diversity, Anesthesiology, Surgery

* Correspondence: karsten.bartels@ucdenver.edu
[1]Department of Anesthesiology, University of Colorado School of Medicine, 12401 E. 17th Avenue Leprino Office Building, 7th Floor, MS B-113, Aurora, CO 80045, USA
Full list of author information is available at the end of the article

Background

Research performance in anesthesiology compared with other medical specialties has historically been low [1]. Accordingly, leaders in the field have called for improvement in academic development opportunities for trainees and junior faculty members [2, 3]. Indeed, professional societies such as the Foundation for Anesthesia Education and Research (FAER), the International Anesthesia Research Society (IARS), and the Anesthesia Patient Safety Foundation (APSF) have committed substantial resources to provide research funding to young investigators in the specialty of anesthesiology [4–6].

In his 2015 *Rovenstine Lecture "Without Science There Is Little Art in Anesthesiology"* at the American Society of Anesthesiologists' annual meeting, Eisenach highlighted the ongoing critical importance of supporting young investigators in anesthesiology [7]. Such support may be especially important to early career women faculty members [8]. Historically, women have lagged behind men in career advancement. A 2008 assessment of the status of women in the field of academic anesthesiology in the United States highlighted the increased participation of women in many aspects of academic anesthesiology in the previous two decades [9]. Yet, the proportion of competitive research grants awarded to women had not changed. The reasons for this lack of improvement were not clear.

Consistent with work by others [10], and to permit an evaluation of another medical specialty represented at the same institutions as anesthesiology departments, we chose to compare National Institutes of Health (NIH) career development awards in anesthesiology departments to such awards in surgery departments from 2006 through 2016. We hypothesized that the two groups differ in terms of overall number of awards as well as gender distribution among principal investigators.

Methods

The Colorado Multi-Institutional Review Board approved this study for exemption (protocol # 17–0304). There was no requirement for informed consent.

The NIH grant-funding database, NIH RePORT [11] was queried for the following career development grant categories: K01 (Mentored Research Scientist Development Award), K08 (Mentored Clinical Scientist Research Career Development Award), and K23 (Mentored Patient-Oriented Research Career Development Award). K08 and K23 awards require a clinical doctoral degree; this is not required for K01-type awards that can be pursued with a research doctoral degree. Given the hybrid nature of K99/R00 "Pathway to Independence Awards" that includes mentored and independent components, we did not include this grant category in our analysis. All awards with an active listing for the years 2006 through 2016 were included using the NIH RePORT filter for department, choosing the identifiers "Anesthesiology" and "Surgery." Only grants with a specified department affiliation "Anesthesiology" or "Surgery" were included in this study. We determined the gender of the principal investigator by the first name and, if required, from faculty listings from departmental websites as described by others [12]. NIH funding opportunity announcements were examined to determine if they were targeted for promotion of underrepresented minorities (URM).

To adjust for the total number of faculty members in academic anesthesiology and surgery departments, respectively, data from the 2016 Association of American Medical Colleges (AAMC) report on "Distribution of U.S. Medical School Faculty by Sex and Rank" [13] were used. Participating U.S. medical schools provide information to the AAMC online or through batch uploads. Faculty members at the instructor and assistant professor ranks were assumed eligible for career development funding. Within-specialty funding rates between women and men were calculated by using the number of 2016 faculty members at the combined assistant professor and instructor level in academic anesthesiology and surgery departments.

Statistical analysis

Funding rates and principal investigator characteristics were analyzed using descriptive statistics, including percentages and ratios. Comparisons were made by department between type of award (K01, K08, K23), gender of principal investigator (PI), and funding opportunity announcements for promotion of URM. Using the AAMC data to determine the number of eligible faculty, funding rates were compared between gender of the PI by department. Comparisons were made using the Fisher's exact test or Chi-square test as appropriate. A P value $<$ 0.05 was considered significant. SPSS, Version 24 (IBM Corporation, Armonk, New York) was used for statistical analysis. Prism 6.0 was used for generation of graphical displays of data (GraphPad Software, Inc., La Jolla, CA).

Results

In the time period between 2006 and 2016, we identified 88 career development grants awarded to investigators in anesthesiology departments compared to 261 in surgery departments. One hundred one grants were awarded to women and 248 grants were awarded to men. The distribution of NIH institutes awarding grants according to specialty is depicted in Table 1.

Of the identified career development awards, K08 awards were most common in both specialties. The distribution of awards differed globally by specialty ($P = 0.0001$) (Fig. 1).

Table 1 Career development grants in anesthesiology and surgery departments by funding institute/agency

Institute/Agency	Anesthesiology	Surgery	Total
NHLBI	13	64	77
NIGMS	30	36	66
NIDDK	5	49	54
NCI	1	45	46
AHRQ	4	12	16
NIA	6	8	14
NINDS	10	4	14
NICHD	4	7	11
Other	15	36	51
All	88	261	349

AHRQ Agency for Healthcare Research and Quality, *NCI* National Cancer Institute, *NHLBI* National Heart, Lung, and Blood Institute, *NIA* National Institute on Aging, *NICHD* Eunice Kennedy Shriver National Institute of Child Health and Human Development, *NIDDK* National Institute of Diabetes and Digestive and Kidney Diseases, *NIGMS* National Institute of General Medical Sciences, *NINDS* National Institute of Neurological Disorders and Stroke

Of the grantees in the two specialties, 29 (33%) were women in anesthesiology and 72 (28%) in surgery (anesthesiology vs. surgery, $P = 0.344$) (Fig. 2).

Awards to promote URM were identified for two grants (2%) in the anesthesiology cohort and nine grants (3%) in the surgery cohort ($P = 0.737$, Fisher's Exact test).

According to the 2016 AAMC report on "Distribution of U.S. Medical School Faculty by Sex and Rank," there were 2314 (41%) women and 3387 (59%) men at the combined instructor and assistant professor rank in academic anesthesiology departments. For academic surgery departments there were 2281 (30%) women and 5325 (70%) men [13]. Overall, faculty members in surgery were more likely to receive an award than in anesthesiology ($P < 0.0001$, Chi square test). Women were less likely to receive an award than men ($P = 0.026$, Chi square test). When award rates were compared between genders within the respective specialty, the differences in award rates were not significant (anesthesiology: $P = 0.156$, surgery: $P = 0.410$, Chi square test).

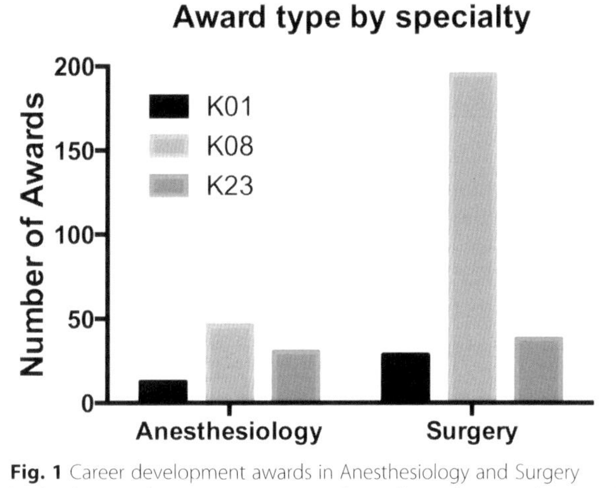

Fig. 1 Career development awards in Anesthesiology and Surgery by funding mechanism. Comparison of award type by specialty using Chi-square test ($P = 0.0001$)

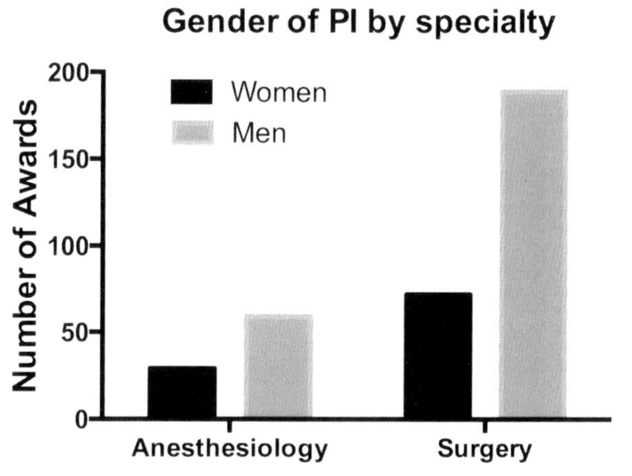

Fig. 2 Career development awards in Anesthesiology and Surgery by gender of principal investigator (PI). There was no difference in the proportion of women grantees between the two specialties. Comparison using Chi square test ($P = 0.344$)

Discussion

The gross number of grants awarded to early career surgery faculty members in the past decade was almost three-fold higher than to anesthesiology faculty members. These findings need to be placed in context of the total number of early career faculty members competing for such grants in the respective specialty. When using the 2016 numbers of faculty members in the assistant professor and instructor ranks as a surrogate for grant-eligible individuals, we found that surgery faculty members were more likely to be awarded funding than anesthesiology faculty members. Although early career women faculty members in both specialties were less likely to receive grant funding than men, this finding was of only marginal statistical significance. Four additional awards towards a women PI in either specialty would have resulted in a non-significant P-value when comparing grant award rates by gender. Finally, funded career development grants geared specifically to promote URM faculty members were extremely uncommon in both specialties.

The relationship between gender and grant support has been examined in other specialties, often showing disadvantageous funding environments for women [14]. In a retrospective analysis of NIH grants awarded to Unites States diagnostic radiology departments, women were found to have received only 15.9% of awards and 13.3% of funding [15]. In a study reporting on 2014 NIH grants to orthopedic surgery departments, 79.5% of grants were awarded to men [16]. Although such findings may not come as a complete surprise, the finding that NIH funding rates for women physician-scientists have recently been decreasing more sharply than for men is concerning [17]. In anesthesiology, early-career grant support from the FAER has been associated with significantly higher academic productivity and subsequent NIH funding [18].

Our study adds to previous reports. Surgery faculty members are more successful in achieving NIH career development funding compared to anesthesiology faculty members. This observation appears to be primarily driven by a higher number of K08 (Mentored Clinical Scientist Research Career Development Awards) awards that often cover basic science-oriented grants submitted by applicants who must hold a clinical doctoral degree. We can only speculate that high numbers of K08-type awards in surgery departments could be due to more favorable existing departmental research infrastructure but possibly also different interests of surgery versus anesthesiology faculty members engaged in research and even in part driven by lack of anesthesiology expertise on NIH study sections. It should be noted that significant protected time for research is a core component of many surgical residencies. In a survey of 18 surgical residency programs in New England, 61% of respondents planned or had already engaged in a research elective, with the majority of residents pursuing research for 2 years or more [19]. In another survey study the University of Washington surgical residency found that 27 of 33 (82%) graduates who performed 2–3 years of research during residency were successful in obtaining NIH funding if they applied for it [20]. Also, in a 2010 analysis of career choices of 1621 MD PhD program graduates, 50 (3.1%) had chosen anesthesiology, whereas 116 (7.2%) had chosen surgery, possibly indicating a higher propensity of MD PhD graduates to choose careers in surgery [21]. When assessing combined award rates for both anesthesiology and surgery, women faculty members are only marginally less likely to be awarded funding compared to men. This finding is important since K-type funding is a critical stepping-stone to independent NIH funding [22].

Observed funding success differences between women and men following career development awards indicate less favorable long-term funding outcomes for women [23]. Culley reported 30% of anesthesiology chair persons have a history of NIH funding, compared to 62% in surgery [10]. Hence, our finding that, regardless of gender, faculty members in anesthesiology departments are less likely to obtain career development funding compared to surgery may not come as a surprise. The reasons for this finding, however, remain uncertain. We can only speculate that junior faculty members in surgery departments are receiving better support and mentoring or that the observed differences are also based on diverse baseline characteristics of men and women choosing anesthesiology versus surgery as a career.

Our study has several limitations. First, we only included funding awarded through the NIH and the Agency for Healthcare Research and Quality and not from foundations such as the FAER or IARS. However, given that we wanted to include the comparison group of surgical career development grant funding, it was necessary to choose a funding agency to which both specialties have access. Second, we could only determine gender through the principal investigator's first name and, if required, by searching on departmental faculty webpages. While self-identified gender determination would be preferable, our approach is consistent with published approaches for gender determination in database research [12]. We did not recognize other genders than men and women in our study. Third, while we assessed the grants for funding opportunity announcements geared to faculty members with URM background, we could not ascertain ethnicity and race for individual principal investigators. Given that the assessment for URM status included only the funding opportunity announcement (NIH career development awards to promote diversity), but not the characteristics of the principle investigators or applicants, our findings do not permit any conclusions on URM status of grant applicants or awardees. Fourth, the denominator used for the gender-specific funding rates was based on AAMC data for the year 2016, not 2006–2016. This was done intentionally, as K-type career development grants usually span 3–5 years and our intent was to provide a relative, but not absolute, comparator to adjust for the difference in faculty members represented in each specialty [13]. In addition, the AAMC-based denominator does not account for the number of grant applications submitted relative to the number of grants awarded, which may differ between specialties.

Conclusions

Based on the 2016 AAMC number of eligible faculty members, faculty members in surgery were more likely to receive an award than faculty members in anesthesiology, but the funding rates for women and men in both departments were only marginally different. Future efforts should focus on identifying the reasons for such differences in award rates to inform initiatives to boost opportunities for junior faculty members to successfully compete for NIH career development funding.

Abbreviations

AAMC: Association of American Medical Colleges; APSF: Anesthesia Patient Safety Foundation; FAER: Foundation for Anesthesia Education and Research; IARS: International Anesthesia Research Society; NIH: National Institutes of Health; URM: Underrepresented minorities

Funding
This work was supported by an American Society of Anesthesiologists Mentoring Program grant from the Committee on Professional Diversity to Lena M. Mayes and by National Institutes of Health grant #K23DA040923 to Karsten Bartels. The aforementioned funding bodies had no role in the design of the study and collection, analysis, and interpretation of data, writing of the manuscript or the decision to submit it for publication.

Authors' contributions
LMM secured funding for the study, contributed to the study design, data collection, interpretation of the results, and manuscript preparation. CAW contributed to the interpretation of the results and manuscript preparation. AFB contributed to the interpretation of the results and manuscript preparation. SZ contributed to the interpretation of the results and manuscript preparation. KB secured funding for the study, contributed to the study design, data analysis, interpretation of the results, and manuscript preparation. All authors read and approved the final manuscript.

Competing interests
The authors declare that they have no competing interests.

Author details
[1]Department of Anesthesiology, University of Colorado School of Medicine, 12401 E. 17th Avenue Leprino Office Building, 7th Floor, MS B-113, Aurora, CO 80045, USA. [2]Department of Anesthesia, University of Iowa Carver College of Medicine, Iowa City, IA, USA. [3]Department of Medicine, University of Colorado School of Medicine, Aurora, CO, USA.

References
1. Reves JG. We are what we make: transforming research in anesthesiology: the 45th Rovenstine lecture. Anesthesiology. 2007;106(4):826–35.
2. Schwinn DA, Balser JR. Anesthesiology physician scientists in academic medicine: a wake-up call. Anesthesiology. 2006;104(1):170–8.
3. Knight PR, Warltier DC. Anesthesiology residency programs for physician scientists. Anesthesiology. 2006;104(1):1–4.
4. Ward DS, Hug CC Jr, Zaidan JR, Sessler AD. What is FAER? The Foundation for Anesthesia Education and Research. Anesthesiology. 2011;115(4):669–70.
5. Ramsay JG, Roizen M. SmartTots: a public-private partnership between the United States Food and Drug Administration (FDA) and the International Anesthesia Research Society (IARS). Paediatr Anaesth. 2012;22(10):969–72.
6. Eichhorn JH. The Anesthesia Patient Safety Foundation at 25: a pioneering success in safety, 25th anniversary provokes reflection, anticipation. Anesth Analg. 2012;114(4):791–800.
7. Eisenach JC. Without science there is little art in anesthesiology: 2015 Rovenstine lecture. Anesthesiology. 2016;124(6):1205–7.
8. Pashkova AA, Svider PF, Chang CY, et al. Gender disparity among US anaesthesiologists: are women underrepresented in academic ranks and scholarly productivity? Acta Anaesthesiol Scand. 2013;57(8):1058–64.
9. Wong CA, Stock MC. The status of women in academic anesthesiology: a progress report. Anesth Analg. 2008;107(1):178–84.
10. Culley DJ, Crosby G, Xie Z, et al. Career National Institutes of Health funding and scholarship of chairpersons of academic departments of anesthesiology and surgery. Anesthesiology. 2007;106(4):836–42.
11. National Institutes of Health Research Portfolio Online Reporting Tools (RePORT). Availavle at: https://projectreporter.nih.gov/reporter.cfm. Last accessed on 1 June 2017.
12. Eloy JA, Svider PF, Kovalerchik O, et al. Gender differences in successful NIH grant funding in otolaryngology. Otolaryngol Head Neck Surg. 2013;149(1):77–83.
13. Association of American Medical Colleges. 2016 Distribution of U.S. Medical School Faculty by Sex and Rank. Available at: https:// http://www.aamc.org/download/475530/data/16table13.pdf. Last accessed on 15 July 2017.
14. Silvestre J, Agarwal D, Lee DI. Analysis of National Institutes of Health funding to departments of urology. Urology. 2016;91:6–11.
15. Franceschi AM, Rosenkrantz AB. Patterns of recent National Institutes of Health (NIH) funding to diagnostic radiology departments: analysis using the NIH RePORTER system. Acad Radiol. 2017;24(9):1162–8.
16. Silvestre J, Ahn J, Levin LS. National Institutes of Health Funding to Departments of Orthopaedic Surgery at U.S. Medical Schools. J Bone Joint Surg Am. 2017;99(2):e5.
17. Cheng MY, Sukhov A, Sultani H, Kim K, Maverakis E. Trends in National Institutes of Health funding of principal investigators in dermatology research by academic degree and sex. JAMA Dermatol. 2016;152(8):883–8.
18. Pagel PS, Hudetz JA. Scholarly productivity and national institutes of health funding of foundation for anesthesia education and research grant recipients: insights from a bibliometric analysis. Anesthesiology. 2015;123(3):683–91.
19. Stewart RD, Doyle J, Lollis SS, Stone MD. Surgical resident research in New England. Arch Surg. 2000;135(4):439–44.
20. Robertson CM, Klingensmith ME, Coopersmith CM. Long-term outcomes of performing a postdoctoral research fellowship during general surgery residency. Ann Surg. 2007;245(4):516–23.
21. Brass LF, Akabas MH, Burnley LD, et al. Are MD-PhD programs meeting their goals? An analysis of career choices made by graduates of 24 MD-PhD programs. Acad Med. 2010;85(4):692–701.
22. Yin HL, Gabrilove J, Jackson R, et al. Sustaining the clinical and translational research workforce: training and empowering the next generation of investigators. Acad Med. 2015;90(7):861–5.
23. Jagsi R, Griffith KA, Jones RD, Stewart A, Ubel PA. Factors associated with success of clinician-researchers receiving career development awards from the National Institutes of Health: a longitudinal cohort study. Acad Med. 2017;92(10):1429–39.

The ultrasound-guided selective nerve block in the upper arm: an approach of retaining the motor function in elbow

Weijuan Zhu[1†], Riyong Zhou[1†], Lulu Chen[1], Yuanqing Chen[1], Lvdan Huang[1], Yun Xia[2], Thomas J. Papadimos[3] and Xuzhong Xu[1*]

Abstract

Background: Proximal brachial plexus blocks can lead to an extended period of motor paralysis and delay the return of motor function. This could influence patient satisfaction, and extend hospitalizations. The aim of the study is to compare a selective distal nerve block of the arm to a proximal axillary block, both ultrasound-guided, in terms of their motor block intensity of the elbow. Our hypothesis is that a selective nerve block of the arm would result in a different motor block of the elbow, compared to the axillary block.

Methods: A sample size of 24 patients who were undergoing elective surgery (ASA I-III) of the wrist, hand or forearm was randomly divided into two groups: Arm Group ($n = 12$) and Axillary Group ($n = 12$). The Arm Group received ultrasound-guided block of the median, ulnar, and medial antebrachial cutaneous nerves at the level of upper-median 1/3 of the arm, and a block of the radial and musculocutaneous nerves at the level of low-median 1/3 of the arm, while the Axillary Group received ultrasound-guided axillary brachial plexus blocks. Both blocks used in combination with general anesthesia.

Results: Our results demonstrated that the incidence of motor block at the elbow in the Arm Group was lower than in the Axillary Group. Compared with the Axillary Group, the duration of motor block at the elbow and the onset time of sensory block in the Arm Group were shortened. The patient satisfaction was increased in the Arm Group. There were no differences in the duration of the sensory block, the effect on postoperative analgesia, or in the duration of the motor block at the shoulder between both groups.

Conclusion: Our study showed that ultrasound-guided selective nerve block in the upper arm allowed improved retention of motor function at the elbow compared to axillary block. Secondarily, the ultrasound-guided selective nerve block seemed to provide similar analgesia after surgery of the hand or forearm with an enhanced patient satisfaction.

Trial registration: Chinese Clinical Trial Registry, ChiCTR-IOR-16008769.

Keywords: Ultrasonography, Nerve block, Upper extremity, Motor activity

* Correspondence: xuzhong@263.net
†Weijuan Zhu and Riyong Zhou are co-first authors.
[1]Department of Anesthesiology, The First Affiliated Hospital of Wenzhou Medical College, 2 Fuxue Road, Wenzhou City, Zhejiang Province 325000, China
Full list of author information is available at the end of the article

Background

Most hand and wrist surgeries can be performed under ultrasound guided regional anesthesia. Interscalene, supraclavicular, axillary and infraclavicular approaches to brachial plexus blockade provide effective anesthesia for surgical procedures [1]. However, proximal brachial plexus blocks may lead to a prolonged period of motor paralysis, i.e. "dead arm." Liebmann et al. [2] recommend that practitioners must be aware that the early return of motor function influences patient satisfaction. Chung importantly indicated that patients who recover rapidly after surgery had shortened hospitalizations and lower total costs [3]. Nonetheless there has been no technique reported thus far that provides both effective analgesia and motor function at the elbow and shoulder during upper limb surgery below the elbow.

We hypothesize that ultrasound-guided block of the median, ulnar, and medial antebrachial cutaneous nerves at the level of upper-median 1/3 of the arm, and a block of the radial and musculocutaneous nerves at the level of low-median 1/3 of the arm could improve the motor function at the elbow. We designed an approach to compare the ultrasound-guided selective nerve block of the upper arm combined general anesthesia with the axillary brachial plexus block combined general anesthesia. Our primary outcome measure was the motor function and the duration of motor blockade of the elbow and shoulder after regional anesthetic blockade. The secondary outcome measures were the anesthetic effect of the block, the onset times, the duration of the sensory blockade, the effect of postoperative analgesia, and patient satisfaction.

Methods

The Ethics Committee at the First Affiliated Hospital of Wenzhou Medical University approved this prospective trial, and the trial was registered at the Chinese Clinical Trial Registry (ChiCTR-IOR-16008769, 2016). Written informed consent was obtained from the participants.

Participants

We recruited 24 patients who were 18 years or older, ASA I to III, and scheduled for elective hand, wrist, and forearm surgery. Exclusion criteria were as follows: local anesthetic allergies, chronic pain, coagulopathy, infection at the planned injection site, peripheral neurologic disease, and inability to comprehend study-related procedures.

Procedure

The 24 patients were randomly divided into two groups: Arm Group and Axillary Group. Ultrasound-guided selective nerve block of the upper arm combined with general anesthesia were used in the Arm Group, while ultrasound-guided axillary brachial plexus block combined general anesthesia were used in the Axillary Group. On arrival in the preoperative room, all patients received standard monitoring, including noninvasive blood pressure, electrocardiogram, and pulse oximetry. A 20-gauge intravenous (IV) catheter was secured in the opposite forearm and midazolam 1 mg and fentanyl 20 μg were administered IV before nerve blockade unless contraindicated.An attending anesthesiologist with > 5 years experience and a case load of at least 200 blocks/year performed all blocks in the preoperative room using an ultrasound machine (SonoSite X-Porte, SonoSite, Bothell, WA, USA) with a linear 38 mm, 15–6 MHz probe, and 5-cm insulated block needles were used to guide a 25 ml injection of ropivacaine 0.375%. Another anesthesiologist recorded the data.

Arm group

Ultrasound-guided selective nerve block in the upper arm combined to general anesthesia was used in the Arm Group. The median, ulnar and medial antebrachial cutaneous were blocked at the upper-median 1/3 of the arm; the radial nerve and the musculocutaneous nerve were blocked at the low-median 1/3 of the arm. The distance from the upper end of the humeral head to the end of olecranon was divided into three equal parts, each defined as one-third of the upper arm.

Upper-median 1/3 approach

The patients were placed in the supine position with one arm in abduction (90°) and externally rotated with the corresponding forearm flexed (90°) (Fig. 1e). A 15–6 MHz high-frequency linear array transducer was placed at the junction of the proximal and the middle third of the arm, perpendicular to the brachial artery. The median was between 12 and 1 o'clock in relation to the humeral artery. The ulnar and medial antebrachial cutaneous nerves were situated at the 3 o'clock position of the basilic vein (Fig. 1g). An 18-gauge, 5-cm needle was advanced along the long axis of the probe from a lateral to medial direction until its tip was positioned at the nerve. After gentle aspiration, 5 ml of ropivacaine 0.375% was injected around each nerve.

Low-median 1/3 approach

The arm was then abducted (Fig. 1a). The ultrasound probe was placed at the junction of the distal and the middle third of the arm. The radial nerve was identified as round with a hyperechoic structure and was located between brachialis and humerus laterally. The musculocutaneous nerve was identified as fusiform with a hyperechoic structure and was located between biceps and brachialis close medially (Fig. 1c). The needle was advanced from a lateral to medial direction using an

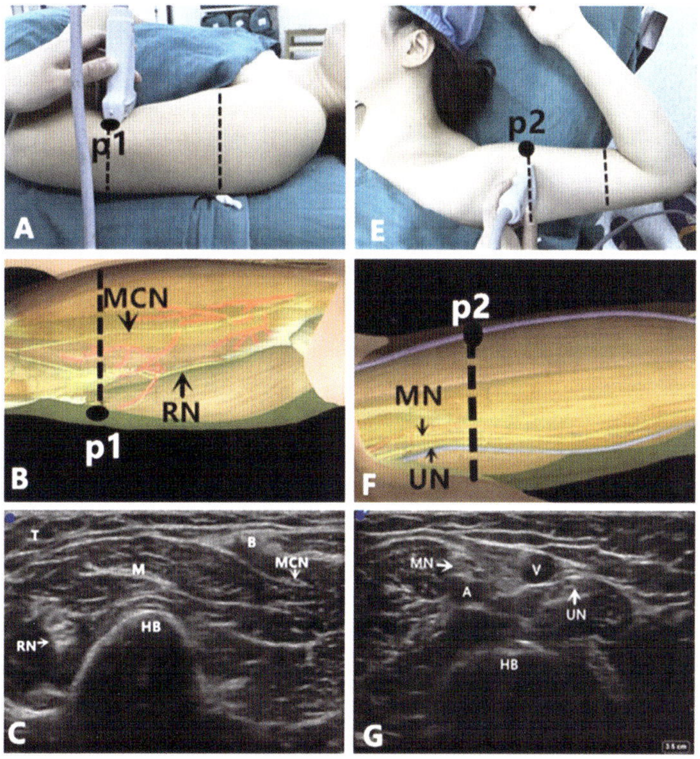

Fig. 1 Position of patient, neuroanatomy and ultrasound imaging at the level of upper-median 1/3 and low-median 1/3 of the arm in the operating room. **a** Position of the patient, the probe, and the needle ("p1") during block of the radial and musculocutaneous nerve. **b** Topography of the radial nerve (RN) and the musculocutaneous nerve (MCN); red = muscular branches; and the black point "p1"denotes the puncture site. The dotted line denotes the probe position. **c** Ultrasound depiction of the radial nerve (RN) and the musculocutaneous nerve (MCN). The blue point is situated at the lateral side of the probe. The RN is round with a hyperechoic structure and is located between brachialis and humerus laterally. The MCN is fusiform with a hyperechoic structure, and is located between biceps and brachialis close medially. Also note the humerus (HB), and the triceps (T), biceps (B), and brachialis (M) muscles. **e** Position of the patient, the probe, and the needle ("p2") during block of the median, ulnar, and medial antebrachial cutaneous nerves. **f** Topography of the median nerve (MN), the ulnar nerve (UN). The black point "p2"denotes the puncture site. The dotted line denotes the probe position. **g** Ultrasound description of the median nerve (MN) and the ulnar nerve (UN). The blue point is situated at the cephalic side of the probe. The MN is between 12 and 1 o'clock in relation to the humeral artery. The UN is situated at the 3 o'clock position of the basilic vein, brachial artery (A), basilic vein (V), and humerus (HB)

in-plane technique until its tip was positioned at the radial nerve. After negative aspiration, 5 ml of ropivacaine 0.375% was injected around the radial nerve. The needle was then redirected toward the musculocutaneous nerve. After negative aspiration, 5 ml of ropivacaine 0.375% was injected around the musculocutaneous nerve. The radial and musculocutaneous nerves floated superiorly after local anesthetic spread and this assisted with identification.

Axillary group

Ultrasound-guided axillary brachial plexus block combined general anesthesia was used in the Axillary Group.

The arm is abducted to 90 degrees and the elbow flexed to 90 degrees (Fig. 2a). The ultrasound probe was placed at the lateral border of pectoralis major muscle. The pulsating axillary artery was visualized, and the probe was maneuvered to locate the individual nerves around the artery (Fig. 2b). After negative aspiration, 5 ml of ropivacaine 0.375% was injected around the median, ulnar, medial antebrachial cutaneous, radial, and musculocutaneous nerves, respectively.

Both blocks were considered successful if after 30 min there was loss of pinprick discrimination. After positioning the patient (Arm Group and Axillary Group) on the surgical table, general anesthesia was induced using propofol and fentanyl and maintained with isoflurane (to maintain a MAC between 0.8 and 1) and nitrous oxide 60% in oxygen via a laryngeal mask.

For postoperative analgesia celecoxib 200 mg po bid was administered for three days postoperatively. If VAS was > 3, Tramadol 100 mg po was administered. If thereafter the VAS was still > 3 intravenous morphine was to be administered.

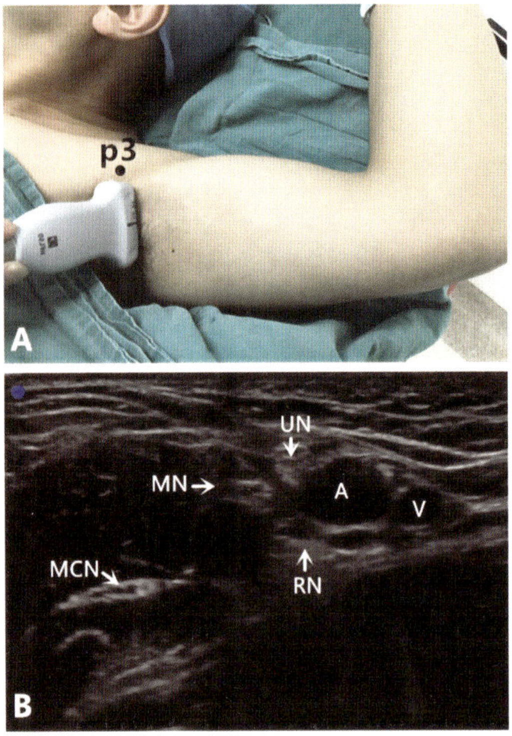

Fig. 2 Position of patient and ultrasound imaging in the operating room when performing the axillary block. **a** Position of the patient, the probe, and the needle ("p3") during the axillary block. **b** Ultrasound depiction of the axillary. Radial nerve (RN), musculocutaneous nerve (MCN), median nerve (MN), ulnar nerve (UN), axillary artery (A) and axillary vein (V) The blue point is situated at the lateral side of the probe

Primary measure

The primary measure of our study was the motor function and the duration of motor blockade of the elbow and shoulder. The duration of motor blockade was defined as time in minutes from the end of local anesthetic administration to the return of normal (or baseline) motor strength in the blocked extremity. Motor block was assessed for flexion and extension of the elbow, adduction and abduction of the shoulder using the following scale: 0 points for no paresis, 1 point for paresis, and 2 points for complete paralysis [4].

Secondary measures

The secondary measures of our study were the onset and the duration of sensory blockade, patients' satisfaction, and the postoperative analgesia. Sensory block onset times were recorded every 2 min from the end of local anesthetic administration, and were evaluated by a pinprick test [4] (using epidural plastic needle). The duration of the sensory blockade was defined as time in minutes from the end of local anesthetic administration until return of pinprick sensation or to the first report of postoperative pain at the surgical site, whichever occurred sooner. The block was identified as successful when VAS = 0 [5].

The effectiveness of postoperative analgesia was determined by the number of patients who still had a VAS > 3 after treatment with Celecoxib and Tramadol. Patients' satisfaction scores were recorded (not satisfied at all [0] to completely satisfied [10]) [6].

Statistical analysis

Our hypothesis is that the incidence of motor blockade with the selective distal arm block will be different from the axillary block. The sample size required for the study was calculated based on a preliminary evaluation using Power Sample Size (PASS 11) software performed in our hospital, where three patients in the Arm Group could flex and extend the elbow while one patient could not; and in the Axillary Group four patients could not flex nor extend the elbow. Thus, a calculated sample size of 6 patients per group was required to provide a statistical power of 0.90 and a type-I error of 0.05 using one-way analysis of variance. We assigned 12 patients to each group to allow for possible dropouts.

The SPSS Statistics for Windows (Version 15; IBM, Armonk, NY) was used to perform the analysis. The normality of data distribution was determined by the Shapiro-Wilk test. The non-normally distributed data (Sensory block onset, Duration time of sensory block, Duration time of motor block in elbow and shoulder, Patients' satisfaction: see Additional file 1) are presented as a median (Q1, Q3) and analyzed with the Mann-Whitney U test. Motor block scale of elbow in Arm Group and Axillary Group are analyzed with the Chi-square test. Statistical significance was considered as $p < 0.05$.

Results

The incidence of motor block of elbow in the Arm Group was lower than in Axillary Group [1/12vs12/12, ($P < 0.001$)] (Table 1). And compared with the Axillary Group, the duration of motor blockade in elbows of the Arm Group was shortened [0(0,0) vs. 600(495,765), $P <$ 0.001]. The onset time of sensory block [Musculocutaneous nerves: 6(4.5,6) vs. 10(10,12), $P < 0.001$; Radial nerve:8(6,8) vs.10(8.5,11.5), $p = 0.002$; Ulnar nerve:

Table 1 Motor block scale of elbow in arm group and axillary group

	0	1	2
Arm group	11	1	0
Axillary group	0	0	12

$P < 0.001$**, 0 points for no paresis, 1 point for paresis, and 2 points for complete paralysis. $n = 12$

10(8,10) vs. 11(10,12), $P = 0.007$; Medial antebrachial cutaneous nerves: 10(8,10) vs. 10(10,10), $P = 0.008$; Median nerve: 10(10,10) vs. 12(10,13.5), $P = 0.032$] in the Arm Group were shortened, while the patients' satisfaction in the Arm Group was increased [10(10,10) vs. 8(7.25,8), $P < 0.001$]. No patients with VAS > 3 were recorded in the postoperative period. There were no differences in the duration of sensory block [540(540,585) vs. 600(540,735), $P = 0.157$] and the duration of motor block of the shoulder [0(0,0) vs. 0(0,0), $P = 1$] between both groups (Table 2).

Discussion

Our study showed that the selective distal ultrasound-guided block of the arm with a volume of 25 ml of ropivacaine preserves the motor function of the elbow, compared with an axillary ultrasound block by the same anesthetic agent. Compared with the Axillary Group, the duration of motor block in elbow and the onset time of sensory block in the Arm Group were shortened, while the patients' satisfaction in the Arm Group was increased.

The ultrasound-guided selective nerve block in the upper arm assists in the retention of the motor function at the elbow whereas the proximal brachial plexus blocks do not. Proximal brachial plexus blocks as axillary may lead to a prolonged period of motor paralysis, i.e. "dead arm". Frizelle [7] reported that the humeral canal approach to the brachial plexus (using stimulation) can provide complete sensory and motor blockade with a 90% rate of success. Carles et al. [8] reported that brachial plexus blocks at the humeral canal, using a neurostimulator, confirm the reliability and safety of this technique. However, motor function at the elbow was still impaired. Guntz et al. [9] reported that ultrasound-guided block of the brachial plexus at the humeral canal could allow the patient to recover the flexion of the forearm while providing effective post-operative analgesia. However in our study, patients could retain flexion and extension of the elbow with effective post-operative analgesia. With the increasing of ambulatory surgery in recent years, selective nerve block in the upper arm is prefer to used, because of its cost saving and reduction of medical resource requirement [3]. Our technique provided for prompt patient recovery and increased patient satisfaction, and it proved to be a basis for early patient discharge.

The radial nerve gives off branches at the level of mid brachium or proximal portion of the upper arm and innervates the triceps brachii, anconeus (extension of elbow), and the partial brachioradialis (flexion of elbow) [10]. Furthermore, the musculocutaneous nerve gives off branches at the level of the middle upper arm and innervates coracobrachiali, biceps brachii and partial brachialis muscles (flexion of elbow) [10]. The medial cutaneous nerve of the forearm gives off branches near the mid brachium; these nerves are so small that ultrasound cannot distinguish them. If an operator blocks the median, ulnar, and medial antebrachial cutaneous nerves at the low-median 1/3 of the arm, the medial antebrachial cutaneous nerves cannot be thoroughly and effectively blocked. Therefore, blocking the median, the ulnar and medial antebrachial cutaneous nerves at the upper-median 1/3 of the arm, along with a second block of the radial and the musculocutaneous nerves at the level of low-median 1/3 of the arm, provides effective analgesia for upper limb surgery below elbow, but also improves retention of the motor function at the elbow and shoulder. In our study, one patient had weak elbow extension (motor block scale = 1). Here, it is possible that the radial never gave off the triceps brachii branch near the level of the junction between the distal and the middle third of the arm.

The blocks in the two groups provided a short onset of action. English [11] reported that one of the main

Table 2 Characteristics of arm group and axillary group ($n = 12$)

	Arm group	Axillary group	P value
Sensory block onset (min)			
Musculocutaneous nerves	6 (4.5,6)	10 (10,12)	$P < 0.001$**
Median nerve	10 (10,10)	12 (10,13.5)	$P = 0.032$*
Radial nerve	8 (6,8)	10 (8.5,11.5)	$P = 0.002$**
Ulnar nerve	10 (8,10)	11 (10,12)	$P = 0.007$**
Medial antebrachial cutaneous nerves	10 (8,10)	10 (10,10)	$P = 0.008$**
Duration time of sensory block (min)	540 (540,585)	600 (540,735)	$P = 0.157$
Duration time of motor block in elbow (min)	0 (0,0)	600 (495,765)	$P < 0.001$**
Duration time of motor block in shoulder (min)	0 (0,0)	0 (0,0)	$P = 1$
Patients' satisfaction	10 (10,10)	8 (7.25,8)	$P < 0.001$**
Types of surgeries(soft-tissue/fractures/internal fixator removal)	7/ 2/ 3	7/ 1/ 4	$P = 1$

*Represent $P < 0.05$, **Represent $P < 0.01$

theories advanced for failure of axillary blockade was the existence of septa within the sheath preventing the spread of agent. Moayeri [12] reported that neural architectural differences and the varying size of adipose tissue compartments around the brachial plexus play an important role in block success. In our study, we did not need to deal with the increased adipose tissue, septa and bundles when using ultrasonography. By blocking peripheral nerves at the level of low-median 1/3 and upper-median 1/3 of the arm, where they are relative thin, allowed easy infiltration of local anesthetics. Therefore, the onset time of the sensory block was shorter and consistent with the work of Guntz [9].

Soberón [13] reported that distal peripheral nerve blocks at forearm may only be applied to wrist and hand surgery. Our approach is applicable to all hand surgeries below the elbow, while distal peripheral nerve blocks are not as appropriate or convenient. Our approach is beneficial to the promotion of ambulatory hand surgery. This study has several limitations. More distal peripheral nerve blocks have been documented to better retain the motor function at the wrist [2], but our study did not demonstrate this. And this study needed two punctures to perform the selective block. The aim of our study was observing the motor function of the elbow, while patient satisfaction was a secondary outcome. Due to the diversity of surgical procedures there may be some element of confounding in our results when measuring duration of sensory blockade. Also, as general anesthesia was used for all cases, a control group that did not receive general anesthesia was not included.

Conclusion

In conclusion, this study showed that an ultrasound-guided block of the median, ulnar, and medial antebrachial cutaneous nerves at the level of upper-median 1/3 of the arm, and a block of the radial and musculocutaneous nerves at the level of low-median 1/3 of the arm, allowed improved retention of motor function at the elbow compared to axillary block. Secondarily, the ultrasound-guided selective nerve block seemed to provide similar analgesia after surgery of the hand or forearm with an enhanced patient satisfaction.

Abbreviations

ASA: American Society of Anesthesiologists; IV: Intravenous; MAC: Minimal alveolar concentration; MHz: Mega Hertz

Acknowledgements

We would like to thank Kejian Shi of The First Affiliated Hospital of Wenzhou Medical College for revising the manuscript.

Author contributions

WZ Contribution: Design the study, conduct the study, analyse the data, and write the manuscript. RZ Contribution: Design the study, conduct the study and write the manuscript. LC, YC, LH Contribution: Conduct the study and data collection. YX Contribution: Design the study and write the manuscript. TP Contribution: Write the manuscript and did the critical manuscript review, writing and preparation. XX Contribution: Design the study, analyze the data, and write the manuscript. All authors read and approved the final manuscript.

Funding

This work was supported by the item from Science & Technology Bureau (No. Y20170654) Wenzhou, Zhejiang, China.

Competing interests

The authors declare that they have no competing interests.

Author details

[1]Department of Anesthesiology, The First Affiliated Hospital of Wenzhou Medical College, 2 Fuxue Road, Wenzhou City, Zhejiang Province 325000, China. [2]Department of Anesthesiology, The Ohio State University Medical Center, Columbus, OH, USA. [3]Department of Anesthesiology, The University of Toledo College of Medicine and Life Sciences, Toledo, OH, Spain.

References

1. Neal JM, Gerancher JC, Hebl JR. Upper extremity regional anesthesia: essentials of our current understanding, 2008. Reg Anesth Pain Med. 2009;34(2):134–70.
2. Liebmann O, Price D, Mills C. Feasibility of forearm ultrasonography-guided nerve blocks of the radial, ulnar, and median nerves for hand procedures in the emergency department. Ann Emerg Med. 2006;48(5):558–62.
3. Chung F. Recovery pattern and home-readiness after ambulatory surgery. Anesth Analg. 1995;80(5):896–902.
4. Rodríguez J, Taboada-Muñiz M, Bárcena M. Median versus musculocutaneous nerve response with single-injection infraclavicular coracoid block. Reg Anesth Pain Med. 2004;29(6):534–8.
5. Bharti N, Bhardawaj N, Wig J. Comparison of ultrasound-guided supraclavicular, infraclavicular and below-C6 interscalene brachial plexus block for upper limb surgery: a randomised, observer-blinded study. Anaesth Intensive Care. 2015;43(4):468–72.
6. Fredrickson MJ, Wolstencroft PJ, Chinchanwala S. Does motor block related to long-acting brachial plexus block cause patient dissatisfaction after minor wrist and hand surgery? A randomized observer-blinded trial. Br J Anaesth. 2012;109(5):809–15.

7. Frizelle HP. Technical note: the humeral canal approach to the brachial plexus. Yale J Biol Med. 1998;71(6):585–9.
8. Carles M, Pulcini A, Macchi P. An evaluation of the brachial plexus block at the humeral canal using a neurostimulator (1417 patients): the efficacy, safety, and predictive criteria of failure. Anesth Analg. 2001;92(1):194–8.
9. Guntz E, Van den Broeck V, Dereeper E. Ultrasound-guided block of the brachial plexus at the humeral canal. Can J Anaesth. 2009;56(2):109–14.
10. Richard L, Drake A, Vogl W, Mitchell AWM. Gray's anatomy for students. 3th ed. Philadelphia: Churchill Livingstone; 2005. p. 717–62.
11. English MJ, Shutt LE. Axillary brachial plexus block: choice of technique. Br J Anaesth. 1990;64:224–31.
12. Moayeri N, Bigeleisen PE, Groen GJ. Quantitative architecture of the brachial plexus and surrounding compartments, and their possible significance for plexus blocks. Anesthesiology. 2008;108(2):299–304.
13. Soberón JR, Crookshank JW, Nossaman BD. Distal peripheral nerve blocks in the forearm as an alternative to proximal brachial plexus blockade in patients undergoing hand surgery: a prospective and randomized pilot study. J Hand Surg Am. 2016;41(10):969–77.

16

Efficacy of different doses of dexmedetomidine as a rapid bolus for children: a double-blind, prospective, randomized study

Fang Chen[1,2], Chengyu Wang[2], Yi Lu[2], Mengmeng Huang[2] and Zhijian Fu[1*]

Abstract

Background: Dexmedetomidine (DEX), a highly sensitive α_2-adrenoceptor agonist that possesses anxiolytic, sedative, and analgesic effects, has been documented as a preventative and treatment for emergence agitation (EA). The therapeutic should be given as a loading dose that is infused during a 10 min period, but if a rapid bolus injection is deemed to be hemodynamically appropriate, it would be a more opportune route of administration. So we studied the efficacy of different doses of DEX as a rapid bolus for children to prevent and treat EA.

Methods: One hundred patients were enrolled and randomly divided into five groups: the control group (group D_1), the 0.25 μg/kg DEX group (group D_2), the 0.5 μg/kg DEX group (group D_3), the 0.75 μg/kg DEX group (group D_4), and the 1 μg/kg DEX group (group D_5). Heart rate (HR), mean blood pressure (MBP) and blood oxygen saturation (SaO_2) were recorded immediately before the study drug injection (baseline) and every minute for 5 min thereafter and at the time points of the skin cut and hernial sac pull. EA and pain were assessed in the post -anesthesia care unit, and any complementary medicine and adverse events were recorded too.

Results: The incidence of EA was significantly decreased in group D_4 and group D_5 compared with D_1.All groups exhibited similar baseline HR and MBP. After administered, HR and MBP were significantly decreased in all DEX group compared with group D_1.In groups D_3, D_4 and D_5, the minimal HR was decreased significantly compared with the groups D_1 and duration time of minimal HR significantly prolonged in group D_5, but no patient needed treatment. As the dosage increased, the recovery time was significantly prolonged. There were no significant differences in occurrence time of minimal HR, the incidence of complementary medicine and adverse events among groups.

Conclusion: Rapid intravenous injection (IV) bolus administration of 0.75 and 1.0 μg/kg of DEX could improve the recovery profile by reducing the incidence of EA in children. Although its use resulted in a transient decreases in HR and MBP, DEX was clinically well-tolerated in children.

Keywords: Dexmedetomidine, Children, Rapid injection, Emergence agitation

* Correspondence: zhijian_fu@163.com
[1]Department of Pain Management, Shandong Provincial Hospital affiliated to Shandong University, 324 Jingwu Road, Jinan 250021, China
Full list of author information is available at the end of the article

Background

Dexmedetomidine (DEX), a highly selective α_2-adrenoreceptor agonist, offers anxiolytic, sedative, and analgesic effects with negligible respiratory depression [1–3].DEX has been approved for use in adults, but the US Food and Drug Administration has not approved the drug for children. However, DEX has been documented in pediatric patients as a premedication, a sedative in the pediatric intensive care unit, in conjunction with inhaled anesthetic agents, and as a therapeutic for the prevention and treatment of emergence agitation (EA) following general anesthesia [4–6]. EA, particularly in children, presents a great challenge to good patient care [7, 8]. While 2-, 5-, or 10-min DEX infusions lower the occurrence of EA in pediatric patients [9, 10], it is typically not convenient to administer a bolus infusion in the clinical area of an elevated-turnover work-intensive pediatric anesthesiology unit. A quickly administered bolus injection, if deemed to be hemodynamically appropriate, would be a more opportune route of administration to avert and treat EA. Jooste EH et al. [11] had observed that rapid IV bolus administration of DEX in 12 children who underwent heart

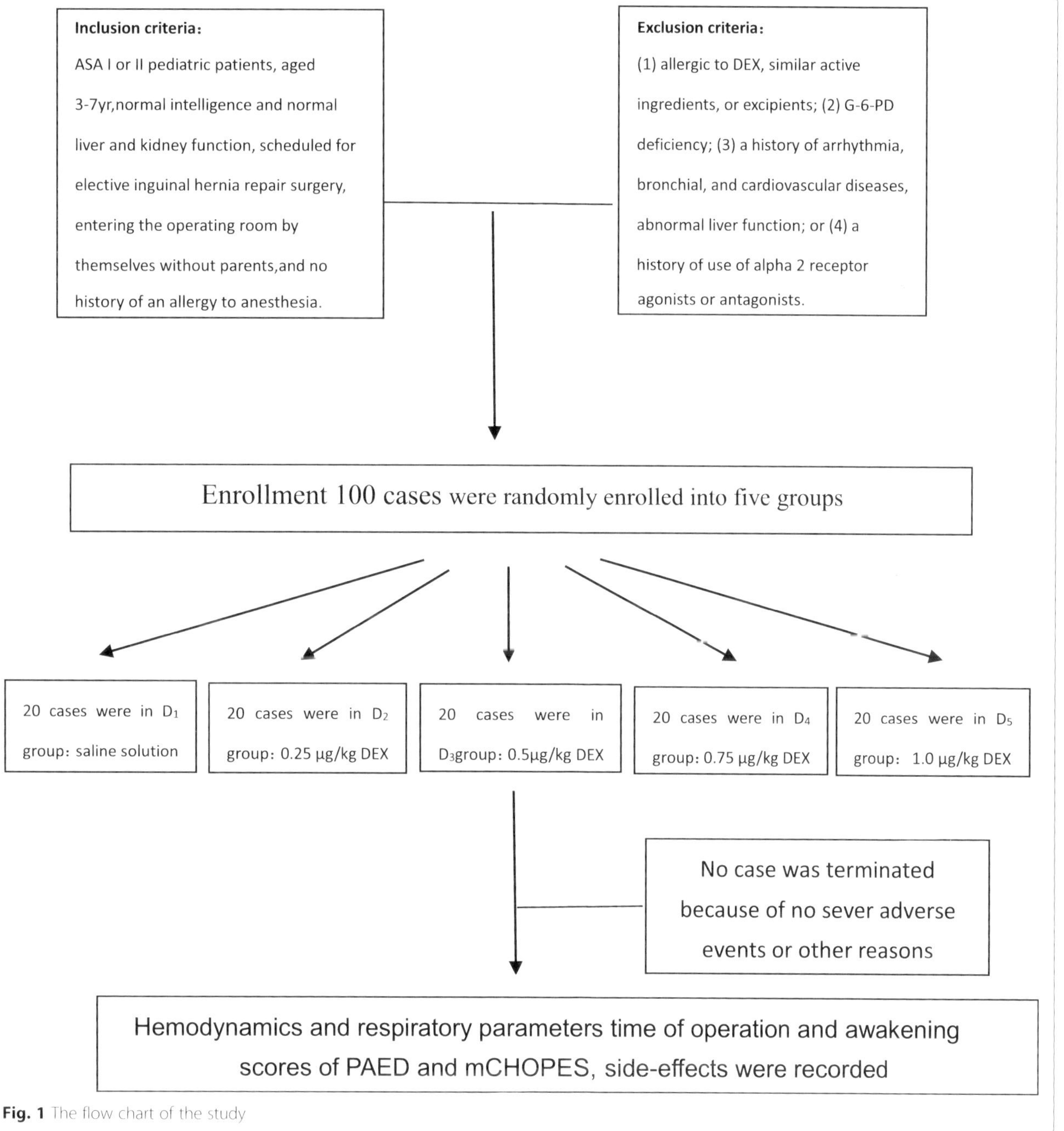

Fig. 1 The flow chart of the study

Table 1 Demographic and surgical characteristics of patients

Variable	Group D_1	Group D_2	Group D_3	Group D_4	Group D_5
Age, median (IQR), yr	4 (4–5)	5 (3–6)	4 (3.5–5)	4 (3–4.5)	4 (3–5)
Male/Female, No./No.	17/3	17/3	16/4	16/4	16/4
Weight, median (IQR), kg	17.0 (16.0–20.0)	18.3 ± 3.95	17.0 (15.0–17.75)	16.4 ± 3.28	18.5 ± 3.76
Duration of surgery, median (IQR), min	14.4 ± 5.95	11.5 (10.0–14.5)	12.0 (9.5–14.0)	11.0 (9.5–20.5)	11.5 (9.0–13.0)

There were no statistically significant differences ($P > 0.05$) among the groups

transplants was clinically well-tolerated, although its use resulted in a transient but significant increase in systemic and pulmonary blood pressure and a decrease in heart rate (HR). In addition, Hauber JA et al. [12] documented that fast IV bolus administration of 0.5 μg/kg DEX improved pediatric patients' recuperation profile by lowering the occurrence of EA. Although a statistically significant change in hemodynamics was observed, no patient required intervention for hemodynamic changes. However, the aforementioned studies used either a small sample study or only one dose. DEX is often used to avert and treat postoperative agitation in dosages of 0.25–1 μg/kg, and many clinical institutions now commonly administer DEX as a rapid (under 5 s) IV bolus. Therefore, our study examined the efficacy of different doses of DEX as a rapid bolus for prevention and treating EA in pediatric patients.

Methods

Design and setting

We conducted a double-blind randomized controlled trial in 100 patients in the 2nd Affiliated Hospital & Yuying Children's Hospital of WenZhou Medical University.

Patient selection

According to the preliminary experimental results, two groups with the smallest difference in the five groups were analyzed with a = 0.05, b = 0.2, and the difference between groups was 0.4.The calculated sample size was 16 cases per group. Considering the 20% sample exfoliate rate, we need 20 cases per group, a total of 100 cases sample size.

This clinical trial was registered at http://www.chictr.org.cn (No. ChiCTR-IPR-17010658), and conducted from April 2017 to October 2017. After obtaining informed written consent from parent of each child, 100 ASA I or II pediatric patients, aged 3–7 yr., were randomly (Random number method) enrolled into five groups: the control group (group D_1), the 0.25 μg/kg DEX group (group D_2), the 0.5 μg/kg DEX group (group D_3), the 0.75 μg/kg DEX group (group D_4), and the 1 μg/kg DEX group (group D_5). Inclusion criteria were: normal intelligence and normal liver and kidney function, scheduled for elective inguinal hernia repair surgery, entering the operating room by themselves without parents, and no history of an allergy to anesthesia.

Patients were excluded if they met any of the following criteria: (1) allergic to DEX, similar active ingredients, or excipients; (2) G-6-PD deficiency; (3) a history of arrhythmia, bronchial, and cardiovascular diseases, abnormal liver function; or (4) a history of use of alpha $_2$ receptor agonists or antagonists (Fig. 1).

Table 2 Incidence of Emergence Agitation (PAED > 12)

Groups	Number	Incidence (%)	P value*
Group D_1	6	30%	
Group D_2	1	5%	$P = 0.096$
Group D_3	1	5%	$P = 0.096$
Group D_4	0	0%	$P < 0.001$
Group D_5	0	0%	$P < 0.001$

*Compared with Group D_1

Medication

No premedication was administered. A peripheral venous catheter was inserted approximately 2 h prior to surgery (while in the unit). EMLA cream (lidocaine 2.5% and prilocaine 2.5%, Astra Zeneca Inc., Sweden) was used to ease venous cannulation. HR, noninvasive arterial blood pressure, blood oxygen saturation (SaO2), electrocardiogram (ECG), and bispectral index (BIS) were monitored. After preoxygenation via face mask, anesthesia was induced with propofol 2–3 mg/kg and inhalation of 6 vol% sevoflurane. After the pupils were fixed, the laryngeal mask airway (LMA) was inserted and the ilioinguinal/iliohypogastric nerve block was performed by ultrasound guidance to relieve postoperative pain. Anesthesia was maintained with 2-3 vol% sevoflurane to maintained BIS from 40 to 60 and retaining spontaneous respiration. After the vital signs were stable, study groups received a rapid bolus injection of different doses of DEX (Jiangsu singch pharmaceutical co., LTD) at a rate of less than 5 s, while patients in the control group received saline in an equal volume. When the surgery was completed, every one of the patients was moved to the post-anesthesia care unit (PACU), and the children naturally regained consciousness.

Data collection

HR, mean blood pressure (MBP), and SaO_2 were recorded immediately before the study drug injection

Table 3 Heart Rate Changes

Groups	Baseline	1 min	2 min	3 min	4 min	5 min	Skin cut	Hernial sac pull
Group D_1 median (IQR)	97.0$^{\triangle}$ (91.0–103.5)	97.5$^{\#\triangle}$ (94.0–103.0)	99.0$^{\triangle}$ (94.0–104.5)	99.0$^{\triangle}$ (93.5–106.5)	99.0$^{\triangle}$ (95.0–107.5)	100.5$^{\triangle}$ (94.5–108.5)	104.5$^{\triangle}$ (95.0–111.0)	112.0$^{\#*}$ (104.0–118.0)
Group D_2 median (IQR)	101.5 (86.5–115.0)	91.0$^{\triangle*}$ (81.5–102.5)	95.0$^{\triangle}$(85.0–106.0)	94.5$^{\triangle}$(85.5–107.0)	98.0$^{\triangle}$(85.0–108.5)	97.5$^{\triangle}$(86.5–108.5)	100.5$^{\triangle}$(90.0–112.5)	103.5$^{\#*}$ (94.5–130.0)
Group D_3 median (IQR)	104.5(91.5–109.0)	88.5$^{*\triangle}$ (79.5–97.0)	93.0$^{*\triangle}$ (85.5–99.0)	95.0$^{*\triangle}$ (85.0–101.0)	97.0$^{*\triangle}$ (86.0–103.5)	97.5$^{\triangle}$ (89.0–105.0)	100.0 (95.0–108.5)	104.5 (93.5–112.5)
Group D_4 mean ± SD	104.0 ± 10.4	89.7 ± 10.2$^{*\triangle}$	93.6 ± 9.4$^{*\triangle}$	96.6± 7.6*	97.5 ± 7.5*	97.4 ± 7.5*	97.1 ± 9.6	102.0 ± 8.7
Group D_5 median (IQR)	99.0 (93.5–102.0)	84.0$^{*\triangle}$ (79.5–90.5)	88.0* (86.0–95.5)	89.0* (87.5–96.5)	90.0* (86.5–97.0)	89.0* (86.0–96.0)	88.5 (84.0–97.0)	95.5 (89.0–99.5)

*Compared with baseline, $^{\triangle}$compared with the time point of the hernial sac pull, $^{\#}$ Compared with group D_5, $P < 0.05$

(baseline), every minute for 5 min thereafter, and at the time points of the skin cut and hernial sac pull. EA was assessed by the study staff upon arrival in the PACU using the Pediatric Anesthesia Emergence Delirium (PAED) scale (0–20 scale), with a score of > 12 considered to be a diagnosis of EA [12]. Propofol 1 mg/kg was administered via IV for EA if the patient was determined to be pain-free and when the parent or caregiver was unable to comfort the child. Pain was evaluated using the Modified Children's Hospital of Eastern Ontario Pain Scale (m-CHOPES), and intravenous fentanyl 0.5 µg/kg was administered if the score was≥7. The time of operation and awakening, and any side effects, such as respiratory and cardiovascular depression were recorded. Any supplementary postoperative drugs were also recorded. Finally, patients with an Alderete score ≥ 9 were sent back to the ward.

Statistical analysis

All of the data are presented as mean ± standard deviation (SD), median (interquartile range), or number (%), as appropriate. The measurement data was analyzed by Shapiro-Wilk. The normal distribution data which satisfied the homogeneity test of variance was tested by ANOVA, if not, by Kruskal-Wallis. The abnormal distribution data was analyzed by Kruskal-Wallis to compare among groups. Pearson's chi-squared test was used to assess the comparison among groups in count data. The repeated measurement data (MAP and HR) was analyzed by two-way ANOVA, and the comparisons of intra-group and among groups were analyzed by bonferroni. Data were analyzed using SPSS software (SPSS 16.0, SPSS, Inc., Chicago, IL, USA). A p value of less than 0.05 was considered to be a significant difference.

Results

There were 100 pediatric patients who were enrolled and randomly divided into five groups. As seen in Table 1, there were no significant demographic and surgical characteristic differences among the groups.

The incidence of EA was significantly lower in groups D_4 and D_5, and a trend of fewer was observed in group D_2 and D_3 (Table 2).

There were no significant differences in the basal HR among the five groups. In group D_1, there were no significant differences among the basal HR and every minute for 5 min thereafter, but the HR at the point of the hernial sac pull was increased significantly compared with the baseline. In group D_2, the HR was decreased at 1 min compared with the baseline, and then returned to the baseline at 2, 3, 4 and 5 min, and the points of skin cut, but the HR at the point of the hernial sac pull was increased significantly compared with the baseline. In group D_3, the HR was decreased at 1, 2,3 and 4 min compared with the baseline, and the HR returned to the baseline at 5 min, the points of skin cut and hernial sac pull. In groups D_4 and D_5, the HR was decreased at 1, 2, 3, 4 and 5 min compared with the baseline, and the HR returned to the baseline at the time point of the skin cut and hernial sac pull (Table 3).

The minimal HR of groups D_3, D_4, and D_5 were decreased significantly compared with groups D_1. And the duration time of minimal HR was significantly prolonged in group D_5 compared with group D_1. There were no significant differences in occurrence time of minimal HR among groups (Table 4).

There were no significant differences in the basal MBP among the five groups. In group D_1, there were no significant differences among the basal MBP and every minute for 5 min thereafter, but the MBP at the point of the hernial sac pull was increased significantly compared with the baseline. In group D_2, the MBP was decreased at 2, 3, 4, and 5 min compared with the baseline, and the MBP returned to the baseline at the point of skin cut and hernial sac pull. In group D_3 and D_4, the MBP was decreased at 3, 4, and 5 min compared with the baseline, and the MBP returned to the baseline at the point of skin cut and hernial sac pull. In group D_5, the MBP was decreased at 5 min and the points of the skin cut and hernial sac pull compared with the baseline (Table 5).

There were no significant differences in incidencerate of complementary medicine, adverse events, and bradycardia (we defined bradycardia as HR decrease of ≥30% during the 5-min observation period postdexmedetomidine bolus, compared to predexmedetomidine bolus baseline values). There were eight patients who had a 30% decrease from the baseline of HR, and none of the patients required treatment for bradycardia. Four patients needed propofol to treat EA, and no one needed treatment for bradycardia, pain, or other adverse events, including cough, headache, and vomiting (Table 6). All of the patients with spontaneous respiration could maintain $SaO_2 \geq 98\%$.There were significant differences in the recovery time between every two groups ($P < 0.05$) (Table 7).

Table 4 Minimal Heart Rate

Groups	Minimal	Duration time(s)	Occurrence time(s)
Group D_1	92 ± 12	2.0 (1.0–3.5)	30.0 (20.0–42.5)
Group D_2	88 ± 16	2.0 (2.0–6.0)	42.0 (39.0–49.0)
Group D_3	83 ± 11*	5.0 (3.0–6.5)	38.5 (35.0–43.0)
Group D_4	84 ± 11*	3.0 (2.0–5.0)	41.0 (34.5–50.0)
Group D_5	81 ± 8*	6.0 (2.0–9.0)*	41.0 (32.5–49.0)

*Compared with group D_1 respectively, $P < 0.05$

Table 5 MBP Changes [median (IQR)]

Groups	Baseline	1 min	2 min	3 min	4 min	5 min	Skin cut	Hernial sac pull
Group D_1	58.0$^{\wedge}$ (56.5–62.0)	58.0 (57.0–62.5)	58.0$^{\wedge}$ (56.0–61.5)	58.0$^{\wedge}$ (56.0–61.0)	57.0$^{\wedge}$ (56.0–58.5)	57.5$^{\wedge}$ (55.0–59.5)	61.5 (56.0–64.5)	64.5* (60.0–69.5)
Group D_2	60.0 (53.5–66.5)	58.5 (51.5–65.0)	57.0$^{*\wedge}$ (49.5–61.0)	58.0* (50.0–60.5)	57.0* (48.0–60.5)	57.0$^{*\wedge}$ (49.5–60.5)	57.0$^{\wedge}$ (52.0–60.0)	62.0 (55.0–70.5)
Group D_3	58.0 (55.5–60.5)	58.0 (55.5–61.5)	55.5$^{\wedge}$ (52.0–58.0)	53.0* (51.0–56.5)	53.0$^{*\wedge}$ (51.0–55.5)	53.0* (51.0–56.0)	54.5 (51.0–57.5)	58.5 (53.5–61.5)
Group D_4	59.0 (55.0–65.5)	59.5 (57.5–67.0)	56.5 (53.0–61.0)	55.0* (51.5–60.0)	53.5* (50.0–58.5)	55.0$^{*\wedge}$ (49.5–59.0)	57.5 (50.5–61.0)	59.5 (56.5–64.0)
Group D_5	57.0 (54.0–63.0)	61.5$^{\wedge}$ (57.5–68.0)	54.5 (51.0–65.0)	54.0 (49.0–60.0)	53.0 (49.5–60.5)	52.5* (50.0–56.5)	53.5* (49.5–59.0)	52.5* (48.5–59.0)

*Compared with Baseline, $^{\wedge}$compared with the time point of hernial sac pull, $P < 0.05$

Discussion

Even without a pediatric label, additions to the literature on pediatric applications of DEX have risen in the last few years [4]. DEX has numerous properties that make it beneficial as a sedative and anesthetic; it has been documented to sedate in a manner that is similar to natural sleep, and it is used as an anxiolytic, analgesic, and sympatholytic [1, 2, 13]. In addition, it has an anesthetic-sparing impact with negligible respiratory depression, and it can be used to avert and treat postoperative EA [13]. The hemodynamic reactions of DEX are related to the rate of infusion and dose [5]. Although it is recommended that DEX is infused as a bolus over 10 min, the BP and HR response are still present [2, 14]. As doses of DEX get larger, hypotension and transient hypertension are greater. While there are many clinical encounters in the rapid bolus injection of DEX, there is minimal efficacy data that are accessible [11, 12, 15].

In our study, we found that 0.75 and 1.0 μg/kg DEX rapid infusion could significantly reduce the incidence of EA, while 0.25 and 0.5 μg/kg DEX had the fewer trend. Hauber JA et al. [12] had found that 0.5 μg/kg DEX rapid infusion could reducing the incidence of EA. The difference may because different subjective evaluation of the score of PAED and the smaller sample size. In addition, 0.5, 0.75 and 1.0 μg/kg DEX could reduce the surgical stress of the hernial sac pull. As the dosage increased, the recovery time was significantly prolonged, but there were no significant differences in the incidence of total adverse events. EA is a traumatic experience for children and their parents, and it can result in injury [16]. DEX has been well reported as an effective agent for EA, and the rapid bolus administration of DEX for the treatment of EA is more practical and timely than a 10-min infusion.

DEX could significantly decrease HR and MBP. The minimal HR was significantly lower after the administration of DEX in the dose of 0.5, 0.75 and 1 μg/kg, and the duration time was significantly prolonged after 1.0 μg/kg DEX infusion, but no one needed treatment. In human and animal models, DEX has a biphasic blood pressure impact: a preliminary but transitory elevation in blood pressure accompanied by a long-lasting hypotensive effect that is induced by peripheralα_2-adrenoreceptor and then central α_2 adrenoreceptor stimulation [11, 12, 17]. Therefore DEX should be administered as a loading dose during a 10-min period to diminish the dose-dependent, biphasic, hemodynamic reaction. In our study, hypertension was not seen, this could have happened since the rapid infusion of DEX eradicated the time differential between the stimulation of the peripheral and central α_2-adrenoreceptor.

Table 6 Comparison of complementary medicine, adverse events, and bradycardia [No. (%)]

Groups	Complementary Medicine	Adverse events	Bradycardia[a]
Group D_1	3 (15%)	0	0
Group D_2	0	0	1 (5%)
Group D_3	1 (5%)	3 (15%)	3 (15%)
Group D_4	0	1 (5%)	2 (10%)
Group D_5	0	1 (5%)	2 (10%)

There were no statistically significant differences ($P > 0.05$) among the groups
[a]Bradycardia was defined as HR decrease of ≥30% during the 5-min observation period postdexmedetomidine bolus, compared to predexmedetomidine bolus baseline values

Table 7 Recovery time (mean ± SD)

Groups	Recovery time (min)
Group D_1	21.3 ± 7.1
Group D_2	30.3 ± 8.6
Group D_3	40.7 ± 8.2
Group D_4	49.5 ± 6.4
Group D_5	60.4 ± 21.1

There were significant differences in the recovery time between every two groups ($P < 0.05$)

The general agreement seems to be that DEX is linked to minimal respiratory depression [1, 5, 17, 18]. Our study found that the rapid injection of DEX can cause a decrease in tidal volume, but it does not affect SaO_2 without special handling. This may because deep sedation and oral/pharyngeal anatomic frequently happened in deep sleep after the administration of DEX.

Conclusion

In conclusion, rapid infusion of DEX at dose of 0.75, and 1.0 μg/kg DEX could prevent EA. Even though the use of DEX resulted in transient decreases in HR and MBP, the drug is well-tolerated in pediatric patients. Our study provides a new clinical application for the rapid intravenous injection of DEX for the prevention and treatment of EA.

Abbreviations

BIS: Bispectral index; DEX: Dexmedetomidine; EA: Emergence agitation; ECG: Electrocardiogram; HR: Heart rate; IV: Intravenous injection; LMA: Laryngeal mask airway; MBP: Mean blood pressure; m-CHOPES: Modified Children's Hospital of Eastern Ontario Pain Scale; PACU: Post-anesthesia care unit; PAED: Pediatric Anesthesia Emergence Delirium; SaO_2: Blood oxygen saturation; SD: Standard deviation

Acknowledgements

We would like to thank the following team members for their contributions to the success of this trial.

Funding

The research was funded by Wenzhou City Public Welfare Science and Technology Project of China (Y20170139).

Authors' contributions

FC analyzed and interpreted the patient data regarding the MBP, HR, ED, adverse events, bradycardia and recovery time. CYW analyzed demographic and surgical characteristics of patients. YL and MMH were a major contributor in writing the manuscript. All authors read and approved the final manuscript.

Competing interests

The authors declare that they have no competing interests.

Author details

[1]Department of Pain Management, Shandong Provincial Hospital affiliated to Shandong University, 324 Jingwu Road, Jinan 250021, China. [2]Department of Anesthesiology, Critical Care and Pain Medicine, The 2nd Affiliated Hospital & Yuying Children's Hospital of WenZhou Medical University, Wenzhou, China.

References

1. Su X, Meng ZT, Wu XH, et al. Dexmedetomidine for prevention of delirium in elderly patients after non-cardiac surgery: a randomised, double-blind, placebo-controlled trial. Lancet. 2016;388:1893–902.
2. Riker RR, Shehabi Y, Bokesch PM, et al. Dexmedetomidine vs midazolam for sedation of critically ill patients: a randomized trial. JAMA. 2009;301:489–99.
3. Linares SB, García CMA, Ramírez CIL, et al. Pre-anesthetic medication with intranasal dexmedetomidine and oral midazolam as an anxiolytic. A clinical trial. An Pediatr (Barc). 2014;81:226–31.
4. Mason KP, Kelhoffer ER, Prescilla R, et al. Feasibility of measuring memory response to increasing dexmedetomidine sedation in children. Br J Anaesth. 2017;118:254–63.
5. Mason KP, Lerman J. Review article: Dexmedetomidine in children: current knowledge and future applications. Anesth Analg. 2011;113:1129–42.
6. Su F, Gastonguay MR, Nicolson SC, et al. Dexmedetomidine pharmacology in neonates and infants after open heart surgery. Anesth Analg. 2016;122:1556–66.
7. Vlajkovic GP, Sindjelic RP. Emergence delirium in children: many questions, few answers. Anesth Analg. 2007;104:84–91.
8. Cole JW, Murray DJ, McAllister JD, et al. Emergence behaviour in children: defining the incidence of excitement and agitation following anaesthesia. Paediatr Anaesth. 2002;12:442–7.
9. Sato M, Shirakami G, Tazuke-Nishimura M, et al. Effect of single-dose dexmedetomidine on emergence agitation and recovery profiles after sevoflurane anesthesia in pediatric ambulatory surgery. J Anesth. 2010;24:675–82.
10. Ibacache ME, Muñoz HR, Brandes V, et al. Single-dose dexmedetomidine reduces agitation after sevoflurane anesthesia in children. Anesth Analg. 2004;98:60–3. table of contents
11. Jooste EH, Muhly WT, Ibinson JW, et al. Acute hemodynamic changes after rapid intravenous bolus dosing of dexmedetomidine in pediatric heart transplant patients undergoing routine cardiac catheterization. Anesth Analg. 2010;111:1490–6.
12. Hauber JA, Davis PJ, Bendel LP, et al. Dexmedetomidine as a rapid bolus for treatment and prophylactic prevention of emergence agitation in anesthetized children. Anesth Analg. 2015;121:1308–15.
13. Mahmoud M, Mason KP. Dexmedetomidine: review, update, and future considerations of paediatric perioperative and periprocedural applications and limitations. Br J Anaesth. 2015;115:171–82.
14. Xia ZQ, Chen SQ, Yao X, et al. Clinical benefits of dexmedetomidine versus propofol in adult intensive care unit patients: a meta-analysis of randomized clinical trials. J Surg Res. 2013;185:833–43.
15. Dawes J, Myers D, Görges M, et al. Identifying a rapid bolus dose of dexmedetomidine (ED50) with acceptable hemodynamic outcomes in children. Paediatr Anaesth. 2014;24:1260–7.
16. Makkar JK, Bhatia N, Bala I, et al. A comparison of single dose dexmedetomidine with propofol for the prevention of emergence delirium after desflurane anaesthesia in children. Anaesthesia. 2016;71:50–7.
17. Hall JE, Uhrich TD, Barney JA, et al. Sedative, amnestic, and analgesic properties of small-dose dexmedetomidine infusions. Anesth Analg. 2000;90:699–705.
18. Shimotori H, Kawano M. Anesthetic management with Dexmedetomidine in patients with serious mental and physical disabilities undergoing dental treatment. Masui. 2016;65:414–7.

17

A method for addressing right upper lobe obstruction with right-sided double-lumen endobronchial tubes during surgery: a randomized controlled trial

Wei Yu, Zijian Wang, Dapeng Gao, Wei Zhang, Wen Jin, Xuesong Ma and Sihua Qi*

Abstract

Background: A right-sided double-lumen tube (R-DLT) tends to obstruct the right upper lobe intraoperatively due to anatomical distortion during surgery. If the R-DLT is poorly matched with the patient's airway anatomy, it will not be possible to correctly replace the tube with a fiberoptic bronchoscope (FOB). In our study, we aimed to explore an efficient method for difficult repositioning caused by right upper lobe occlusion during surgery: repositioning the R-DLT from the right main bronchus into the left main bronchus. The current study was designed to assess the efficacy and safety of this method.

Methods: Sixty adult patients scheduled to undergo left-sided thoracic surgery were randomly assigned to two groups. With the patient in the right lateral position during surgery, the R-DLT was pulled back to the trachea while being rotated 90° clockwise; it was then either rotated 90° clockwise for placement into the left main bronchus (Group L) or rotated 90° anticlockwise and returned to the right main bronchus (Group R) using FOB guidance. The primary outcomes included clinical performance, which was measured by intubation time, and the quality of lung collapse. A secondary outcome was safety, which was determined according to bronchial injury and vocal cord injury.

Results: The median intubation time (IQR [range]) required for placement of a R-DLT into the left main bronchus was shorter than the time required for placement into the right main bronchus (15.0 s [IQR, 12.0 to 20.0 s]) vs 23.5 s [IQR, 14.5 to 65.8 s], P = 0.005). The groups showed comparable overall results for the quality of lung collapse during the total period of one-lung ventilation (P = 1.000). The numbers of patients with bronchial injuries or vocal cord injuries were also comparable between groups (Group R, 11/30 vs. Group L 8/30, P = 0.580 for bronchus injuries; Group R, 15/30 vs. Group L 13/30, P = 0.796 for vocal cord injuries).

Conclusions: Repositioning a R-DLT from the right main bronchus into the left main bronchus had good clinical performance without causing additional injury. This may be an efficient method for the difficult repositioning of a R-DLT due to right upper lobe occlusion during surgery.

Keywords: airway management methods, one-lung ventilation, adverse effects, intubation

* Correspondence: qisihua2007@163.com
Department of Anaesthesiology, Fourth Affiliated Hospital of Harbin Medical University, 37 Yiyuan Road, Harbin 150001, Heilongjiang Province, China

Background

In left-sided thoracic surgery, one-lung ventilation (OLV) can generally be achieved by placing a right- or left-sided double-lumen tube (R-DLT or L-DLT). A R-DLT has a smaller margin of safety for correct placement than a L-DLT [1]. The main problem with using a R-DLT is that it is prone to cause right upper lobe obstruction and collapse [2–4]. Nevertheless, many clinicians choose a R-DLT for left-sided thoracic surgery because the consensus is that the thoracic surgical procedure may change at any time, and for some procedures, using a R-DLT is absolutely indicated, such as in sleeve resection and left-sided pneumonectomy [5]. However, it has been found that during some operations, a R-DLT is not actually necessary.

A R-DLT has a tendency to become malpositioned intraoperatively [6] due to anatomical distortion that may occur during lateral positioning of the patient [7]. If a R-DLT is poorly matched with the anatomy of the patient's airway, it will not be possible to replace the R-DLT correctly using a fiberoptic bronchoscope (FOB) even with repeated attempts, and multiple attempts to replace a R-DLT can lead to severe airway injury. Although these problems can be corrected by exchanging a R-DLT with a L-DLT or by using an endobronchial blocker, exchanging a DLT with the patient in the lateral position is not only difficult but also risks losing access to the airway.

The distance between the branching point of the left upper lobe orifice and the carina is approximately 4.5 cm in women and 5.0 cm in men [1, 8]. For most patients, the size of the left main bronchus is long enough to hold the tip of a R-DLT without occluding the left upper lobe orifice. Thus, transferring a R-DLT from the right main bronchus into the left main bronchus may be a feasible method for instances where R-DLT repositioning is difficult due to right upper lobe occlusion during surgery. Because the performance of this method is controversial, we performed a prospective, randomized controlled trial to test the efficacy and safety of moving a R-DLT from the right main bronchus into the left main bronchus with patients in the lateral position during surgery.

Methods

Patients and groups

This single-center, controlled, randomized, single-blinded study was approved by the Ethics Committee of The Fourth Affiliated Hospital of Harbin Medical University, Harbin, China (Chairperson Prof Changjiu Zhao) (No. YLXJS.2015.02) on 30 July 2015. The study protocol was registered with the Chinese Clinical Trial Registry (ChiCTR-IPR-15006933).

After providing written informed consent, adult patients with American Society of Anesthesiologists physical status classifications of 1 to 3 and aged 18–75 years were enrolled in our study. All of the patients underwent left-sided video-assisted thoracoscopic surgery (VATS) (e.g., lung biopsy, lobectomy, segmentectomy, pleural decortication) requiring OLV. We excluded patients for which we anticipated difficulties in tracheal intubation (e.g., a Mallampati score ≥ 3), a Cormack score of 3 or 4, the presence of a tracheostomy, pre-existing sore throat or hoarseness, or recent respiratory infection (< 1 month).

All of the recruited patients were allocated 1:1 into two groups using computer-generated randomization, and the group allocation number was hidden in opaque envelopes. To ensure blinding, three anesthesiologists were involved in the study. The first anesthesiologist performed anesthesia and the first bronchial intubation with the patient in the dorsal decubitus position. The second anesthesiologist opened the opaque envelope and performed the second tracheal intubation with the patient in the lateral decubitus position. The third anesthesiologist evaluated and recorded all of the parameters. Only the second anesthesiologist knew the group allocation of the study.

Anesthetic management

The patients, who were not given any premedication, were transferred to the operating room. A catheter was placed in the radial artery for arterial blood gas analysis and continuous monitoring of blood pressure. All of the patients received a thoracic epidural catheter at the level of T_{4-5} or T_{5-6} for postoperative pain management.

After the induction of anesthesia with injections of 0.3 $\mu g \cdot kg^{-1}$ sufentanil, 0.2 $mg \cdot kg^{-1}$ cisatracurium, and 1.5–2.5 $mg \cdot kg^{-1}$ propofol, all patients were preoxygenated with 100% oxygen for 3 min. A laryngeal mask airway (LMA) was inserted after lubricating the cuff with a water-based jelly. A bronchoscope was advanced down the LMA, and then, a pulmonologist observed the airway condition and measured the length of the left main bronchus with the bronchoscope. A video was also obtained for subsequent analysis and comparison [4].

After removal of the LMA, the Cormack-Lehane classification was used for quantification via direct laryngoscopy [9]. A disposable polyvinyl chloride R-DLT (Mallinckrodt Medical, Inc., Athlone, Ireland) without a carinal hook was used for tracheal intubation, and the size was selected according to patient gender, height and chest CT scan by a separate anesthetist. After the bronchial tip passed the vocal cords, the stylet was removed. The tube was rotated 90° clockwise and advanced until the estimated depth of insertion was reached. The accuracy of R-DLT placement was assessed with a FOB. The pressure of the R-DLT cuffs was measured with a noninvasive manometer (Endotest; Rüsch, Kernen, Germany) and maintained below 30 mmHg.

Anesthesia was maintained with sevoflurane (2–4% end-tidal concentration) and 0.25–1.0 $\mu g{\cdot}kg^{-1}{\cdot}min^{-1}$ remifentanil. In addition, 0.5–2 $\mu g{\cdot}kg^{-1}{\cdot}min^{-1}$ cisatracurium was continuously administered i.v. to maintain muscular blockade, and neuromuscular blockade was assessed by train-of-four monitoring. Volume-controlled mode was used with the following parameters: the tidal volume was 5–7 $ml{\cdot}kg^{-1}$ (ideal body weight) during OLV and 8 $ml{\cdot}kg^{-1}$ (ideal body weight) during two-lung ventilation, and respiration rates were regulated according to the end-tidal carbon dioxide tension within 35–45 mmHg. The inspired oxygen concentration was 100% before OLV initiation and was gradually reduced to maintain an oxygen saturation (SaO_2) greater than 95%.

After performing two-lung ventilation for 15 min with the patient in the supine position, the following variables were recorded as the basal values: mean arterial pressure, heart rate, arterial blood oxygen tension, and pulmonary mechanics (peak pressure, plateau pressure, and dynamic compliance). After the bronchial cuff was deflated, the patient was move into the right lateral position, and the head was fixed in place. Then, the R-DLT was pulled back 6 cm to the trachea while being rotated 90° clockwise in the right lateral position (rotating the tip of the bronchial lumen towards the posterior side of the trachea). A FOB was advanced down the bronchial lumen. Then, the R-DLT was either rotated 90° clockwise while being guided via the FOB to the left main bronchus (left intubation group) or rotated 90° anticlockwise while being guided via the FOB back to the right main bronchus (right intubation group). The anesthesiologist was at the patient's head, and the descriptions referring to clockwise/anticlockwise are relative to the orientation of the bronchoscopist. The placement of the R-DLT was adjusted with a FOB, and the resistance while placing the R-DLT was recorded. After completing the intubation procedure, we recommended leaving the R-DLT free to rotate to a lower rotation resistance. In our preliminary experiments, we found that the rotation resistance was high when the tube was rotated with the tip facing the anterior wall, which may more easily cause the DLT to twist in the airway or damage the airway during rotation. The reasons for the high rotation resistance that occurred might be best explained as follows. The R-DLT was initially rotated 90° clockwise after the bronchial tip passed the vocal cords. If the rotation direction was not consistent with the first rotation direction, it was more likely to lead to distortion of the R-DLT and increase rotation resistance. After the initiation of OLV, the pulmonary mechanics were recorded at 5 min, 15 min, and 30 min, and the arterial blood gas values were recorded before and 10 min after lung collapse.

After completing the surgery, the R-DLT was removed, and the laryngeal mask was inserted again. A bronchoscope was advanced down the LMA, and the pulmonologist re-assessed the airway condition with a bronchoscope to check for injuries caused by the R-DLT. Vocal cord injuries were recorded with video and assessed by an otolaryngologist. Airway injuries were defined according to methods described by Knoll [10–12]. For postoperative pain therapy, a mixture of 0.125% ropivacaine and 0.25 $\mu g{\cdot}ml^{-1}$ sufentanil was given by epidural patient-controlled analgesia.

Intubation variables and efficacy of the R-DLT

The following intubation-related variables were evaluated and recorded by the anesthesiologist: visualization of glottic exposure (Cormack-Lehane grade); time for the first tracheal intubation with the patient in the supine position, defined as the time from when the laryngoscope was placed into the mouth until the end-tidal carbon dioxide level was detected; time for the second tracheal intubation with the patient in the lateral position, which was the primary outcome of the study and was defined as the time from the beginning of tube withdrawal from the bronchial lumen to the trachea until successful intubation; and the number of intubation attempts. In addition, the ease of R-DLT placement (easy/difficult/very difficult) was also recorded for the second tracheal intubation.

According to the anatomy and pulmonary mechanics, the tube position was evaluated, and the observations were grouped into four categories: optimal, which consisted of a clear and unobstructed view of the main carina and subcarina; suboptimal, which consisted of unobstructed airways (without increased peak inspiratory pressure) and partly visible main carina or subcarina; misplaced, which consisted of acceptable mechanical ventilation and a nonvisible main carina or subcarina; and unsatisfactory, which consisted of inadequate complete mechanical ventilation and a nonvisible main carina or subcarina. The surgeon, who was blinded to the group allocation of the study, assessed the extent of lung collapse [4]: 1, excellent (complete collapse); 2, fair (some residual air); and 3, poor (no collapse or residual air interfering with surgical exposure).

Assessment of postoperative hoarseness and sore throat

Hoarseness was defined as acoustic quality assessed according to the difference relative to the patient's previous voice quality [12]. This variable was graded as mild (as deemed by the patient), moderate (as noticed by the observer), or severe (aphonia). Sore throat was defined as continuous pain in the throat [3, 13] and was rated as follows: mild (pain with swallowing), moderate (continuous pain and increased pain while swallowing), or severe (pain interfering with eating and requiring painkillers). The anesthesiologist asked each patient specific questions regarding his or her postoperative sore throat and hoarseness at 1 h after emergence from anesthesia and at 24 h, 48 h, and 72 h [12, 14].

Statistical analysis

The sample size was calculated based on the intubation time. We defined a clinically important difference in intubation time as 10 s; therefore, using a standard deviation of 12 s based on a pilot study, an $\alpha = 0.05$ and $\beta = 0.2$, 46 patients (23 patients in each group) were required. Considering potential dropouts, 30 patients were included in each group.

Continuous variables were tested for a normal distribution using the Kolmogorov–Smirnov test. Normally distributed continuous data, presented as the mean (standard deviation), were compared using independent Student's *t*-tests. Non-normally distributed continuous data, presented as the median (interquartile range, IQR), were analyzed using the Mann–Whitney rank sum test. Numbers (%) for categorical variables were compared using Fisher's exact test. The results were considered statistically significant when P was less than 0.05. Statistical analysis was performed using SPSS Statistics 18.0 (IBM Corp., Armonk, NY).

Results

During the period from August 2015 to June 2016, 79 patients were initially assessed for eligibility. Nineteen patients were excluded, and 60 patients were randomized (30 patients in each group) and completed the study (Fig. 1). Demographic and surgical data for the groups are summarized in Table 1.

Factors related to tracheal intubation did not differ significantly between the study groups for the initial tracheal intubation when in the dorsal decubitus position (Additional file 1: Table S1). For the second tracheal intubation in the lateral decubitus position, placement of the R-DLT into the left bronchus required a median duration of 15.0 s (IQR, 12.0 to 20.0 s), and placement of the R-DLT to the right bronchia required a median duration of 23.5 s (IQR, 14.5 to 65.8 s) ($P = 0.005$). Compared with right bronchial intubation, R-DLT placement into the left bronchus was rated as easier by the anesthesiologist with the patient in the lateral decubitus position ($P < 0.001$) (Table 2). Only 70% of right bronchial intubations and 26.7% of left bronchial intubations were initially placed in an optimal position. However, the total number of intubations in the proper position (optimal and suboptimal positions) without the need for repositioning were comparable in both groups (Group R, 26/30 vs. Group L, 27/30; $P = 1.000$) (Table 2). Additionally, the values for blood gas parameters, pulmonary

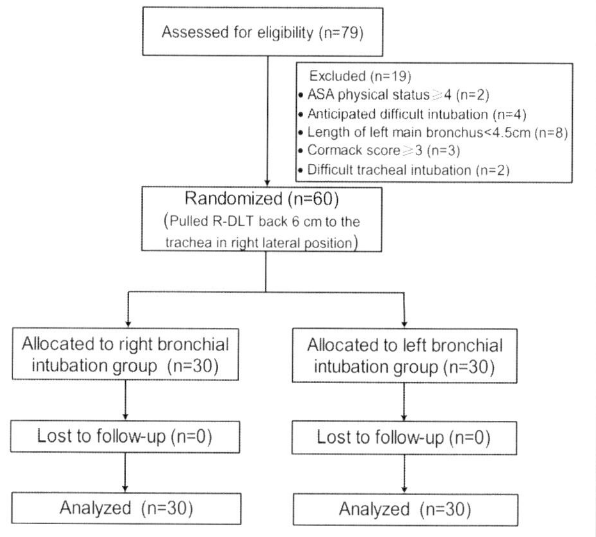

Fig. 1 Experimental Flowchart. Study flow chart. ASA, American Society of Anesthesiologists physical status; R-DLT, right-sided double-lumen tube

mechanics, and quality of collapse were similar between the groups and are summarized in Table 3 and Additional files 2 and 3: Tables S2 and S3.

The overall incidence of bronchial injury was 32% (19 patients) for Group R and Group L combined. The intensity of bronchial injury did not differ significantly between the groups (Table 4) ($P = 0.824$). The number of patients with vocal cord injuries did not significantly differ between the two groups ($P = 0.796$). The overall incidence of vocal cord injury was 47% (28 patients), and the majority of the vocal cord injuries included redness (16 patients) and edema (9 patients) (Table 4).

The overall incidence of postoperative hoarseness was 27% (16 patients) at 1 h, 17% (10 patients) at 24 h, 13% (8 patients) at 48 h, and 5% (3 patients) at 72 h (Table 5), and these last 3 patients recovered from hoarseness on postoperative day 4. The presence of sore throat was similar between Group R and Group L: 11 patients vs. 14

Table 1 Patient characteristics and surgical data

	Group R ($n = 30$)	Group L ($n = 30$)
Age (years)	56.8 (9.8)	59.9 (8.8)
Male	19	21
Weight (kg)	65.5 (11.1)	64.6 (11.9)
Height (cm)	169.1 (5.9)	168.7 (8.1)
ASA physical status (I/II/III)	6/21/3	7/20/3
Smoking, Y/N	14/16	12/18
Cormack-Lehane view (1/2)	25/5	22/8
DLT size (FG), 35/37/39	12/16/2	14/13/3
Duration of surgery (min)	198.9 (54.2)	175.8 (37.0)

ASA American Society of Anesthesiologists physical status

Table 2 Factors related to the second tracheal intubation in the lateral decubitus position

	Group R ($n = 30$)	Group L ($n = 30$)	*P* value
Time required for tracheal intubation and R-DLT positioning(s)	23.5 (14.5–65.8)	15.0 (12.0–20.0)	0.005[a]
Position after intubation (optimal/suboptimal/ misplaced/ unsatisfactory)	21/5/4/0	8/19/2/1	> 0.001[b]
Number of tracheal intubation attempts (1/2/3)	25/4/1	27/2/1	0.832[b]
Ease of placing the R-DLT (easy/difficult/very difficult)	19/8/3	27/3/0	> 0.001[b]
Number of repositions (0/1/2/3)	22/6/1/1	24/3/1/2	0.794[b]
Patients[c]	26	27	1.000[b]

[a]Median (IQR) of the non-normal variables (Kolmogorov–Smirnov test, $P < 0.05$); significance tested by the Mann–Whitney rank sum test
[b]Numbers for the categorical variables; significance tested by Fisher's exact test
[c]Number of patients with optimal or suboptimal positioning of the bronchial tubes

patients experienced this outcome ($P = 0.601$) (Table 5). The overall incidences of sore throat were highest at 1 h and decreased thereafter. No patients suffered from sore throat on postoperative day 5.

Discussion

The use of a R-DLT is related to a high risk of right upper lobe obstruction and collapse [2–4]. However, there are also some absolute indications for using a R-DLT, such as for treating left endobronchial tumors, disruption of the left mainstem bronchus, left lung transplantation, sleeve resection, left-sided pneumonectomy, and left bronchial compression of a thoracic aortic aneurysm. Due to the uncertainty in surgical procedures and patient conditions, a R-DLT is initially preferred for left-sided thoracic surgery in a number of clinical institutions. To the best of our knowledge, only a few case reports have described attempts at right bronchial intubation using a left-sided double-lumen tube [13, 15]. There are no previous prospective investigations that evaluated the efficiency and safety of repositioning a R-DLT from the right main bronchus into the left main bronchus with patients in the lateral position during surgery. Therefore, we designed a study to assess the efficiency and safety of this bronchial intubation technique.

Table 3 Quality of collapse

	Group R ($n = 30$)	Group L ($n = 30$)	*P* value
Quality of collapse after 10 min, n			0.430[a]
Excellent	10	14	
Fair	19	16	
Poor	1	0	
Quality of collapse overall, n			1.000[a]
Excellent	25	26	
Fair	5	4	
Poor	0	0	

[a]Numbers for the categorical variables; significance tested by Fisher's exact test

The procedure for placement of a R-DLT in the left mainstem bronchus was rated as being easier and faster than that for placement in the right mainstem bronchus, mainly because R-DLT placement requires proper positioning of the R-DLT, with the ventilation slot opening directly into the bronchial orifice of the right upper lobe. Placement of R-DLTs is easy in most patients but can be troublesome in a subset of patients. After successful bronchial intubation when in the dorsal decubitus position, some patients are moved into the right lateral decubitus position, with R-DLT malpositioning detected via FOB, indicating a lack of alignment between the right upper lobe R-DLT ventilation slot and the origin of the right upper bronchus. It is sometimes not possible to replace a R-DLT correctly despite many attempts, and multiple attempts may cause serious airway damage. At the same time, subsequent operative procedures may not require a R-DLT. In these situations, the use of a R-DLT would still provide adequate surgical conditions if the R-DLT is repositioned into the left main bronchus.

Only 26.7% of left bronchial intubations were positioned optimally after the second tracheal intubation with the patient in the lateral decubitus position. The reasons for the high rate of malpositioning reported here might be best explained as follows. First, when the R-DLT was rotated 180° clockwise and guided to the left main bronchus via the FOB, the tube was prone to rotate slightly clockwise due to the distal curve of the structure. To lower rotation resistance, we recommend leaving the R-DLT free to rotate. Second, the more stringent definition of DLT malpositioning used here may be responsible for the higher malposition rates. Even in cases where malpositioning was noted, it was not always the case that left bronchial intubation using a R-DLT during OLV exhibited poor clinical performance. Retrospectively, most cases of R-DLT malpositioning were attributable to a position in which the carina is partly visible or to bronchial cuff herniation, which did not affect the mechanical ventilation. In addition, the malpositioning could be corrected easily and rapidly via bronchoscopy. Unlike other studies, we did not apply suction to R-DLTs [12].

A secondary outcome of our study was safety, which was determined according to damage to the airway. Risk factors for vocal cord and bronchial injury include physical contact with the tube and the cuff [12]. In our study,

Table 4 Incidence of bronchial injuries and vocal cord injuries

	Group R ($n = 30$)	Group L ($n = 30$)	P value
Bronchial injuries			0.824[a]
None	19	22	
Redness	8	6	
Edema	2	1	
Hematoma	1	1	
Patients[b]	11	8	0.580[a]
Vocal cord injuries			0.176[a]
None	15	17	
Redness	9	7	
Edema	5	4	
Hematoma	1	2	
Patients[b]	15	13	0.796[a]

[a]Numbers for the categorical variables; significance tested by Fisher's exact test
[b]Number of patients with bronchial injuries or vocal cord injuries

the numbers of patients with bronchial injuries or vocal cord injuries were comparable in both groups, and most airway injuries were minor. For example, tracheal redness could be observed at the site where the angled tip of the R-DLT touched the wall during bronchial insertion. When the lateral wall pressure of the bronchial cuffs is greater than the mean capillary perfusion pressure, bronchial mucosa injury may occur in a few hours [12]. In our study, to lower the pressure of the bronchial cuffs, we used a stethoscope to listen to the trachea for air leaks and injected the smallest amount of air necessary to achieve an adequate tracheal seal; we also monitored cuff pressure.

The incidences of postoperative sore throat and hoarseness were not significantly different between the groups receiving right- or left-side bronchial intubation with a R-DLT, mainly because we left the R-DLT free to rotate to reduce the pressure in the throat. In addition, when a R-DLT is inserted into a patient's airway, body heat may decrease the stiffness of the DLT. In a previous study, warming the distal part of the DLT appeared to be effective for reducing some airway complications [16, 17] . A previous study reported that 3% of the patients were

Table 5 Incidence and intensity of postoperative hoarseness and sore throat

	Hoarseness			Sore throat		
	Group R ($n = 30$)	Group L ($n = 30$)	P Value	Group R ($n = 30$)	Group L ($n = 30$)	P value
At 1 h			0.481			0.491[a]
No complaints	23	21		21	18	
Mild	3	2		3	5	
Moderate	3	5		4	5	
Severe	1	2		2	2	
At 24 h			0.154			0.503[a]
No complaints	27	23		24	22	
Mild	2	3		3	3	
Moderate	1	4		2	3	
Severe	0	0		1	2	
At 48 h			0.445			0.666[a]
No complaints	27	25		28	27	
Mild	2	3		0	1	
Moderate	1	2		1	1	
Severe	0	0		1	1	
At 72 h			0.557			0.57[a]
No complaints	29	28		29	28	
Mild	1	2		0	1	
Moderate	0	0		1	1	
Severe	0	0		0	0	
Patients[b]	9	10	1.000	11	14	0.601[a]

[a]Numbers for the categorical variables; significance tested by Fisher's exact test
[b]Numbers of patients with postoperative hoarseness and sore throat

hoarse for more than 5 postoperative days [18]. In our study, no patient had hoarseness on the 4th day after the operation, although the limited size of our study might explanation the lack of patients with long-lasting hoarseness.

This study has certain limitations. First, we cannot completely exclude the possibility that sore throat might be caused by the laryngeal mask and the flexible bronchoscope itself. In our study, experienced pulmonologists and anesthesiologists performed all of the procedures to minimize airway injury. Second, numerous patients refused to undergo postoperative flexible bronchoscope examination. Thus, vocal cord injuries and bronchial injuries were assessed only immediately after extubation. Third, in our study, the sample size was too small to detect rare cases of severe airway damage (e.g., serious tracheal wall rupture).

Conclusions

In conclusion, repositioning R-DLTs from the right main bronchus into the left main bronchus showed good clinical performance without causing additional injury with patients in the lateral position during surgery. Thus, this approach may offer a solution to right upper lobe occlusion by a R-DLT during surgery.

Abbreviations

FOB: fiberoptic bronchoscope; L-DLT: left -sided double-lumen tube; OLV: one-lung ventilation; R-DLT: right-sided double-lumen tube

Acknowledgements

The authors thank Qing Dong, Department of Department of Cardiothoracic Surgery, the Fourth Affiliated Hospital of Harbin Medical University, Harbin, Heilongjiang Province, China, for his assistance with this study.

Funding

The study was funded only by the Natural Science Foundation of China (No. 81271456). No external funding and no competing interests are declared.

Authors' contributions

WY and SQ designed the study, collected data, and wrote and revised the manuscript. DG helped perform the study, interpreted and analyzed the data, performed statistical analyses, and revised subsequent drafts of the manuscript. JW and WJ collected data and wrote and revised the manuscript. WZ and SM revised the manuscript critically for important intellectual content. All authors approved the final manuscript.

Competing interests

The authors declare that they have no competing interests.

References

1. Benumof JL, Partridge BL, Salvatierra C, Keating J. Margin of safety in positioning modern double-lumen endotracheal tubes. Anesthesiology. 1987;67:729–38.
2. Yoo JY, Kim DH, Choi H, Kim K, Chae YJ, Park SY. Disconnection technique with a bronchial blocker for improving lung deflation: a comparison with a double-lumen tube and bronchial blocker without disconnection. J Cardiothorac Vasc Anesth. 2014;28:904–7.
3. Cohen E. Con: right-sided double-lumen endotracheal tubes should not be routinely used in thoracic surgery. J Cardiothorac Vasc Anesth. 2002; 16:249–52.
4. Mourisse J, Liesveld J, Verhagen A, van Rooij G, van der Heide S, Schuurbiers-Siebers O, et al. Efficiency, efficacy, and safety of EZ-blocker compared with left-sided double-lumen tube for one-lung ventilation. Anesthesiology. 2013;118:550–61.
5. Campos JH, Gomez MN. Pro: right-sided double-lumen endotracheal tubes should be routinely used in thoracic surgery. J Cardiothorac Vasc Anesth. 2002;16:246–8.
6. Slinger P. The clinical use of right-sided double-lumen tubes. Can J Anaesth. 2010;57:293–300.
7. Bussieres JS, Lacasse Y, Cote D, Beauvais M, St-Onge S, Lemieux J, et al. Modified right-sided Broncho-Cath double lumen tube improves endobronchial positioning: a randomized study. Can J Anaesth. 2007;54: 276–82.
8. Campos JH. Update on tracheobronchial anatomy and flexible fiberoptic bronchoscopy in thoracic anesthesia. Curr Opin Anaesthesiol. 2009;22:4–10.
9. Cormack RS, Lehane J. Difficult tracheal intubation in obstetrics. Anaesthesia. 1984;39:1105–11.
10. Mencke T, Echternach M, Kleinschmidt S, Lux P, Barth V, Plinkert PK, et al. Laryngeal morbidity and quality of tracheal intubation: a randomized controlled trial. Anaesthesiology. 2003;98:1049–56.
11. Peppard SB, Dickens JH. Laryngeal injury following short-term intubation. Ann Otol Rhinol Laryngol. 1983;92:327–30.
12. Knoll H, Ziegeler S, Schreiber JU, Buchinger H, Bialas P, Semyonov K, et al. Airway injuries after one-lung ventilation: a comparison between double-lumen tube and endobronchial blocker: a randomized, prospective, controlled trial. Anesthesiology. 2006;105:471–7.
13. McHardy FE, Chung F. Postoperative sore throat: cause, prevention and treatment. Anaesthesia. 1999;54:444–53.
14. Capan LM, Bruce DL, Patel KP, Turndorf H. Succinylcholine-induced postoperative sore throat. Anaesthesiology. 1983;59:202–6.
15. Higgins PP, Chung F, Mezei G. Postoperative sore throat after ambulatory surgery. Br J Anaesth. 2002;88:582–4.
16. Seo JH, Cho CW, Hong DM, Jeon Y, Bahk JH. The effects of thermal softening of double-lumen endobronchial tubes on postoperative sore throat, hoarseness and vocal cord injuries: a prospective double-blind randomized trial. Br J Anaesth. 2016;116:282–8.
17. Schneider B, Schickinger-Fischer B, Zumtobel M, Mancusi G, Bigenzahn W, Klepetko W, et al. Concept for diagnosis and therapy of unilateral recurrent laryngeal nerve paralysis following thoracic surgery. Thorac Cardiovasc Surg. 2003;51:327–31.
18. Jones MW, Catling S, Evans E, Green DH, Green JR. Hoarseness after tracheal intubation. Anaesthesia. 1992;47:2130–6.

18

Peep titration based on the open lung approach during one lung ventilation in thoracic surgery: a physiological study

Michela Rauseo[1,5*], Lucia Mirabella[1], Salvatore Grasso[2], Antonella Cotoia[1], Savino Spadaro[3], Davide D'Antini[1], Franca Valentino[1], Livio Tullo[1], Domenico Loizzi[4], Francesco Sollitto[4] and Gilda Cinnella[1]

Abstract

Background: During thoracic surgery in lateral decubitus, one lung ventilation (OLV) may impair respiratory mechanics and gas exchange. We tested a strategy based on an open lung approach (OLA) consisting in lung recruitment immediately followed by a decremental positive-end expiratory pressure (PEEP) titration to the best respiratory system compliance (C_{RS}) and separately quantified the elastic properties of the lung and the chest wall. Our hypothesis was that this approach would improve gas exchange. Further, we were interested in documenting the impact of the OLA on partitioned respiratory system mechanics.

Methods: In thirteen patients undergoing upper left lobectomy we studied lung and chest wall mechanics, transpulmonary pressure (P_L), respiratory system and transpulmonary driving pressure (ΔP_{RS} and ΔP_L), gas exchange and hemodynamics at two time-points (a) during OLV at zero end-expiratory pressure ($OLV_{pre\text{-}OLA}$) and (b) after the application of the open-lung strategy ($OLV_{post\text{-}OLA}$).

Results: The external PEEP selected through the OLA was 6 ± 0.8 cmH_2O. As compared to $OLV_{pre\text{-}OLA}$, the PaO_2/FiO_2 ratio went from 205 ± 73 to 313 ± 86 ($p = .05$) and C_L increased from 56 ± 18 ml/cmH_2O to 71 ± 12 ml/cmH_2O ($p = .0013$), without changes in C_{CW}.
Both ΔP_{RS} and ΔP_L decreased from 9.2 ± 0.4 cmH_2O to 6.8 ± 0.6 cmH_2O and from 8.1 ± 0.5 cmH_2O to 5.7 ± 0.5 cmH_2O, ($p = .001$ and $p = .015$ vs $OLV_{pre\text{-}OLA}$), respectively. Hemodynamic parameters remained stable throughout the study period.

Conclusions: In our patients, the OLA strategy performed during OLV improved oxygenation and increased C_L and had no clinically significant hemodynamic effects. Although our study was not specifically designed to study ΔP_{RS} and ΔP_L, we observed a parallel reduction of both after the OLA.

Keywords: One lung ventilation, Recruitment maneuver, Thoracic surgery, Open lung approach

* Correspondence: michela.rauseo@hotmail.it
[1]Department of Anesthesia and Intensive care, University of Foggia, Viale Pinto, 1-71100 Foggia, Italy
[5]Interdepartmental Division of Critical Care Medicine, University of Toronto, Toronto, ON, Canada
Full list of author information is available at the end of the article

Background

During one-lung ventilation (OLV) in the lateral decubitus position for thoracic surgery, hypoxemia may occur in almost 10% of patients [1–3], due to the total collapse of the non-dependent lung and, eventually, to atelectasis in the ventilated, dependent lung [4, 5]. We recently demonstrated [6] that a recruitment strategy applied to the dependent lung followed by a moderate PEEP level results in significant alveolar recruitment, increased arterial oxygenation and reduction of the respiratory system elastance (E_{RS}), without hemodynamic impairment. Our data are in agreement with reports from several physiological studies [7–10], however little is still known on how to perform recruitment and set PEEP in this context. Recent physiological data suggest that immediately after the recruitment maneuver (RM), PEEP should be titrated through a decremental trial, in order to optimize respiratory mechanics while minimizing alveolar over distension [11]. This approach, originally proposed for patients with Acute Respiratory Distress Syndrome (ARDS), is designated as the "open lung approach" (OLA). Its physiological rationale is that alveolar recruitment is a pan-inspiratory phenomenon, so that a maximal inflation is needed to reverse lung atelectasis. Furthermore, due to the hysteresis between the inspiratory and expiratory volume-pressure curve, in the OLA approach, PEEP is titrated in the expiratory limb of the respiratory system volume-pressure curve, immediately after obtaining the maximal recruitment [11, 12].

A key point in understanding the effects of the OLA strategy is the partitioning between lung and chest wall mechanical properties, through the measurement of transpulmonary pressure (P_L), i.e. the lung distending pressure: in clinical conditions, P_L allows to evaluate the influence of chest wall mechanics on lung volumes and airway pressures. For a given airway opening pressure (P_{AO}), pleural pressure (P_{PL}) varies depending on the amount of lung compression exerted by the chest wall [13]. Therefore, when the chest wall compression rises, P_L drops and lungs may be underinflated, independently from the level of P_{AO} [14]. We recently demonstrated that OLA applied during laparoscopic surgery was associated with a significant increase in P_L and improvement in gas exchange, suggesting that PEEP and transpulmonary pressure are important determinants of respiratory mechanics [15].

The measurement of lung and chest wall response to the OLA may thus be of interest during OLV, since a multiplicity of factors may account for the alveolar derecruitment that usually develops in the dependent lung during OLV, such as the underlying lung parenchymal disease, the loss of chest wall elastic recoil, the lateral decubitus usually with a 15–20° posterior rotation of the coxa [2], the surgical manoeuvres [4], the mediastinum weight and the ventilatory set up used [16–18].

Our study was thus launched to evaluate the effect on oxygenation and on lung and chest wall mechanics of the OLA applied on the dependent lung during thoracic surgery.

Methods

After approval of the local ethics committee and written informed consent from each patient, the study was performed in consecutive patients scheduled to undergo elective lung lobectomy or resection through thoracotomy requiring OLV in the right lateral position, from February to November 2012 (ClinicalTrials.gov: NCT03435523). Inclusion criteria were age > 18 years, surgery and OLV lasting ≥60 min. Exclusion criteria were lung reduction surgery, pneumonectomy, patients with severe COPD with preoperative forced expiratory volume in 1 s (FEV_1) to forced vital capacity (FVC) ratio, expressed as a percentage (FEV_1/FVC%) < 60%, presence of large bullae, pleural diseases and/or acute or chronic uncompensated cardiac disease.

Upon their arrival in the operating room, patients were pre-medicated with midazolam 0.03–0.04 mg/kg. After applying standard monitoring device [electrocardiogram and pulse oximeter (Intellivue MP40 monitor, Philips, Boeblingen, Germany)], radial artery was cannulated (Radial Artery Catheterization Set, Arrow International, Reading, PA, USA) and the cannula was connected to the FloTrac™ sensor and the Vigileo™ monitor (Edwards Life Sciences LLC, Irwine, CA, USA, software version 01.10), which, in addition to arterial pressure transduction, allowed stroke volume (SV) and stroke volume variation (SVV) estimation from the arterial pressure waveform. The level of anesthesia was assessed through bi-spectral index (BIS) monitoring (Aspect A-2000 ®; Aspect Medical System, Newton, MA). Patients were given a bolus of 8 ml/kg of normal saline IV before the induction of anesthesia and were then maintained with 5 ml/kg/h of normal saline solution. A standardized protocol for hemodynamic management was applied in order to assure fluid volume optimization [16, 17]. Briefly, if SVV was lower than 13%, no additional fluids were given whereas if SVV was higher 13%, additional boluses of 250 ml of artificial colloid were infused over 15–20 min. After each bolus SVV was re-evaluated, and a further bolus was administered if SV increased by more than 10%, until reaching a SVV lower than 13%.

Anesthesia was induced with propofol 2 mg*kg $^{-1}$, fentanyl 3 γ*kg $^{-1}$, and succinylcholine 1 mg*kg $^{-1}$. Anesthesia was maintained with an infusion of propofol 150 200 γ*kg $^{-1}$*min $^{-1}$, remifentanil 0.1 0.2 γ*kg $^{-1}$*min $^{-1}$and cisatracurium 1.5 γ*kg $^{-1}$*min $^{-1}$. The infusion rate of propofol was varied in order to target a BIS value between 50 and 60.

After induction, the trachea and left bronchus were intubated with a left double lumen tube (DLT) of the appropriate size (Rushelit Rush AG lab, Waiblingen, Germany). Correct DLT position was checked using fiber optic bronchoscopy and confirmed after turning the patients in the lateral position. At OLV time, the lumen of the non-ventilated lung was left open to atmosphere. The lungs were ventilated using a Fabius GS Premium (Drager, Lubeck, Germany) with a square flow waveform. Ventilation was set for a tidal volume (Vt) of 6–8 ml*kg $^{-1}$ PBW, respiratory rate (RR) of 12–14 breath/min, inspiratory time (Ti) of 33% without inspiratory pause. Patients were initially ventilated using oxygen in air with an inspiratory oxygen fraction (FiO_2) as needed to maintain the SaO2 > 95%. No PEEP was initially added. During OLV the Vt was reduced by 30% from starting value, increasing respiratory rate as needed, while all the other parameter were kept constant [6].

Study protocol (Fig.1)

When OLV was started, after assuring that patients were hemodynamically stable (i.e. mean arterial blood pressure, mBP $\geq$ 80 mmHg, HR $\geq$ 60 b/min) and that the preload index continued to be adequate (i.e. SVV ≤ 13%), the recruitment manoeuver was applied selectively to the ventilated lung as already described [6, 13, 18, 19]. In summary, the ventilator was switched to pressure-control ventilation with an inspiratory pressure of 20 cmH_2O above PEEP. After a 3 min equilibration, PEEP was applied in steps of 5,10,15 and 20 cmH_2O every five respiratory breaths; the maximal *recruiting pressure of 40 cmH_2O (20 PEEP/20 driving pressure) was applied for six breaths.* Subsequently, after setting an inspiratory pressure of 15 cmH_2O above PEEP, PEEP was stepwise reduced, starting from 15 cmH_2O, by 2 cmH_2O every 2 min. During the decremental PEEP trial, static C_{RS} was measured at every step, through end inspiratory and end expiratory occlusions. The PEEP level corresponding to highest C_{RS} during the decremental trial was identified as the "best PEEP". Subsequently, the lungs were recruited again and the "best" PEEP was applied. The ventilator was then switched to volume-control ventilation maintaining the baseline settings, except that for the "best" PEEP level. This setting was maintained until the end of surgery.

Hemodynamic, gas exchange and respiratory mechanics measurements were obtained in two steps, before surgery, with the chest wall closed: a) on OLV in the lateral decubitus before applying the open lung approach ($OLV_{pre\text{-}OLA}$), and, b) 20 min after applying the open lung approach ($OLV_{post\text{-}OLA}$).

Measurements

Blood pressure (BP) was measured through a radial catheter connected to the pressure transducer of the MP40 monitor. Hemodynamic parameters obtained through the Vigileo included SV, cardiac output (CO), and stroke volume variation (SVV) whereas stroke volume index (SVI) and cardiac index (CI) were calculated using standard formulae. All intravascular pressure measurements were zeroed to the mid-axillary line. Analysis of arterial blood gases was performed (ABL 330; Radiometer, Copenaghen, Denmark).

Respiratory mechanics parameters were recorded, digitized and collected on a personal computer through a 12-bit analog-to digital converter board (DAQCard 700; National Instrument, Austin, TX) at a sample rate of 200 Hz (ICU Lab, KleisTEK Engineering, Bari, Italy).

Flow was measured with a heated pneumotachograph (Fleisch no.2; Fleisch, Lausanne, Switzerland), connected to a differential pressure transducer (Diff-Cap, ± 1cmH20; Special Instruments, Nordlingen, Germany) inserted between the Y-piece of the ventilator circuit and the endotracheal tube. The pneumotachograph was linear over the experimental range of flow. Volume was obtained by numerical integration of the flow signal. P_{AO} was measured proximal to the endotracheal tube with a pressure transducer (Special Instruments Digima-Clic ±100 cmH20; Nordlingen, Germany). The difference between the level of the PEEP set on the ventilator (read as the P_{AO} value at the end of a regular breath) ($PEEP_{external}$) and the pressure in P_{AO} during a 3–5 s end-expiratory occlusion ($PEEP_{TOT,\ RS}$) was measured and regarded as the static intrinsic PEEP of the respiratory system ($PEEPi_{RS}$) according to Pepe [14].

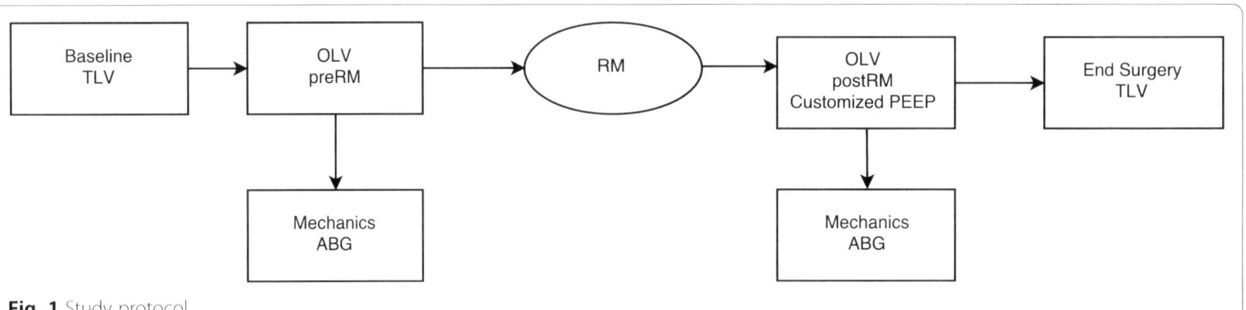

Fig. 1 Study protocol

P_{PL} was estimated by measurement of esophageal pressure (P_{eso}), by a thin latex balloon-tipped catheter connected via a polyethylene catheter to a pressure transducer (Special Instrument DigimaClic ±100 cmH2O; Nordlingen, Germany). The esophageal balloon was filled with 1–1.5 ml of air and the correct position of the probe was verified on the computer software of recording and analysis (ICU Lab, KleisTEK Engineering, Bari, Italy) according to the literature [20–24].

The end-inspiratory and end-expiratory occlusions were performed through the inspiratory and expiratory holds on the Fabius GS Premium ventilator.

Total positive end expiratory pressure ($PEEP_{TOT}$), P_{AO}, P_{PLAT}, P_L, C_{RS}, C_L, C_{CW}, ΔP_{RS} and ΔP_L were measured as previously described [15].

Statistical analysis

A sample size calculation was performed using data from our previous study [6] on the effects of recruiting maneuvers on C_{RS} and PaO_2/FiO_2 in patients undergoing OLV for thoracic surgery. Based on these data, the significant change in C_{RS} before and after the recruitment maneuver was designated as a 25% C_{RS} increase with a SD of 8.9 and the improvement in PaO_2/FiO_2 as a ratio increase of 115 with a SD of 120. The larger sample size of 13 patients resulted from the P/F ratio and was used for patients' enrollment. The α and β errors for the sample size were chosen as 0.05 and 0.90 respectively [25, 26]. Statistical comparison of respiratory mechanics, hemodynamic and gas exchange data was performed between the two study steps: data were tested for normal distribution by the Kolmogorov-Smirnov goodness- of –fit test and presented as mean (±SD). Paired T-test analysis was performed between $OLV_{pre\text{-}OLA}$ and $OLV_{post\text{-}OLA}$ to evaluate the effect of the recruitment maneuvers on respiratory mechanics, hemodynamic and gas exchange. A p value < 0.05 was considered statistically significant. Data are presented as mean ± SD. Statistical analysis was performed using the software Statistica 10.0 (Statsoft Italia srl 2011).

Results

Thirteen out of 24 patients initially evaluated for enrolment were included in the study. The enrolment flow diagram is reported in Fig. 2. The mean external PEEP

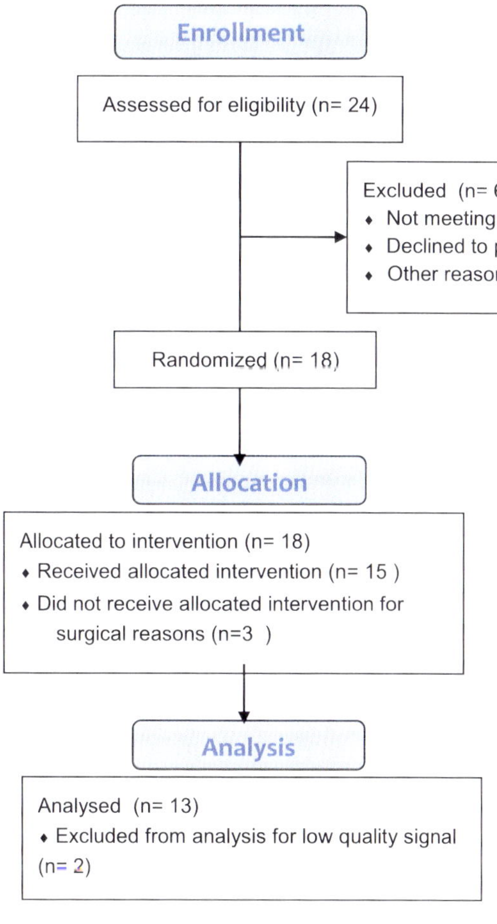

Fig. 2 CONSORT flow chart

resulting from the decremental PEEP titration after the RM was 6 ± 0.8 cmH_2O (range 5–8 cmH_2O).

Demographic characteristics and baseline spirometric data of the population studied are presented in Table 1. The study was completed successfully in all the patients without protocol-related complications or adverse events.

None of the patients was affected by postoperative pulmonary complications.

Hemodynamic parameters remained unchanged throughout the study despite a transient decrease in CI and MAP during the RM (Table 2).

Table 3 shows the main respiratory mechanics and gas exchange parameters throughout the study (data are expressed as mean ± SD). On $OLV_{pre\text{-}OLA}$ the PaO_2/FiO_2 ratio was 205 ± 73 and improved to 313 ± 86 ($p = 0.05$) on $OLV_{post\text{-}OLA}$ while $PaCO_2$ and pH remained unchanged.

Both C_{RS} and C_L significantly increased from 45 ± 11 ml/cmH_2O to 62 ± 13 ml/cmH_2O and from 56 ± 18 ml/cmH_2O to 71 ± 12 ml/cmH_2O ($p = 0.001$, $p = 0.0013$, vs $OLV_{pre\text{-}OLA}$, respectively), while C_{CW} did not change.

Airway resistance (Raw) went from 11.24 ± 3.72 cmH_2O/L/s to 7.42 ± 4.21 cmH_2O/L/s. ΔP_{RS} and ΔP_L decreased after the OLA from 9.2 ± 0.4 cmH_2O to 6.9 ± 0.6 cmH_2O and from 8.1 ± 0.5 cmH_2O to 5.7 ± 0.5 cmH_2O respectively ($p = 0.001$ and $p = 0.015$ vs $OLV_{pre\text{-}OLA}$).

Discussion

The main result of the present study is that during OLV in lateral decubitus, the application of an open lung strategy consisting in a RM followed by a decremental PEEP titration significantly improves oxygenation and lung mechanical properties without significant hemodynamic effects.

It is well acknowledged that OLV in lateral decubitus may induce a "multiple-hit" mechanism for lung injury: on one side the dependent lung is prone to mechanical damage due to intratidal cyclic parenchymal opening and closing, compression by mediastinal structures, surgical manipulations and loss of elastic recoil, on the other there is the collapse and re-expansion of the non dependent lung [27]. Moreover, the reduction of aerated lung capacity may worsen the ventilation-to-perfusion matching that could result in a significant gas exchange impairment [28, 29]. The common ventilatory setting to counterbalance hypoxemia during OLV used to include Vt as high as during two-lungs ventilation (i.e. 8 to 10 ml/Kg) [7, 30–32] and PEEP as a rescue therapy in case of severe hypoxemia, in selected patients. Recent studies, however, demonstrated that large Vts do exacerbate the risk for Ventilator-Induced Lung Injury (VILI) through the enhancement of oxidative and inflammatory reactions [33], whereas a lung-protective ventilatory strategy with smaller Vt and PEEP applied after appropriate lung recruitment on the dependent lung during OLV minimizes VILI, resulting in less postoperative lung complications [34–38], and increases oxygenation [9, 18, 19, 28]. However, very low Vts as the one suggested for ventilating the dependent lung during OLV (4–5 ml/Kg) may per se induce alveolar de-recruitment unless an "adequate" PEEP level is set. Unfortunately, there is no agreement on the correct PEEP setting in the OLV context. In a recent study, Spadaro and coworkers documented the physiological interplay between very low Vts and two PEEP levels (5 and 10 cmH_2O) on oxygenation, respiratory mechanics and ventilation/perfusion

Table 1 Patients demographic characteristics

Patient No	Age (yr)	Sex	BMI (Kg/m^2)	ASA	pH	PaO_2 (mmHg)	$PaCO_2$ (mmHg)	FEV_1 (% Pred)	FEV_1/FVC (%)	Surgery	Duration (min)
1	60-69	2	21.6	2	7.31	73	53	42	67	Left upper lobectomy	75
2	50-59	2	19.64	4	7.43	76	43	55	67	Left upper lobectomy	65
3	60-70	2	20.83	3	7.42	82	38	65	77	Left upper lobectomy	80
4	50-60	2	22.18	3	7.42	108	24	87	88	Left upper lobectomy	70
5	60-70	2	25.75	3	7.42	81	48	50	60	Left upper lobectomy	70
6	50-60	2	16.86	2	7.38	73	43	115	108	Left upper lobectomy	60
7	50-60	2	22.05	2	7.42	89	47	98.2	77	Left upper lobectomy	85
8	50-60	1	20.83	3	7.4	73	42	42	67	Left upper lobectomy	90
9	40-50	2	25.75	3	7.41	89	50	69	78	Left upper lobectomy	95
10	70-80	2	22.41	2	7.38	84	38	96	99	Left upper lobectomy	105
11	60-70	2	23.33	2	7.38	113	40	57	107	Left upper lobectomy	110
12	60-70	1	19.39	4	7.4	97	43	82	71	Left upper lobectomy	85
13	50-60	2	26.36	2	7.45	63	49	108	114	Left upper lobectomy	90
Mean	59		22.07		7.4	86.4	42.6	86.6	82.3		83.1
SD	6.8		2.75		0.03	16.2	6.15	22.5	19.43		17.35

BMI body mass index, *FEV_1* forced expiratory volume in 1 s, *% pred* percentage of the predicted value, *FVC* forced vital capacity; FiO2 during the ABG was 21%

Table 2 Hemodynamic parameters during the different experimental conditions

	TLV Baseline	OLV_{preOLA}	During RM	$OLV_{postOLA}$	TLV end	ANOVA
HR (b/m)	76 ±14	77± 12	80 ±11	76 ±13	75± 12	N.S.
MAP (mmHg)	91 ±12	86 ±15	82 ±10 *	88 ±14	90 ±11	$P < 0.05$
CI (l/m^2)	2.7 ±0.4	3.1 ±0.9	2.4± 0.3 *	2.8± 0.4	3.0± 0.2	$P< 0.05$
SVV (%)	12± 2	13 ±1	13± 2	13± 2	14 ±1	N.S.

ANOVA *$P<0.05$ TLV baseline vs RM
HR heart rate, *MAP* mean arterial blood pressure, *CI* cardiac index, *SVV* stroke volume variation, *TLV* two-lung ventilation, *OLV* one-lung ventilation, *RM* recruitment manoeuvre. Data are expressed as mean ± SD

mismatch during OLV. Their findings were that in this setting only a relatively high PEEP level (10 cmH_2O) guarantees improvement of gas exchange, shunt reduction and improvement of respiratory mechanics [39]. In the present study we found that lower PEEP levels, i.e. 6 ± 0.8 cmH_2O (range 5–8 cmH_2O) were able to improve oxygenation and lung mechanics. The apparent discrepancy between ours and Spadaro's data could be explained by the different design of the two studies. Indeed, we applied a complete lung recruitment and individualized PEEP titration strategy whereas Spadaro studied two fix PEEP levels were applied without previous maximal lung recruitment. Our study seems to confirm that in the OLV context, similarly than in early ARDS, a decremental PEEP titration trial is required to keep the lung fully opened after a maximal lung recruitment maneuver [40].

Table 3 Breathing pattern and gas exchange parameters during the different experimental conditions

	$OLV_{pre\text{-}OLA}$	$OLV_{post\text{-}OLA}$	*p*-value
V_T (ml/Kg PBW)	5.9±0.9	5.9±0.7	0.47
RR (breaths/min)	18±1	18±1	0.77
$P_{AO,\ PLAT}$ (cmH_2O)	12.8±1.6	16.7±2.2*	0.003
$PEEP_{ext}$ (cmH_2O)	0	6±0.8	0.3
$PEEP_{TOT,\ RS}$ (cmH_2O)	3.6±1.4	9.8±1.2*	0.0001
ΔP_{RS} (cmH_2O)	9.24±0.4	6.88±0.6*	0.001
ΔP_L (cmH_2O)	8.1±0.5	5.7±0.5*	0.015
C_{RS} (ml/cmH_2O)	45±11.3	62±13.4*	0.001
C_L (ml/cmH_2O)	56.17±18.18	71.06 ±12.25*	0.0013
C_{CW} (ml/cmH_2O)	310±15.4	312±14.2	NS
Raw ($cmH_2O/L/s$)	11.24±3.72	7.42±4.21*	0.004
pH	7.37±0.05	7.37±0.03	NS
$PaCO_2$ (mmHg)	44±2.9	43±3.8	NS
PaO_2/FiO_2(mmHg)	205±73	313±86*	0.004

Pared T-test was used for the comparison of continuous variables. Data are expressed as mean ± SD
C_{RS} respiratory system compliance, C_L lung compliance, C_{CW} chest wall compliance, ΔP_{RS} respiratory system driving pressure, ΔP_L transpulmonary driving pressure, FiO_2 inspiratory oxygen fraction, PaO_2 arterial oxygen tension, $PaCO_2$ arterial carbon dioxide tension, *PEEP* positive end expiratory pressure, $PEEP_{ext}$ external PEEP, $PEEP_{TOT,RS}$ respiratory system total PEEP, $P_{AO,PLAT}$ respiratory system plateau airways pressure, *RR* respiratory rate, V_T tidal volume
statistical significant when compared to $OLV_{pre\text{-}OLA}$

In a previous report, our group demonstrated that, besides the positive effect on gas exchange, the application of a RM followed by a standard PEEP of 5 mmHg during OLV induces a reduction in E_{RS} [6]. Recently, Ferrando et al. [11], showed that the improvement in C_{RS}, dead space and oxygenation during OLV was more noticeable in patients undergoing a PEEP titration after the RM. Actually, individualizing the level of PEEP required to maintain the lung open after the RM, is presently considered superior to the "one-size-fit-all" method of standardized PEEP in order to match that particular patients respiratory mechanical properties [41]. Currently, the appropriate method to select PEEP remains unclear, however the decremental PEEP titration method that we used in the present study and that lead to an average PEEP level of 6 ± 0.8 cmH_2O, is widely studied and relatively easy to perform at the bedside, even during anesthesia [11, 18, 19]. When compared to Ferrando et al. [11], we used the same recruitment maneuver and observed an improvement in gas exchange and C_{RS}. The novelty of our study is that we partitioned lung and chest wall mechanics response to the OLA strategy, which allowed to highlight how this response is attributable mainly to the lung component. In literature, an amount of data confirm that the dependent hemithorax is compressed in lateral position: actually, the static P/V curve of the lungs has a rightward horizontal shift in lateral decubitus as compared to the upright position (i.e. about15% less compliant), with a similar slope [42]. By separately measuring the C_{RS} of both hemithoraces, Klingsted et al. [43], in a seminal paper demonstrated that the C_{RS} of the dependent hemithorax is about two-thirds of the contra lateral one when both lungs are ventilated in lateral decubitus (as during differential lung ventilation (DLV)). Interestingly, they also found that when switching to OLV, the static airway P/V curve of the dependent lung (super-syringe method with inflation of 1.5–2 l), is shifted to the left and steeper, as compared to the P/V curve obtained in the same lung during DLV, and therefore demonstrated a greater potential for lung recruitment with the application of selective PEEP. The same was observed for the esophageal P/V curve, which was shifted to the left and steeper, showing a small increase in pressure for the whole volume range.

This suggests that during OLV the elastic recoil of the non-dependent, collapsed lung and the "compression" that it may exert on the dependent lung are lower than the elastic, expanding force in the chest wall. Our results seem to confirm these data. We measured respiratory mechanics on the dependent lung and found that on OLV_{pre}, the chest wall contributed roughly by 30% to total respiratory system elastance whereas the lung contributed by 70%. After implementing the OLA strategy, the absolute chest wall elastance did not change and therefore the decrease in total respiratory system elastance was due essentially to the decrease in lung elastance.

The reduction in inspiratory resistances observed, further suggests a more even distribution of Vt within the lung following the opening up of collapsed alveoli. Moreover, it seems reasonable to hypothesize that patients lateral position per se (surgical bed tilted in mild reverse Trendelenburg to allow a better surgical exposure, and consequent reduced abdominal content's backpressure against the diaphragm [38]), keeps chest wall mechanics invariable, as demonstrated by the unchanged E_{CW} absolute average value after the OLA.

An additional result of the present study is the reduction of both airways and transpulmonary driving pressure following the OLA strategy. Our study protocol was not specifically designed to study driving pressures: PEEP titration was indeed performed in order to obtain the highest C_{RS} and not the lowest ΔP. In that case, actually, different PEEP level would probably have been reached, anyway we believe that this unanticipated result does deserve some considerations.

An increasing amount of data in literature suggests that driving pressure is a predictor of mortality in ARDS patients [44, 45], and a key mediator of the effects of various ventilatory interventions [5, 6, 15]. ΔP is the tidal change in static trans-respiratory pressure, measured as P_{PlatRS}-$PEEP_{tot}$, in response to a volume-controlled breath and expresses the ratio between Vt and respiratory system compliance Vt/C_{RS} [45]. Many data show that reducing the alveolar cyclic collapse and reopening (atelectrauma) may protect lungs from VILI [44, 45]. Therefore, a ventilatory setting aimed at obtaining the lowest ΔP is suggested as method for personalizing ventilation to individual lung physiology. The reduction in ΔP following recruitment manoeuvres and/or PEEP application is also regarded as a realistic target for ventilatory adjustments. Moreover, measuring the tidal change of the real lung-distending pressure, i.e. ΔP_L, is suggested as a useful tool to understand how much of the ΔP is due to the lungs and how much to chest wall elastance [45]. The relationship between the two driving pressures is not thoroughly clarified; however, in our patients the parallel reduction of both driving pressures measured during volume-controlled ventilation after the OLA as compared to the ones measured before the OLA, may suggests its efficacy in terms of alveolar recruitment and, if confirmed by further studies, could corroborate the usefulness of ΔP monitoring.

We also confirm that a correct hemodynamic management during the OLA strategy, does allow a safe maneuver: indeed, once the volemic status was optimized through the SVV, the OLA did not affect hemodynamic, if one excludes transient and not clinically relevant decrease in CI and PAM during the RM.

This study has nonetheless a few limitations. Firstly, we could not measure recruited volume, since we needed to keep respiratory mechanics measurement as short as possible in order not to prolong surgery. As regards esophageal pressure measurement, its pro and cons as a surrogate for transpulmonary pressure have been widely debated in literature [21–24], and any further discussion is beyond the scope of the present study. Nonetheless, the feasibility of P_{es} and the signal quality could be questioned when switching from supine to lateral position, since the heart, the mediastinum, and the weight of the surrounding parenchyma could compress and modify the balloon's shape. However, we believe that these shortcomings should have been counterbalanced by having P_{es} waveforms always collected by the same operator (MR), and the Baydur test and the filling volume test repeatedly performed within the duration of the surgery.

Although the sample population size was small, as is the rule for physiologically oriented cross over studies like ours, our data suggest that the OLA strategy could optimize oxygenation and lung mechanics during OLV. However, physiological improvements not necessarily translate in improvements in clinically meaningful outcome parameters. Recently, a large RCT in patients undergoing major abdominal surgery was not able to show any advantage of a perioperative OLA strategy over standard treatment in terms of a composite endpoint of postoperative pulmonary and systemic complications [46]. Nevertheless, due to the peculiarities of OLV, the potential impact of OLA during OLV in a large RCT is worth to investigate and the ongoing PROTHOR study (will hopefully add more definitive knowledge in this field (clinicaltrials.gov ID NCT02963025).

Conclusions

The results of our study provide evidence that decremental PEEP titration on the best C_{RS}, immediately after maximal lung recruitment, improves oxygenation and lung mechanics. Beyond these clear physiological benefits, the eventual impact of the OLA strategy on patients outcome is yet unknown and warrants further clinical studies.

Abbreviations

% pred: percentage of the predicted value; ARDS: Acute Respiratory Distress Syndrome; BIS: Bi-spectral index; BMI: Body mass index; BP: Blood pressure; CI: Cardiac index; C_L: Lung compliance; CO: Cardiac output; C_{RS}: Respiratory system compliance; FEV_1: Forced expiratory volume in 1 s; FiO_2: Inspiratory oxygen fraction; FVC: Forced vital capacity; HR: Heart rate; mBP: Mean arterial blood pressure; OLA: Open lung approach; OLV: One lung ventilation; $PaCO_2$: arterial carbon dioxide tension; $P_{AO,PLAT}$: Respiratory system plateau airways pressure; PaO_2: arterial oxygen tension; PEEP: Positive end expiratory pressure; P_{eso}: esophageal pressure; P_L: Transpulmonary pressure; RM: Recruitment maneuvers; RR: Respiratory rate; SV: Stroke volume; SVV: Stroke volume variation; VILI: Ventilator induced lung injury; V_T: Tidal volume; ΔP_{RS} and ΔP_L: Respiratory system and transpulmonary driving pressure

Acknowledgements

None.

Funding

The study was funded by a project grant from the University of Foggia, Italy (n. 85/2009). None of the paper authors received honorarium from Companies involved in the study.

Authors' contributions

All authors have read and approved the final version. MR: Conception and design of the study, acquisition of data, analysis and interpretation of data, participated in drafting and revising the manuscript. LM: Revised the manuscript critically for important intellectual content. SG: Revised the manuscript critically for important intellectual content. AC: Participated in drafting the manuscript. SS: Participated in drafting the manuscript, analysis and interpretation of data. DD'A: Acquisition of data. FV: Acquisition of data. LT: Participated in drafting the manuscript. DL: Acquisition of data. FS: Acquisition of data. GC: Conception and design, interpretation of data, gave final approval of the version to be submitted.

Competing interests

The authors Savino Spadaro and Gilda Cinnella are Associate Editors for BMC Anesthesiology.

Author details

[1]Department of Anesthesia and Intensive care, University of Foggia, Viale Pinto, 1-71100 Foggia, Italy. [2]Department of Anesthesia and Intensive care, University of Bari, Bari, Italy. [3]Department of Anesthesia and Intensive care, University of Ferrara, Ferrara, Italy. [4]Department of Thoracic Surgery, University of Foggia, Foggia, Italy. [5]Interdepartmental Division of Critical Care Medicine, University of Toronto, Toronto, ON, Canada.

References

1. Park SH, Jeon YT, Hwang JW, Do SH, Kim JH, Park HP. A preemptive alveolar recruitment strategy before one-lung ventilation improves arterial oxygenation in patients undergoing thoracic surgery: a prospective randomised study. Eur J Anaesthesiol. 2011;28(4):298–302.
2. Ng A, Swanevelder J. Hypoxaemia associated with one-lung anaesthesia: new discoveries in ventilation and perfusion. Br J Anaesth. 2011;106(6):761–3. https://doi.org/10.1093/bja/aer113.
3. Lohser J. Evidence-based Management of one-Lung Ventilation. Anesthesiology Clin. 2008;26:241–72. https://doi.org/10.1016/j.anclin.2008.01.011.
4. Hoftman N, Canales C, Leduc M, Mahajan A. Positive end expiratory pressure during one-lung ventilation: selecting ideal patients and ventilator settings with the aim of improving arterial oxygenation. Ann Card Anaesth. 2011;14(3):183–7. https://doi.org/10.4103/0971-9784.83991.
5. Borges JB, Senturk M, Ahlgren O, Hedenstierna G, Larsson A. Open lung in lateral decubitus with differential selective positive end-expiratory pressure in an experimental model of early acute respiratory distress syndrome. Crit Care Med. 2015;43(10):e404–11. https://doi.org/10.1097/CCM.0000000000001143.
6. Cinnella G, Grasso S, Natale C, Sollitto F, Cacciapaglia M, Angiolillo M, Pavone G, Mirabella L, Dambrosio M. Physiological effects of a lung-recruiting strategy applied during one-lung ventilation. Acta Anaesthesiol Scand. 2008;52:766–75. https://doi.org/10.1111/j.1399-6576.2008.01652.x.
7. Gama de Abreu M, Heintz M, Heller A, Széchényi R, Albrecht DM, Koch T. One-lung ventilation with high tidal volumes and zero positive end-expiratory pressure is injurious in the isolated rabbit lung model. Anesth Analg. 2003;96:220–8.
8. Slinger P. Pro: low tidal volume is indicated during one-lung ventilation. Cardiovasc Anesth. 2006;103:2. https://doi.org/10.1213/01.ane.0000223701.24874.c8.
9. Unzueta C, Tusman G, Suarez-Sipmann F, Bohm S, Moral V. Alveolar recruitment improves ventilation during thoracic surgery: a randomized controlled trial. Br J Anaesth. 2006;108(3):517–24. https://doi.org/10.1093/bja/aer415.
10. Michelet P, Blayac D, Vincent A, D'journo X-B, Perrin G, Badier M, Thomas P, Bregeon F. How do COPD and healthy-lung patients tolerate the reduced volume ventilation strategy during OLV ventilation. Acta Anaesthesiol Scand. 2010;54:1128–36. https://doi.org/10.1111/j.1399-6576.2010.02281.x.
11. Ferrando C, Mugarra A, Gutierrez A, Carbonell JA, García M, Soro M, Tusman G, Belda FJ. Setting individualized positive end-expiratory pressure level with a positive end-expiratory pressure decrement trial after a recruitment maneuver improves oxygenation and lung mechanics during one-lung ventilation. Anesth Analg. 2014;118:657–65.
12. Slinger PD, Kruger M, McRae K, Winton T. Relation of the static compliance curve and positive end-expiratory pressure to oxygenation during one-lung ventilation. Anesthesiology. 2001;95:1096–102.
13. Gattinoni L, Caironi P, Cressoni M, Chiumello D, Ranieri VM, Quintel M, Russo S, Patroniti N, Cornejo R, Bugedo G. Lung recruitment in patients with the acute respiratory distress syndrome. N Engl J Med. 2006; 27;354(17):1775–86.
14. Pepe PE, Hudson LD, Carrico CJ. Early application of positive end-expiratory pressure in patients at risk for the adult respiratory-distress syndrome. N Engl J Med. 1984;311(5):281–6.
15. Cinnella G, Grasso S, Spadaro S, Rauseo M, Mirabella L, Salatto P, De Capraris A, Nappi L, Greco P, Dambrosio M. Effects of Recruitment Maneuver and Positive End-expiratory Pressure on Respiratory Mechanics and Transpulmonary Pressure during Laparoscopic Surgery. Anesthesiology. 2013;118:114–22.
16. Garutti I, Martinez G, Cruz P, Piñeiro P, Olmedilla L, de la Gala F. The Impact of Lung Recruitment on Hemodynamics During One-Lung Ventilation. J Cardiothorac Vasc Anesth. 2009;23(4):506–8. https://doi.org/10.1053/j.jvca.2008.12.023.
17. Benes J, Chytra I, Altmann P, Hluchy M, Kasal E, Svitak R, Pradl R, Stepan M. Intraoperative fluid optimization using stroke volume variation in high risk surgical patients: results of prospective randomized study. Crit Care. 2010; 14(3):R118. https://doi.org/10.1186/cc9070.
18. Tusman G, Böhm SH, Melkun F, Staltari D, Quinzio C, Nador C, Turchetto E. Alveolar recruitment strategy increases arterial oxygenation during one-lung ventilation. Ann Thorac Surg. 2002;73:1204–9.
19. Tusman G, Bohm SH, Sipmann FS, Maisch S. Lung recruitment improves the efficiency of ventilation and gas exchange during one-lung ventilation anesthesia. Anesth Analg. 2004;98:1604–9.
20. Talmor D, Sarge T, Malhotra A, O'Donnell CR, Ritz R, Lisbon A, Novack V, Loring SH. Mechanical ventilation guided by esophageal pressure in acute lung injury. N Engl J Med. 2008;359:2095–104. https://doi.org/10.1056/NEJMoa0708638.

21. Akoumianaki E, Maggiore SM, Valenza F, Bellani G, Jubran A, Loring SH, Pelosi P, Talmor D, Grasso S, Chiumello D, Guérin C, Patroniti N, Ranieri VM, Gattinoni L, Nava S, Terragni PP, Pesenti A, Tobin M, Mancebo J, Brochard L. PLeUral pressure working Group (PLUG—Acute Respiratory Failure section of the European Society of Intensive Care Medicine). The application of esophageal pressure measurement in patients with respiratory failure. Am J Respir Crit Care Med. 2014;189:520–31.
22. Chiumello D, Cressoni M, Colombo A, Babini G, Brioni M, Crimella F, Lundin S, Stenqvist O, Gattinoni L. The assessment of transpulmonary pressure in mechanically ventilated ARDS patients. Intensive Care Med. 2014;40(11): 1670–8. https://doi.org/10.1007/s00134-014-3415-4.
23. Chiumello D, Consonni D, Coppola S, Froio S, Crimella F, Colombo A. The occlusion tests and end-expiratory esophageal pressure: measurements and comparison in controlled and assisted ventilation. Ann Intensive Care. 2016; 6(1):13.
24. Mauri T, Yoshida T, Bellani G, Goligher EC, Carteaux G, Rittayamai N, Mojoli F, Chiumello D, Piquilloud L, Grasso S, Jubran A, Laghi F, Magder S, Pesenti A, Loring S, Gattinoni L, Talmor D, Blanch L, Amato M, Chen L, Brochard L, Mancebo J. PLeUral pressure working Group (PLUG—Acute Respiratory Failure section of the European Society of Intensive Care Medicine). Esophageal and transpulmonary pressure in the clinical setting: meaning, usefulness and perspectives. Intensive Care Med. 2016;42(9):1360–73. https://doi.org/10.1007/s00134-016-4400-x.
25. Bland JM, Altman DG. Measuring agreement in method comparison studies. Stat Methods Med Res. 1999;8:135–60.
26. Bland JM, Altman DG. Statistical methods for assessing agreement between two methods of clinical measurement. Lancet 1986; 8;1(8476):307–10.
27. Benumof JL. Conventional and differential lung management of one-lung ventilation. In: Benumof JL, editor. Anesthesia for thoracic surgery. Philadelphia: WB Saunders; 1995. p. 406–31.
28. Kozian A, Schilling T, Schütze H, Senturk M, Hachenberg T, Hedenstierna G. Ventilatory protective strategies during thoracic surgery: effects of alveolar recruitment maneuver and low-tidal volume ventilation on lung density distribution. Anesthesiology. 2011;114:1025–35.
29. Schilling T, Kozian A, Huth C, et al. The pulmonary immune effects of mechanical ventilation in patients undergoing thoracic surgery. Anesth Analg. 2005;101:957–65.
30. Shen Y, Zhong M, Wu W, Wang H, Feng M, Tan L, Wang Q. The impact of tidal volume on pulmonary complications following minimally invasive esophagectomy: a randomized and controlled study. J Thorac Cardiovasc Surg. 2013;146:1267–73.
31. Wrigge H, Uhlig U, Zinserling J, Behrends-Callsen E, Ottersbach G, Fischer M, Uhlig S, Putensen C. The effects of different ventilatory settings on pulmonary and systemic inflammatory responses during major surgery. Anesth Analg. 2004;98:775–81.
32. Végh T, Juhász M, Szatmári S, Enyedi A, Sessler DI, Szegedi LL, Fülesdi B. Effects of different tidal volumes for one-lung ventilation on oxygenation with open chest condition and surgical manipulation: a randomised cross-over trial. Minerva Anestesiol. 2013;79:24–32.
33. Michelet P, D'Journo XB, Roch A, Doddoli C, Marin V, Papazian L, Decamps I, Bregeon F, Thomas P, Auffray JP. Protective ventilation influences systemic inflammation after esophagectomy: a randomized controlled study. Anesthesiology. 2006;105:911–9.
34. Sutherasan Y, D'Antini D, Pelosi P. Advances in ventilator-associated lung injury: prevention is the target. Expert Rev Respir Med. 2014;8(2):233–48. https://doi.org/10.1586/17476348.2014.890519.
35. Qutub H, El-Tahan MR, Mowafi HA, El Ghoneimy YF, Regal MA, Al Saflan AA. Effect of tidal volume on extravascular lung water content during one-lung ventilation for videoassisted thoracoscopic surgery: a randomised, controlled trial. Eur J Anaesthesiol. 2014;31:466–73.
36. Verhage RJ, Boone J, Rijkers GT, Cromheecke GJ, Kroese AC, Weijs TJ, Borel Rinkes IH, van Hillegersberg R. Reduced local immune response with continuous positive airway pressure during one-lung ventilation for oesophagectomy. Br J Anaesth. 2014;112:920–8.
37. Fujiwara M, Abe K, Mashimo T. The effect of positive endexpiratory pressure and continuous positive airway pressure on the oxygenation and shunt fraction during one-lung ventilation with propofol anesthesia. J Clin Anesthesia. 2001;13:473–7.
38. Lohser J, Slinger P. Lung injury after one-lung ventilation: a review of the pathophysiologic mechanisms affecting the ventilated and the collapsed lung. Anesth Analg. 2015;121(2):302–18. https://doi.org/10.1213/ANE.0000000000000808.
39. Spadaro S, Grasso S, Karbing DS, Fogagnolo A, Contoli M, Bollini G, Ragazzi R, Cinnella G, Verri M, Cavallesco NG, Rees SE, Volta CA. Physiologic evaluation of ventilation perfusion mismatch and respiratory mechanics at different positive end-expiratory pressure in patients undergoing protective one-lung ventilation. Anesthesiology. 2018 Mar;128(3):531–8. https://doi.org/10.1097/ALN.0000000000002011.
40. Cinnella G, Grasso S, Raimondo P, D'Antini D, Mirabella L, Rauseo M, Dambrosio M. Physiological effects of the open lung approach in patients with early, mild, diffuse acute respiratory distress syndrome: an electrical impedance tomography study. Anesthesiology. 2015 Nov;123(5):1113–21. https://doi.org/10.1097/ALN.0000000000000862.
41. Nieman GF, Satalin J, Andrews P, Aiash H, Habashi NM, Gatto LA. Personalizing mechanical ventilation according to physiologic parameters to stabilize alveoli and minimize ventilator induced lung injury (VILI). Intensive Care Med Exp. 2017;5(1):8. https://doi.org/10.1186/s40635-017-0121-x.
42. Washko GR, O'Donnell CR, Loring SHJ. Volume-related and volume-independent effects of posture on esophageal and transpulmonary pressures in healthy subjects. Appl Physiol (1985). 2006;100(3):753–8.
43. Klingstedt C, Baehrendtz S, Bindslev L, Hedenstierna G. Lung and chest wall mechanics during differential ventilation with selective PEEP. Acta Anaesthesiol Scand. 1985;29(7):716–21.
44. Serpa Neto A, Hemmes SN, Barbas CS, Beiderlinden M, Fernandez-Bustamante A, Futier E, Hollmann MW, Jaber S, Kozian A, Licker M, Lin WQ, Moine P, Scavonetto F, Schilling T, Selmo G, Severgnini P, Sprung J, Treschan T, Unzueta C, Weingarten TN, Wolthuis EK, Wrigge H, Gama de Abreu M, Pelosi P, Schultz MJ. PROVE Network investigators. Incidence of mortality and morbidity related to postoperative lung injury in patients who have undergone abdominal or thoracic surgery: a systematic review and meta-analysis. Lancet Respir Med. 2014;2(12):1007–15. https://doi.org/10.1016/S2213-2600(14)70228-0.
45. Amato MB, Meade MO, Slutsky AS, Brochard L, Costa EL, Schoenfeld DA, Stewart TE, Briel M, Talmor D, Mercat A, Richard JC, Carvalho CR, Brower RG. Driving pressure and survival in the acute respiratory distress syndrome. N Engl J Med. 2015;372:747–55. https://doi.org/10.1056/NEJMsa1410639.
46. Ferrando C, Soro M, Unzueta C, Suarez-Sipmann F, Canet J, Librero J, Pozo N, Peiró S, Llombart A, León I, India I, Aldecoa C, Díaz-Cambronero O, Pestaña D, Redondo FJ, Garutti I, Balust J, García JI, Ibáñez M, Granell M, Rodríguez A, Gallego L, de la Matta M, Gonzalez R, Brunelli A, García J, Rovira L, Barrios F, Torres V, Hernández S, Gracia E, Giné M, García M, García N, Miguel L, Sánchez S, Piñeiro P, Pujol R, García-Del-Valle S, Valdivia J, Hernández MJ, Padrón O, Colás A, Puig J, Azparren G, Tusman G, Villar J, Belda J. Individualized PeRioperative Open-lung VEntilation (iPROVE) Network. Individualised perioperative open-lung approach versus standard protective ventilation in abdominal surgery (iPROVE): a randomised controlled trial. Lancet Respir Med. 2018;6(3):193–203. https://doi.org/10.1016/S2213-2600(18)30024-9 Epub 2018 Jan 19.

19

Positive end-expiratory pressure improves elastic working pressure in anesthetized children

Pablo Cruces[1,2], Sebastián González-Dambrauskas[3], Federico Cristiani[4], Javier Martínez[3], Ronnie Henderson[4], Benjamin Erranz[5] and Franco Díaz[5,6,7*]

Abstract

Background: Positive end-expiratory pressure (PEEP) has been demonstrated to decrease ventilator-induced lung injury in patients under mechanical ventilation (MV) for acute respiratory failure. Recently, some studies have proposed some beneficial effects of PEEP in ventilated patients without lung injury. The influence of PEEP on respiratory mechanics in children is not well known. Our aim was to determine the effects on respiratory mechanics of setting PEEP at 5 cmH_2O in anesthetized healthy children.

Methods: Patients younger than 15 years old without history of lung injury scheduled for elective surgery gave informed consent and were enrolled in the study. After usual care for general anesthesia, patients were placed on volume controlled MV. Two sets of respiratory mechanics studies were performed using inspiratory and expiratory breath hold, with PEEP 0 and 5 cmH_2O. The maximum inspiratory and expiratory flow (Q_I and Q_E) as well as peak inspiratory pressure (PIP), plateau pressure (P_{PL}) and total PEEP (tPEEP) were measured. Respiratory system compliance (C_{RS}), inspiratory and expiratory resistances (RawI and RawE) and time constants (K_{TI} and K_{TE}) were calculated. Data were expressed as median and interquartile range (IQR). Wilcoxon sign test and Spearman's analysis were used. Significance was set at $P < 0.05$.

Results: We included 30 patients, median age 39 (15–61.3) months old, 60% male. When PEEP increased, PIP increased from 12 (11,14) to 15.5 (14,18), and C_{RS} increased from 0.9 (0.9,1.2) to 1.2 (0.9,1.4) $mL \cdot kg^{-1} \cdot cmH_2O^{-1}$; additionally, when PEEP increased, driving pressure decreased from 6.8 (5.9,8.1) to 5.8 (4.7,7.1) cmH_2O, and Q_E decreased from 13.8 (11.8,18.7) to 11.7 (9.1,13.5) $L \cdot min^{-1}$ (all $P < 0.01$). There were no significant changes in resistance and Q_I.

Conclusions: Analysis of respiratory mechanics in anesthetized healthy children shows that PEEP at 5 cmH_2O places the respiratory system in a better position in the P/V curve. A better understanding of lung mechanics may lead to changes in the traditional ventilatory approach, limiting injury associated with MV.

Keywords: Positive end-expiratory pressure, Mechanical ventilation, Respiratory mechanics, Pediatrics

* Correspondence: francodiazr@gmail.com
[5]Unidad de Cuidados Intensivos Pediátricos, Clínica Alemana de Santiago, Avda. Vitacura, 5951 Santiago, Chile
[6]Facultad de Medicina Clínica Alemana Universidad del Desarrollo, Santiago, Chile
Full list of author information is available at the end of the article

Table 1 Clinical characteristics of children included in the study

Number	Age (mo)	Weight (kg)	Height (cm)	Surgery	Comorbidities
1	40–50	17.5	105	Inguinal hernia	none
2	40–50	16.7	105	Umbilical hernia	none
3	30–40	13	90	Cryptorchid	none
4	10–20	5.1	67	CVL placement	Short bowel insufficiency
5	30–40	15	94	Anorectoplasty	Partial anomalous venous return
6	40–50	15	94	Inguinal hernia	Asthma
7	20–30	11.2	82	Epigastric hernia	none
8	10–20	9.2	70	Enterostomy closure	Imperforated anus
9	50–60	18	101	Enterostomy closure	Colostomy
10	60–70	14.2	104	Esophageal dilatation	Esofageal coloplasty
11	50–60	26	114	Abdominal tumor	none
12	30–40	22	99	Hidrocele	none
13	50–60	19	90	Fimosis	none
14	30–40	23	103	Cryptorchid	none
15	20–30	11.9	81	Inguinal hernia	none
16	70–80	24.6	120	Cryptorchid	none
17	3–10	7	63	Inguinal hernia	none
18	10–20	10.4	77	Inguinal hernia	none
19	10–20	13.5	80	Cryptorchid	none
20	120–130	25.8	132	Colecystectomy	none
21	3–10	5.7	62	Inguinal hernia	none
22	140–150	40	154.5	Thyroidectomy	none
23	3–10	4.9	N/A	Eventration repair	Traumatic eventration
24	80–90	19.7	116	Enterostomy closure	Hirschprung's Disease
25	80–90	27	118	Enterostomy closure	Hirschprung `sDisease
26	110–120	29	129.5	Anoplasty	Anorectal Malformation
27	100–110	21	116	CVL placement	Astrocytoma
28	10–50	14	103	Anoplasty	Anorectal malformation
29	1–10	4.6	56.5	Exploratory laparoscopy	none
30	10–20	7.3	77	CVL placement	Lymphoblastic leukemia

mo months old, *CVL* central venous line, *N/A* non-available

that changes in PEEP that resulted in an increase in ΔP were associated with more postoperative pulmonary complications. It is not surprising that in these studies, ΔP was the best predictor of unfavorable outcomes. We believe that the best performance of this parameter is because it integrates the set tidal volume and the patient's compliance, thus giving a more precise idea of the individual conditions of each patient.

In our patients, we observed a 14.8% (CI95% 9.3,20.3%) reduction of ΔP when PEEP of 5 cmH_2O was applied. The range of improvement was very wide and only one patient had a significant increase in ΔP (greater than 10%). These results are in accordance with a study by Wirth et al. They elegantly showed, with electric impedance tomography in 30 anesthetized children, that changing PEEP from 2 cmH_2O to 5 cmH_2O homogenizes regional lung ventilation [30]. One of our patients had a significant increase of ΔP. This a very good example that ventilatory settings need to be tailored individually, because adding 5 cmH_20 of PEEP probably led to overdistension in this patient. We maintained the set V_T after applying PEEP of 5 cmH_2O; thus, the reduction of ΔP was dependent on the improvement in C_{RS}. The improvement in C_{RS} and EELV may be seen as minor, but we believe that even these small changes may have significant consequences during and after surgery, reducing lung inflammation, alteration of gas exchange, among others. Experimental and clinical data have shown that injurious ventilatory parameters can generate detrimental effects, even when applied for short periods of time [1, 2, 31, 32].

Table 2 Ventilatory parameters and respiratory system mechanics of children under general anesthesia with ZEEP and PEEP of 5 cmH_2O

	ZEEP (n = 30)		PEEP 5 (n = 30)		P value
	MEDIAN	P25, P75	MEDIAN	P25, P75	
FiO_2	0.40	0.36, 0.50	0.40	0.36, 0.50	1.000
V_{TE}	6.79	6.18, 7.36	6.53	5.97, 7.20	0.290
RR	24	21, 26	24	21, 26	1.0
IT	0.85	0.72, 1.02	0.85	0.72, 1.03	1.00
PIP	12	11, 14	15.5	14.0, 18.5	< 0.01
P_{PL}	7.9	7.2, 9.18	10.95	9.7, 12.6	< 0.01
Paw	4.1	3.6, 4.9	8.5	7.9, 9.8	< 0.01
Q_I	11	8.1, 13.1	11	8.1, 13.1	0.317
Q_E	13.8	11.8, 13.1	11.7	9.1, 13.5	< 0.01
RawI	25.7	18.6, 34.3	26.4	20.1, 33.1	0.447
RawE	28.9	21.9, 39.4	29.3	22.3, 42.1	0.629
C_{RS}	0.96	0.89, 1.22	1.19	0.94, 1.39	< 0.01
K_{TI}	0.36	0.31, 0.48	0.45	0.38, 0.59	0.004

ZEEP PEEP 0 cmH_2O, *FiO_2* fraction of inspired oxygen, *V_{TE}* expiratory tidal volume ($mL{\cdot}kg^{-1}$), *RR* respiratory rate (breath per minute), *IT* inspiratory time (s), *PIP* peak inspiratory pressure (cmH_2O), *P_{PL}* plateau pressure (cmH_2O), *Paw* mean airway pressure (cmH_2O), *Q_I* peak inspiratory flow ($L{\cdot}min^{-1}$), *Q_E* peak expiratory flow, ($L{\cdot}min^{-1}$), *RawI* inspiratory airway resistance ($cmH_2O{\cdot}L^{-1}{\cdot}s^{-1}$), *RawE* expiratory airway resistance ($cmH_2O{\cdot}L^{-1}{\cdot}s^{-1}$), *$C_{RS}$* static respiratory system compliance ($mL{\cdot}cmH_2O^{-1}{\cdot}kg^{-1}$), *$K_{TI}$* inspiratory time constant (s)

The prolongation of K_{TI} and K_{TE} with PEEP of 5 cmH_2O probably reflects mathematical coupling of changes on C_{RS} without modifications on airway resistance. In the same way, the observed lower expiratory flow is related to the lower ΔP. These parameters are indirect markers of improvement on respiratory system mechanics and more protective ventilation.

Our study has some limitations. Respiratory mechanics measurements were done before the surgery, after a short period of applied PEEP; thus, we cannot extrapolate these findings to other surgical timings, e.g., during pneumoperitoneum, when the effect of PEEP preventing lung collapse could be even higher. Due to small size of patients, we did not measure pleural pressure, so we could not determine the contribution of the chest wall to C_{RS}. Included patients were heterogeneous and age range is wide, so in the absence of normal reference data, we cannot generalize these results to all pediatric patients (i.e., younger patients have higher chest compliance, being at higher risk for derecruitment of the lung on ZEEP). Finally, we have to acknowledge that setting of MV parameters can directly modify the component of the equation of motion (i.e., Q_I, RR, I:E ratio), but we tried to standardize the ventilatory setting during measurements. Despite these limitations, we consider our observation of the effect of PEEP in anesthetized

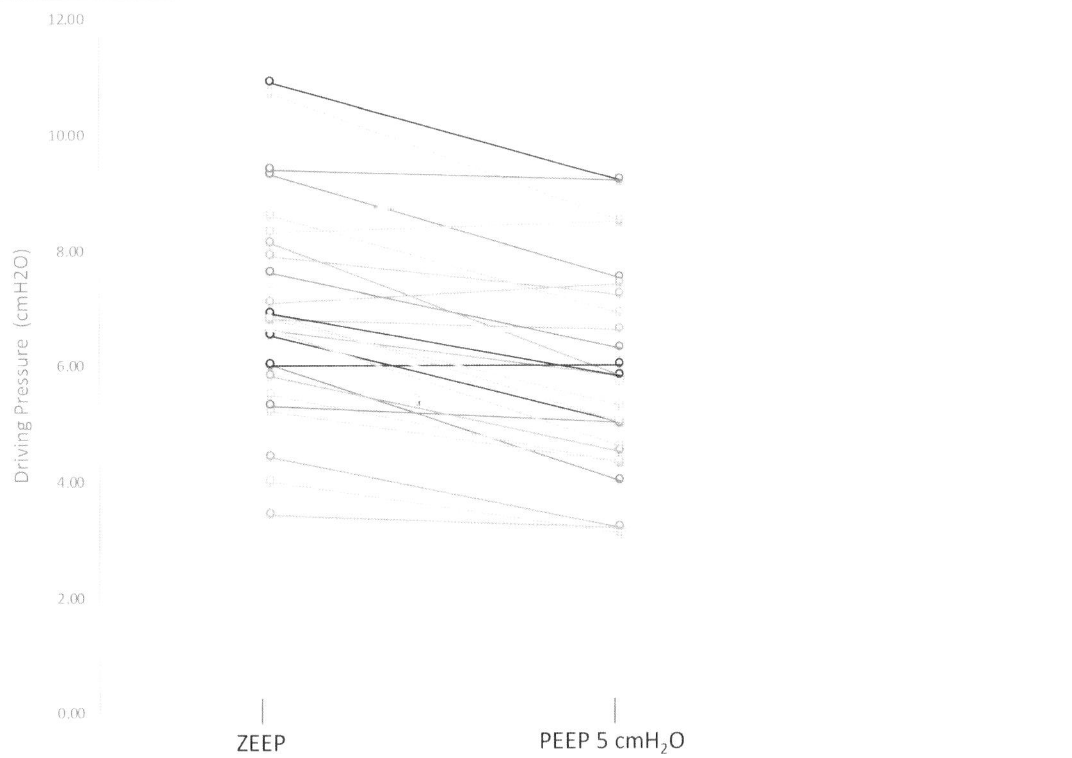

Fig. 1 Individual value plot of driving pressure (cmH_2O) with ZEEP and PEEP at 5 cmH_2O in anesthetized healthy children

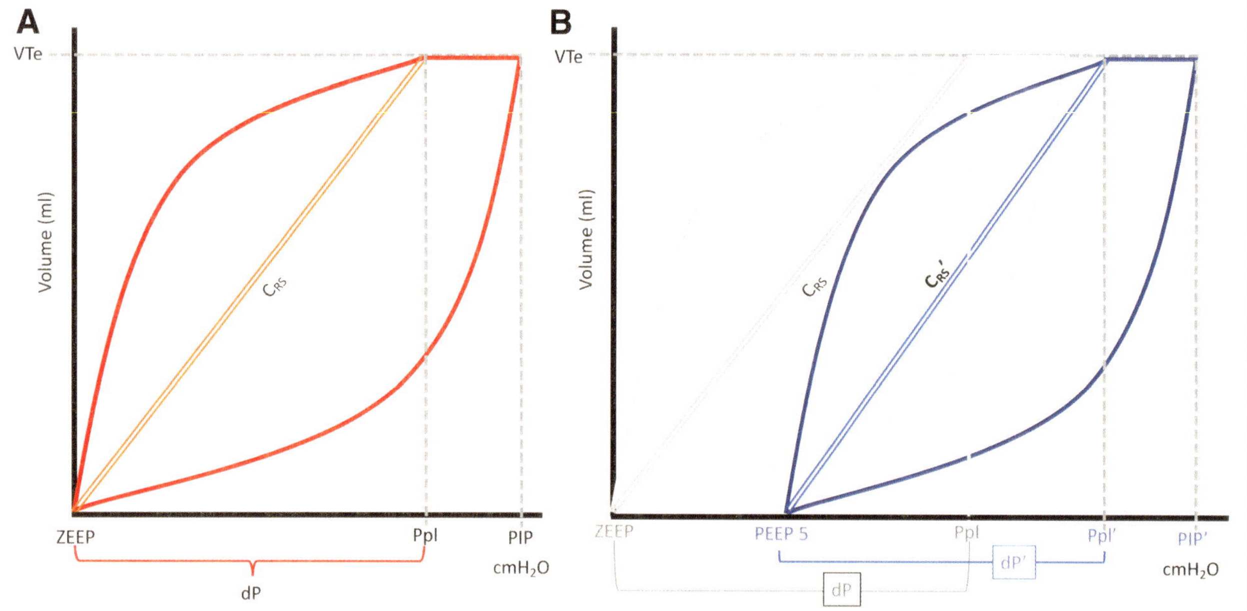

Fig. 2 Pressure – Volume loop (P/V curve) sketch summarizing findings of the study: Anesthetized children with ZEEP (panel **a**) and after setting PEEP at 5 cmH_2O (panel **b**). PIP, P_{PL} and Paw increased after addition of PEEP of 5 cmH_2O (PIP', P_{PL}',Paw'), but dP decreased (dP'). Given the same V_T, C_{RS}, represented as the angle of the diagonal line between PEEP and P_{PL}, increased (C_{RS}'). All of them are sign of a more efficient working pressures of the respiratory system better position in P/V curve. On (panel **b**) respiratory mechanics with ZEEP was added in gray tone as reference

children under mechanical ventilation important in terms of a pathophysiological approach to reduce VILI.

Conclusion

Setting PEEP at 5 cmH_2O in children during general anesthesia improved elastic working pressure of the respiratory system, decreasing driving pressure and intrinsic PEEP. These findings are indirect signs of lungs in a better position in pressure/volume curve, suggesting that the addition of a low level of PEEP improves respiratory mechanics. These findings may be measured with usual mechanical ventilators and anesthesia machines, analyzing respiratory system mechanics after an inspiratory and expiratory hold. Future studies in infants are needed to address respiratory mechanics during anesthesia, ideally in a specific age group and pathologies with high-risk postoperative complications. A better understanding of respiratory system mechanics in children during general anesthesia may lead to a better titration of mechanical ventilation, preventing VILI.

Abbreviations

ARDS: Acute respiratory distress syndrome; C_{RS}: Compliance respiratory system; CT: Computed tomography; EELV: End expiratory lung volume; iPEEP: Intrinsic positive pressure at the end of exhalation; K_{TE}: Expiratory time constant; K_{TI}: Inspiratory time constant; MV: Mechanical ventilation; Paw: Airway pressure; PEEP: Positive pressure at the end of exhalation; PIP: Peak inspiratory pressure; P_{PL}: Plateau pressure; Q_E: Maximum expiratory flow; Q_I: Maximum inspiratory flow; RawE: Resistance expiratory airway; RawI: Resistance inspiratory airway; RR: Respiratory rate; tPEEP: Total positive pressure at the end of exhalation; VILI: Ventilator induced lung injury; V_T: Tidal volume; ZEEP: Positive pressure at the end of exhalation set at 0 cmH_2O; ΔP: Driving pressure

Acknowledgements

'Not applicable'.

Funding

This work was supported by CONICYT #1160631 (Dr. Cruces) and CONICYT. #11160463 (Dr. Diaz) grants. These grants were involved in design of the study, collection of data, writing the manuscript and manuscript language edition services.

Authors' contributions

Study design: PC, SG, FC, JM, RH, FD; Measurements of respiratory mechanics: SG, FC, JM, RH; Statistic analysis: PC, BE, FD, SG; Writing the manuscript: PC,

SG, BE, FD; Review of the manuscript: All authors. All authors read and approved the final manuscript.

Competing interests

The authors declare that they have no competing interests.

Author details

[1]Pediatric Intensive Care Unit, Hospital El Carmen de Maipú, Santiago, Chile. [2]Centro de Investigación de Medicina Veterinaria, Escuela de Medicina Veterinaria, Facultad de Ecología y Recursos Naturales, Universidad Andres Bello, Santiago, Chile. [3]Pediatric Intensive Care Unit, Centro Hospitalario Pereira Rossell, Montevideo, Uruguay. [4]Department of Anesthesiology, Centro Hospitalario Pereira Rossell, Montevideo, Uruguay. [5]Unidad de Cuidados Intensivos Pediátricos, Clínica Alemana de Santiago, Avda. Vitacura, 5951 Santiago, Chile. [6]Facultad de Medicina Clínica Alemana Universidad del Desarrollo, Santiago, Chile. [7]Area de Cuidados Críticos, Hospital Padre Hurtado, Santiago, Chile.

References

1. Slutsky AS, Ranieri VM. Ventilator-induced lung injury. N Engl J Med. 2013; 369:2126–36.
2. Donoso A, Cruces P. Daño pulmonar inducido por ventilación mecánica y estrategia ventilatoria convencional protectora. Rev Chil Pediatr. 2007;78: 241–52.
3. Bein T, Grasso S, Moerer O, Quintel M, Guerin C, Deja M, et al. The standard of care of patients with ARDS: ventilatory settings and rescue therapies for refractory hypoxemia. Intensive Care Med. 2016;42:699–711.
4. Imai Y, Kawano T, Miyasaka K, Takata M, Imai T, Okuyama K. Inflammatory chemical mediators during conventional ventilation and during high frequency oscillatory ventilation. Am J Respir Crit Care Med. 1994;150:1550–4.
5. Tusman G, Böhm SH, Warner DO, Sprung J. Atelectasis and perioperative pulmonary complications in high-risk patients. Curr Opin Anaesthesiol. 2012;25:1–10.
6. Vargas M, Sutherasan Y, Gregoretti C, Pelosi P. PEEP role in ICU and operating room: from pathophysiology to clinical practice. ScientificWorldJournal. 2014;2014:852356.
7. Futier E, Constantin JM, Paugam-Burtz C, Pascal J, Eurin M, Neuschwander A, et al. IMPROVE study group. A trial of intraoperative low-tidal-volume ventilation in abdominal surgery. N Engl J Med. 2013;369:428–37.
8. Wolthuis EK, Choi G, Dessing MC, Bresser P, Lutter R, Dzoljic M, et al. Mechanical ventilation with lower tidal volumes and positive end-expiratory pressure prevents pulmonary inflammation in patients without preexisting lung injury. Anesthesiology. 2008;108:46–54.
9. Barbosa FT, Castro AA. de Sousa-Rodrigues CF. positive end-expiratory pressure (PEEP) during anaesthesia for prevention of mortality and postoperative pulmonary complications. Cochrane Database Syst Rev. 2014;6:CD007922.
10. Severgnini P, Selmo G, Lanza C, Chiesa A, Frigerio A, Bacuzzi A, et al. Protective mechanical ventilation during general anesthesia for open abdominal surgery improves postoperative pulmonary function. Anesthesiology. 2013;118:1307–21.
11. Wahba RW. Perioperative functional residual capacity. Can J Anaesth. 1991; 38;384–400.
12. Fletcher ME, Stack C, Ewart M, Davies CJ, Ridley S, Hatch DJ, et al. Respiratory compliance during sedation, anesthesia, and paralysis in infants and young children. J Appl Physiol. 1985;70:1977–82.
13. Dobbinson TL, Nisbet HI, Pelton DA, Levison H. Functional residual capacity (FRC) and compliance in anaesthetized paralysed children. II. Clinical results. Can Anaesth Soc J. 1973;20:322–33.
14. Serafini G, Cornara G, Cavalloro F, Mori A, Dore R, Marraro G, et al. Pulmonary atelectasis during paediatric anaesthesia: CT scan evaluation and effect of positive end-expiratory pressure (PEEP). Paediatr Anaesth. 1999;9:225–8.
15. Trachsel D, Svendsen J, Erb TO. von Ungern-Sternberg BS. Effects of anaesthesia on paediatric lung function. Br J Anaesth. 2016;117:151–63.
16. Feldman JM. Optimal ventilation of the anesthetized pediatric patient. Anesth Analg. 2015;120:165–75.
17. Wanderer JP, Ehrenfeld JM, Epstein RH, Kor DJ, Bartz RR, Fernandez-Bustamante A, et al. Temporal trends and current practice patterns for intraoperative ventilation at U.S. academic medical centers: a retrospective study. BMC Anesthesiol. 2015;15:40.
18. Kneyber MC. Intraoperative mechanical ventilation for the pediatric patient. Best Pract Res Clin Anaesthesiol. 2015;29:371–9.
19. Erranz B, Díaz F, Donoso A, Salomón T, Carvajal C, Torres MF, et al. Decreased lung compliance increases preload dynamic tests in a pediatric acute lung injury model. Rev Chil Pediatr. 2015;86:404–9.
20. Díaz F, Erranz B, Donoso A, Carvajal C, Salomón T, Torres M, Cruces P. Surfactant deactivation in a pediatric model induces hypovolemia and fluid shift to the extravascular lung compartment. Paediatr Anaesth. 2013;23:250–7.
21. Feldman JM. Optimal ventilation of the anesthetized pediatric patient. Anesth Analg. 2015;120:165–75.
22. Peterson-Carmichael S, Seddon PC, Cheifetz IM, Frerichs I, Hall GL, Hammer J, et al. ATS/ERS working group on infant and young ChildrenPulmonary function testing. An official American Thoracic Society/EuropeanRespiratory society workshop report: evaluation of respiratory mechanics andFunction in the pediatric and neonatal intensive care units. Ann Am Thorac Soc. 2016;13:S1–11.
23. Kaditis AG, Motoyama EK, Zin W, Maekawa N, Nishio I, Imai T, et al. The effect of lung expansion and positive end-expiratory pressure on respiratory mechanics in anesthetized children. Anesth Analg. 2008;106:775–85.
24. Cruces P, González-Dambrauskas S, Quilodrán J, Valenzuela J, Martínez J, Rivero N, et al. Respiratory mechanics in infants with severe bronchiolitis on controlled mechanical ventilation. BMC Pulm Med. 2017;17:129.
25. Jonson B, Richard JC, Straus C, Mancebo J, Lemaire F, Brochard L. Pressure-volume curves and compliance in acute lung injury: evidence of recruitment above the lower inflection point. Am J Respir Crit Care Med. 1999;159:1172–8.
26. Protti A, Maraffi T, Milesi M, Votta E, Santini A, Pugni P, et al. Role of strain rate in the pathogenesis of ventilator-induced lung edema. Crit Care Med. 2016;44:e838–45.
27. Amato MB, Meade MO, Slutsky AS, Brochard L, Costa EL, Schoenfeld DA, et al. Driving pressure and survival in the acute respiratory distress syndrome. N Engl J Med. 2015;372:747–55.
28. Lucangelo U, Bernabé F, Blanch L. Respiratory mechanics derived from signals in the ventilator circuit. Respir Care. 2005;50:55–65.
29. Neto AS, Hemmes SN, Barbas CS, Beiderlinden M, Fernandez-Bustamante A, Futier E, et al. Association between driving pressure and development of postoperative pulmonary complications in patients undergoing mechanical ventilation for general anaesthesia: a meta-analysis of individual patient data. Lancet Respir Med. 2016;4:272–80.
30. Wirth S, Artner L, Broß T, Lozano-Zahonero S, Spaeth J, Schumann S, et al. Intratidal recruitment/derecruitment persists at low and moderate positive end-expiratory pressure in paediatric patients. Respir Physiol Neurobiol. 2016;234:9–13.
31. Rausch SMK, Haberthur D, Stampanoni M, Schittny JC, Wall WA. Local strain distribution in real three-dimensional alveolar geometries. Ann Biomed Eng. 2011;39:2835–43.
32. Webb HH, Tierney DF. Experimental pulmonary edema due to intermittent positive pressure ventilation with high inflation pressures. Protection by positive end-expiratory pressure. Am Rev Respir Dis. 2003;1974:556–65.

20

Programmed intermittent epidural bolus versus continuous epidural infusion for postoperative analgesia after major abdominal and gynecological cancer surgery: a randomized, triple-blinded clinical trial

Thomas Wiesmann*, Lilli Hoff, Lara Prien, Alexander Torossian, Leopold Eberhart, Hinnerk Wulf and Carsten Feldmann

Abstract

Background: Continuous epidural infusion (CEI) is the standard application setting for epidural infusion. A new mode, the programmed intermittent epidural bolus (PIEB) technique, showed reduced local anesthetic (LA) consumption and improved analgesia in obstetric analgesia. Goal of this trial was to evaluate the effects of PIEB versus CEI [combined with patient-controlled bolus (PCEA)] on LA consumption and pain scorings in major abdominal cancer surgery.

Methods: Following ethical approval, patients scheduled for major abdominal cancer surgery under general anesthesia in combination with epidural analgesia were randomized to receive either a PIEB mode of 6 mL/h or a CEI mode set at 6 mL/h of ropivacaine 0.2%, both combined with a PCEA mode set at a 4 mL bolus. LA consumptions and pain scorings were documented until the second postoperative evening.

Results: Eighty-four datasets were analyzed (CEI: $n = 40$, PIEB: $n = 44$). Regarding the primary endpoint, cumulative LA PCEA bolus volumes until day 2 differed significantly between the groups [PIEB 10 mL (2–28 mL) versus CEI, 28 mL (12–64 mL), median (25th–75th percentiles), $p = 0.002$]. Overall, LA consumption volumes were significantly lower in the PIEB group versus in the CEI group [PIEB: 329 mL (291–341 mL) vs. CEI: 350 mL (327–381 mL), $p = 0.003$]. Pain scores were comparable at each time point.

Conclusions: This trial demonstrates reduced needs for PCEA bolus in the PIEB group. There were no clinically relevant benefits regarding morphine consumption, pain scorings, or other secondary outcome parameters.

* Correspondence: wiesmann@med.uni-marburg.de
Department of Anesthesiology and Intensive Care Medicine, Philipps University Marburg, University Hospital Marburg (UKGM - Campus Marburg), Baldinger Strasse, 35033 Marburg, Germany

Background

Major abdominal cancer surgery is regularly linked with intermediate to severe pain following the procedure. Postoperatively, analgesic therapy should be performed by a multimodal combination of systemic analgesics and the use of regional anesthesia techniques such as thoracic epidural analgesia [1, 2]. Additional proven effects of epidural analgesia such as reduced time to the recovery of bowel function are beneficial after abdominal surgery [3]. Epidural infusion is usually administered by an elastomeric or electronic pump delivering continuous local anesthetic (LA) flow via the indwelling epidural catheter, in addition to patient-controlled epidural bolus (PCEA) applications. Recent advances in infusion technology have resulted in the technique of a programmed intermittent epidural bolus (PIEB) at a set interval [4]. In obstetric analgesia, this application mode prompted a significant decrease of LA consumption, [4] potentially due to a better distribution of LA in the epidural space in comparison with the continuous infusion technique. However, this technique has not yet been evaluated for major abdominal surgery.

To our knowledge, this is the first randomized triple-blinded trial (patient blind, researcher blind, blinded statistician) to investigate the effects of PIEB versus continuous epidural infusion (CEI) for postoperative analgesia in combination with PCEA option after major open abdominal and gynecological (i.e., pancreatic, colonic, ovarian, and cervical) cancer surgery on LA consumption (primary endpoint) and postoperative pain management including opioid consumption and potential side effects (secondary endpoints).

Methods

Ethics, consent & permissions

Following approval by the local ethics committee (Ethical Commission, University Hospital Marburg, AZ 119/16) and registration in the ClinicalTrials.gov registry (NCT03378804), this triple-blinded, randomized, and controlled single-center study was performed in accordance with the Declaration of Helsinki. Written informed consent was obtained from all participating subjects prior to enrollment. This manuscript adheres to the applicable CONSORT guidelines.

Patients (ASA classification 1 to 4) scheduled for elective major abdominal (pancreatic and colonic) and gynecological (ovarian and cervical) cancer surgery with scheduled midline laparotomy were screened between January 2017 and November 2017. Exclusion criteria were age < 18 years or > 80 years, an inability to give consent, pregnancy, general contraindications for or an inability to undergo thoracic epidural analgesia techniques, inability to use a patient-controlled epidural analgesia (PCEA) technique, scheduled postoperative mechanical ventilation, and known or suspected allergy to LA.

Predefined dropout criteria were failed epidural anesthesia, revision surgery within the first 24 h and mechanical ventilation during intensive care unit stay.

Anesthesia, surgery, and postoperative analgesia

In the induction area, standard monitoring was applied according to current national guidelines. Insertion of a thoracic epidural catheter (Perifix; B. Braun, Melsungen, Germany), using a loss-of-resistance technique was performed after skin disinfection in the sitting position at the Th8–Th9 or the Th9–Th10 interspaces under mild sedation using 5 μg to 15 μg of intravenous (IV) sufentanil. Following negative aspiration and negative response to a test dose of 3 mL of bupivacaine 0.5% (without epinephrine), the indwelling catheter was fixed using sterile drapings (Tegaderm; 3 M, Maplewood, MN, USA). An initial dose of 15 mL of ropivacaine 0.375% was applied via the indwelling epidural catheter with the patient in the supine position. After 15 min, cold/warm sensibility testing was performed bilaterally to evaluate the appropriate spread (multisegmental sensory blockade) of the epidural block.

Anesthesia induction was performed with sufentanil 0.2 μg kg^{-1} to 0.3 μg kg^{-1}, propofol 2 mg kg^{-1} to 3 mg kg^{-1}, and cisatracurium 0.1 mg kg^{-1} or rocuronium 0.5 mg kg^{-1} to 0.6 mg kg^{-1}. Intraoperatively, a balanced anesthesia technique using desflurane (target bispectral index values of 35 to 55) and remifentanil 0.1 μg kg^{-1} min^{-1} to 0.25 μg kg^{-1} min^{-1} was administered. Intraoperatively, all patients underwent active warming to achieve normothermia. All patients received a standardized IV double antiemetic prophylaxis using dexamethasone 4 mg to 8 mg and granisetrone 1 mg or droperidol 0.625 mg to 1.25 mg with regard to patient-specific conditions [5]. Recovery from neuromuscular blockade was monitored in all patients, a reversal was performed individually at the discretion of the respective anesthetist if the Train-of-Four (TOF) ratio did not reach 4/4 and the Double Burst Stimulation (DBS) showed a residual blockade phenomena. Prior to emergence from anesthesia at the end of the operation, all patients received 15 mg kg^{-1} to 20 mg kg^{-1} metamizole (dipyrone) as a nonopioid analgesic component of our standard multimodal analgesic regimen.

After surgery, patients were extubated in the operation room and transferred either to the postanesthesia care unit (PACU) or—if so scheduled—directly into the intensive care unit for further care.

Intervention groups

At the beginning of the operation, a PCEA pump (AmbIT® PIB PCA; Teleflex, Wayne, PA, USA) with a sterile bag

Results

From January 2017 until November 2017, 182 patients were assessed for eligibility. Of these, 72 patients did not participate in the study (16 patients refused to participate in the study, 25 patients did not meet inclusion criteria, nine patients had medical contraindications, 17 were excluded due to logistic issues such as postponed or cancelled surgery, and five were excluded due to other reasons). Finally, 110 patients were randomized (Fig. 1). Blinded intention-to-treat analysis of 84 patients was performed according to protocol. Details of dropout reasons and relevant protocol violations are given in Fig. 1.

Among the 84 patients analyzed (40 patients in the CEI group and 44 patients in the PIEB group), baseline patient characteristics were found to be similar between the groups (Table 1).

Local anesthetic consumption

Regarding the primary outcome measurement, the applied PCEA bolus volumes were significantly higher in the CEI group [28 mL (12–64 mL)] versus in the PIEB group [10 mL (2–28 ml), $p = 0.004$, Table 2]. Additionally, the differences between the need for additional PCEA bolus were statistically different on POD1 and POD2 but not so from the initial time of surgery until the evening of the same day (Table 2).

A statistically significant difference in overall LA consumption was observed in the PIEB group [329 mL (291–341.1 mL); median 25th–75th percentiles] as compared with in the CEI group [350.3 mL (326.5–380.8 mL), $p = 0.01$] until 48 h postoperatively (POD2). The LA volumes applied by the CEI or PIEB mode alone (without PCEA bolus volumes) were not significantly different between

Table 1 Demographic and perioperative data

	Group CEI (n = 40)	Group PIEB (n = 44)	p-value
Age, y	58 ± 16	63 ± 12	0.09
Sex, (M/F)	9/31	15/29	0.24
Weight, kg	80 ± 21	79 ± 20	0.96
Height, cm	167 ± 8	168 ± 9	0.61
BMI, kg/m^2	29 ± 7	28 ± 7	0.81
ASA status I/II/III	0/23/17	1/28/15)	0.37
Length of hospital stay, d	14 (10–18)	12 (10–16)	0.53
Type of surgery (colonic/pancreatic/gynaecological)	12/09/19	14/10/20	0.84
Length of surgery, min	205 (171–329)	173(135–253)	0.06
Epidural insertion height (lower spinal segment)	Th10 (Th9-Th11)	Th10 (Th9-Th11)	0.60
Epidural catheter performance time, min	12(8–17)	10(7–12)	0.14
Length of epidural catheter therapy, d	5 (5–7)	5 (5–6)	0.33
MAP initial (MAP1), mmHg	107 (91–123)	103 (93–114)	0.46
MAP at initial ropivacaine administration (MAP 2), mmHg	97 (90–116)	100 (89–113)	0.81
MAP 15min after initial ropivacaine administration (MAP 3), mmHg	88 (76–97)	86 (78–98)	0.94
Sufentanil for EDA placement, µg	0 (0–10)	0 (0–5)	0.24
Metamizole intraoperative, g	1.5 (1–1.5)	1.5 (1.5–1.5)	0.76
Metamizole d0, g	2 (1–3.5)	2 (1–3)	0.73
Metamizole d1, g	4 (4–4)	4 (3–4)	0.22
Metamizole d2, g	4 (4–4)	4 (4–4)	0.41
Ibuprofen d0, g	0.8 (0.4–0.8)	0.8 (0.6–0.8)	0.66
Ibuprofen d1, g	1.2 (0.8–1.4)	1.2 (0.6–1.2)	0.83
Ibuprofen d2, g	1.2 (1.2–1.6)	1.2 (1.2–1.8)	0.33
Opioids d0, % (yes/no)	30 (12/28)	36.4 (16/28)	0.54
Opioids d1, % (yes/no)	45 (18/22)	40.1 (18/26)	0.71
Opioids d2, % (yes/no)	67.5 (27/13)	50 (22/22)	0.11
Opiods d0–2, % (yes/no)	75 (30/10)	66 (29/15)	0.37

Values are expressed as the mean ± SD, median (25th–75th percentile), number of patients (n), or absolute numbers (%). *PIEB* programmed intermittent epidural bolus group, *CEI* continuous epidural infusion group, *BMI* body mass index, *ASA* American Society of Anesthesiology, *EDA* epidural anesthesia, *MAP* mean arterial pressure, *LA* local anaesthetic; Statistical significance was tested using Mann-Whitney-U-Testing, T-Testing or Chi-square where appropriate, two-sided p-value. Level of significance $p < 0.05$

Table 2 Local anesthetic consumption

	Group CEI (*n* = 40)	Group PIEB (*n* = 44)	*p*-value	HL-Estimator (95% CI)
LA PCA Bolus d0-d2, ml	28 (12–64)	10 (2–28)	0.002*	16 (4; 28)
LA PIEB/CEI amount d0-d2, ml	323.5(286.6–336.7)	311.4 (263–330.2)	0.161	10.2 (−4; 30.6)
Overall LA consumption d0-d2, ml	350.3 (326.5–380.8)	329 (291–341.1)	0.003	29.55 (10.7;52.1)
LA PCA Bolus d0, ml	0 (0–8)	0 (0–4)	0.046	0 (0; 0)
LA PCA Bolus d1, ml	18 (4–26)	4 (0–14)	0.002*	8 (4; 16)
LA PCA Bolus d2, ml	12 (4–34)	4 (0–12)	0.010*	4 (0; 12)
LA PIEB/CEI amount d0, ml	50.9 (36–55.7)	48 (36–54)	0.238	2.9 (−1,8; 6.8)
LA PIEB/CEI amount d1, ml	140.9 (132.4–145.2)	132.3 (120–141.7)	0.015*	8.3 (1.2; 17.2)
LA PIEB/CEI amount d2, ml	135.2 (110.6–141.4)	131 (109.5–140.1)	0.588	2.3 (−6.6; 11)

LA local anesthetic, *d0* day of operation; *d1/d2* first/second postoperative day; *PIEB* programmed intermittent epidural bolus, *CEI* continuous epidural infusion, *PCA* patient controlled bolus, *HL* Hodges-Lehman. Values are expressed as the median (25th–75th percentiles), Mann-Whitney-U-Testing, two-sided p-value. Uncorrected *p*-values are displayed. Level of significance $p < 0.05$. *, significant

the CEI group [323.5 mL (286.6–336.7 mL)] and the PIEB group [311.4 mL (263–330.2 mL), $p = 0.161$].

Pain scorings and analgesic therapy

NRS value at rest, during cough, and during movement did not differ significantly between the CEI and PIEB groups for each given time point (Table 3). The amounts of ibuprofen and metamizole given as part of our multimodal regimen also did not differ between the groups for the given time points (Table 1). Additionally, overall, the need for opioids (as calculated as IV morphine equivalents) was not significantly different in the CEI group [15 mg [2.5–22.5 mg]] versus in the PIEB group [7.5 mg (0–20 mg), $p = 0.27$] between the end time of the surgery and POD2.

Side effects

Patients in both groups had low needs of necessary norepinephrine therapy in the evening after surgery (3/46 in the CEI group vs. 3/44 in the PIEB group, Table 4). On POD1, one patient in the CEI group and two patients in the PIEB group, respectively, required norepinephrine, whereas, on POD2, no patients required additional norepinephrine.

Table 3 Pain scoring

	Group CEI (*n* = 40)	Group PIEB (*n* = 44)	*p*-value
NRS rest d0	0 (0–0)	0 (0–0)	0.21
NRS rest d1	0 (0–3)	0 (0–2.8)	0.94
NRS rest d2	0.5 (0–3)	0 (0–2.5)	0.34
NRS cough d0	0 (0–3)	0 (0–0)	0.06
NRS cough d1	3 (1–6)	3 (0–5)	0.49
NRS cough d2	2.5 (0.5–5.5)	2.5 (0–6)	0.81
NRS movement d0	0 (0–3)	0 (0–0)	0.32
NRS movement d1	3 (1–5.5)	3 (0–4.5)	0.39
NRS movement d2	3 (0–5)	2 (0–4.5)	0.41
Morphine IV d0, mg	5 (5–7.5)	5 (5–5)	0.03
Morphine IV d1, mg	10 (10–10)	10 (10–10)	0.53
Morphine IV d2, mg	10 (10–15)	10 (10–10)	0.94
Morphine IV d0-d2, mg	15 (2.5–22.5)	7.5 (0–20)	0.27
Opioid need d0, yes / no	12/28	16/28	0.54
Opioid need d1, yes / no	18/22	18/26	0.71
Opioid need d2, yes / no	27/13	22/22	0.11
Opioid need d0-d2, yes / no	30/10	29/15	0.37

Values are expressed as the median (25th–75th percentile and as two-sided p-value of the Mann-Whitney –U test. Uncorrected *p*-values are displayed. Level of significance $p < 0.05$. No significant differences were found after Bonferroni correction. *NRS* numeric rating scale, *d0–3* postoperative day 0–3, *LA* local anaesthetic

Table 4 Side effects / Clinical parameters

	Group CEI (*n* = 40)	Group PIEB (*n* = 44)	*p*-value
Vasopressor need d0, % (yes/no)	7.5 (3/37)	6.8 (3/41)	0.88
Vasopressor need d1, % (yes/no)	2.5 (1/39)	4.5 (2/42)	0.62
Vasopressor need d2, % (yes/no)	0 (0/40)	0 (0/44)	1.00
Nausea d0, % (yes/no)	20 (8/32)	18.2 (8/36)	0.79
Nausea d1, % (yes/no)	22.5 (9/31)	25 (11/33)	0.79
Nausea d2, % (yes/no)	32.5 (13/27)	13.6 (6/38)	0.04
Vomiting d0, % (yes/no)	17.5 (7/33)	11.4 (5/39)	0.40
Vomiting d1, % (yes/no)	20 (8/32)	22.7 (10/34)	0.76
Vomiting d2, % (yes/no)	17.5 (7/33)	15.9 (7/37)	0.85
Satisfaction d0, NRS	10 (10–10)	10 (10–10)	0.15
Satisfaction d1, NRS	10 (10–10)	10 (9–10)	0.19
Satisfaction d2, NRS	10 (8–10)	10 (8–10)	0.84
EDA catheter removal, day	5 (5–7)	5 (5–6)	0.33
Time to first flatus, hours	22.8 (18.6–43.8)	23.1(20.3–45.5)	0.25
Time to first defecation, hours	71.2 (40.8–119)	65.8(32.4–93.5)	0.54

Values are expressed as the median (25th–75th percentiles) or numbers (percents) and as two-sided p-value of the Mann-Whitney –U test or Fisher's exact test when appropriate. Uncorrected p-values are displayed. Level of significance $p < 0.05$. *NRS* numeric rating scale, *d0–3* postoperative day 0–3, *LA* local anaesthetic, *EDA* epidural anesthesia

Time to first passage of flatus was not significantly different in the CEI group [22.8 h (17.6–42.2 h)] as compared with in the PIEB group [23.1 h (20.3–45.5 h), $p = 0.25$]. The time to first passage of feces after surgery was also not significantly different between the CEI group [71.2 h (40.8–119 h)] and the PIEB group [65.8 h (32.4–93.5 h), $p = 0.54$]. Frequencies of nausea and vomiting were not significantly different between groups at the evening of the operation, the first and the second postoperative day. Patient satisfaction at d1 and d2 was not significantly different between groups (Table 4). Additional information regarding sensory spread and motor blockade testing is given in the Additional file 1.

Discussion

To our knowledge, this is the first randomized trial that has investigated different modes of epidural local anesthetic application (continuous vs. programmed intermittent technique) in patients undergoing major abdominal cancer surgery. Our study shows a statistically significant decrease of administered ropivacaine 0.2% until POD2 in patients who experienced PIEB as compared with CEI, both in combination with a patient controlled bolus (PCB) option. Overall pain scores did not differ significantly between the groups at rest, during cough, or during mobilization for each given time point until POD2. Additionally, overall postoperative morphine consumption showed comparable low values. Time to first passage of flatus or feces (stool) were not significantly different between the groups.

Analgesic effects and morphine consumption

Our study results are consistent with previously published obstetric data showing reduced local anesthetic consumption when using a PIEB technique versus a traditional CEI [4, 7–10]. However, the overall reduction of LA consumption between the day of operation and POD2 was approximately 15 mL, resulting in questionable clinical relevance. Again, this is in line with previous reports that showed only mild reductions in LA volumes when the PIEB technique was used. On the other hand, this significant difference is explainable by a reduction of applied PCEA bolus volume as a surrogate of better analgesia. This effect of reduced PCEA bolus consumption in the PIEB group as compared with in the CEI group was consistently shown on POD1 and POD2 but not on the day of the surgery. This may be the result of the large initial bolus of 15 mL of ropivacaine 0.375% that was used for improved sensory testing quality of the epidural technique in the induction area prior to surgery. Pain scores were comparable between the groups, which is explainable by the fact that IV opioids were given as a rescue option in addition to the patient controlled bolus application option of the epidural infusion pump.

Limitations

Our study has several limitations and strengths that need to be addressed.

First, there was a relevant number of dropouts and protocol violations (26 of 110 randomized patients). This was the result of several relevant factors: specifically, reoperations due to early complications as well as unplanned prolonged mechanical ventilation with necessary sedation were classified as severe protocol violations as they potentially interfered with the primary and secondary endpoints of our study. Thus, we decided to exclude patients who experienced these scenarios from our analysis. Additionally, the decision to choose the local anesthetic consumptions as endpoints were problematic in our clinical practice, as some staff members accidentally switched empty LA bags of our study patients and cleared the pump history, which resulted in the loss of the endpoint parameters in several patients.

As a second limitation, the decision to choose local anesthetic consumption as a primary endpoint might be questioned by some colleagues. This surrogate endpoint was selected for use in our study as previous investigations (mainly in obstetric populations) showed no differences in pain scores or rescue opioid use between CEI and PIEB modes. Moreover, from an ethical point of view, it would be inhuman to expose one trial group to higher pain scores by denying rescue opioids just to aim for a difference in pain scorings. Even a difference of 10 mm in the 100 mm visual analogue scale for pain was noted by patients as a relevant difference in pain according to the results of a recent study by Myles et al [11].

Lastly, the optimal PIEB mode has yet to be determined with regard to programmed bolus volume, time interval, local anesthetic, or its concentration [8, 12, 13]. Thus, we chose a pragmatic approach using our standard settings for epidural catheters of 6 mL/h^{-1} for the CEI group and the same volume for the PIEB in the PIEB group. We did not perform an economic analysis of the different types of epidural infusion. PIEB modes are restricted to specific types of commercially available electronic pumps, which potentially might result in higher costs in comparison with other pump systems. Moreover, the programmed intermittent bolus application is applied by the pumps with a higher pressure than in continuous infusion technique, resulting in higher energy consumption as compared with the continuous infusion [14]. When using alkaline batteries, a shorter interval of battery exchange might have a considerable economic and ecologic impact [15]. Thus, if available, A/C adapters or rechargeable batteries should be considered when using PIEB modes, regardless of the specific manufacturer.

Conclusion

In this triple-blinded randomized trial, local anesthetic consumption was significantly lower in patients with a PIEB versus a standard CEI. However, overall pain scores were comparable, as were side effects and patient satisfaction scorings. From a clinical perspective, the overall reduction of local anesthetic consumption was mild comparing the PIEB mode with the CEI mode. Hence, the use of PIEB mode in thoracic epidural analgesia after major abdominal surgery should be further evaluated with regard to optimized programmed bolus volumes and time intervals and outcome before widespread implementation in the clinical setting.

Abbreviations

ASA: American Society of Anesthesiology; CEI: Continuous epidural application; d: Day; EDA: Epidural anesthesia; LA: Local anesthetics; MAP: Mean arterial pressure; ml: Millilitres; NRS: Numeric rating scale; PACU: Postoperative care unit; PCB: Patient controlled bolus; PCEA: Patient controlled epidural analgesia; PIEB: Programmed intermittent epidural bolus; POD: Postoperative day; SD: Standard deviation

Acknowledgements

We thank our staff team in the OR, PACU and the acute pain service for their efforts in performing this study.

Funding

This study was performed with institutional funding.
PCEA pumps were provided by Teleflex Germany (Kernen, Germany).

Authors' contributions

TW: study design, data analysis, interpretation, manuscript draft; LH: data collection & analysis, interpretation, manuscript draft; LP: data collection & interpretation, manuscript draft; AT, study design, data analysis, manuscript draft; LE: study design, data analysis & interpretation; HW: study design, data interpretation, manuscript draft; CF: study design, data collection & interpretation, manuscript draft; All authors read and approved the final manuscript.

Competing interests

Thomas Wiesmann has received speaker fees from B. Braun.
Hinnerk Wulf has received speaker fees from Teleflex Medical, Vygon, B Braun, Pajunk, and Sintetica.
Leopold Eberhart has received honoraria for consulting and speaker fee from Baxter GmbH, Fresenius GmbH, Grunenthal GmbH, and TEVA ratiopharm GmbH.
All other authors have no competing interest to disclose.

References

1. Feldheiser A, Aziz O, Baldini G, Cox BPBW, Fearon KCH, Feldman LS, et al. Enhanced recovery after surgery (ERAS) for gastrointestinal surgery, part 2: consensus statement for anaesthesia practice. Acta Anaesthesiol Scand. 2016;60:289–334.
2. Guay J, Nishimori M, Kopp SL. Epidural local anesthetics versus opioid-based analgesic regimens for postoperative gastrointestinal paralysis, vomiting, and pain after abdominal surgery: a Cochrane review. Anesth Analg. 2016; 123:1591–602.
3. Pöpping DM, Elia N, Van Aken HK, Marret E, Schug SA, Kranke P, et al. Impact of epidural analgesia on mortality and morbidity after surgery: systematic review and meta-analysis of randomized controlled trials. Ann Surg. 2014;259:1056–67.

4. George RB, Allen TK, Habib AS. Intermittent epidural bolus compared with continuous epidural infusions for labor analgesia: a systematic review and meta-analysis. Anesth Analg. 2013;116:133–44.
5. Wiesmann T, Kranke P, Eberhart L. Postoperative nausea and vomiting - a narrative review of pathophysiology, pharmacotherapy and clinical management strategies. Expert Opin Pharmacother. 2015;16(7):1069–770.
6. Berdine HJ, Nesbit SA. Equianalgesic dosing of opioids. J Pain Palliat Care Pharmacother. 2006;20:79–84.
7. Nunes J, Nunes S, Veiga M, Cortez M, Seifert I. A prospective, randomized, blinded-endpoint, controlled study - continuous epidural infusion versus programmed intermittent epidural bolus in labor analgesia. Braz J Anesthesiol. 2016;66:439–44.
8. Wong CA, Ratliff JT, Sullivan JT, Scavone BM, Toledo P, McCarthy RJ. A randomized comparison of programmed intermittent epidural bolus with continuous epidural infusion for labor analgesia. Anesth Analg. 2006;102:904–9.
9. Capogna G, Camorcia M, Stirparo S, Farcomeni A. Programmed intermittent epidural bolus versus continuous epidural infusion for labor analgesia: the effects on maternal motor function and labor outcome. A randomized double-blind study in nulliparous women. Anesth Analg. 2011;113:826–31.
10. McKenzie CP, Cobb B, Riley ET, Carvalho B. Programmed intermittent epidural boluses for maintenance of labor analgesia: an impact study. Int J Obstet Anesth. 2016;26:32–8.
11. Myles PS, Myles DB, Galagher W, Boyd D, Chew C, MacDonald N, et al. Measuring acute postoperative pain using the visual analog scale: the minimal clinically important difference and patient acceptable symptom state. Br J Anaesth. 2017;118:424–9.
12. Zakus P, Arzola C, Bittencourt R, Downey K, Ye XY, Carvalho JC. Determination of the optimal programmed intermittent epidural bolus volume of bupivacaine 0.0625% with fentanyl 2 μg.Ml −1at a fixed interval of forty minutes: a biased coin up-and-down sequential allocation trial. Anaesthesia. 2017;116:133–7.
13. Carvalho B, George RB, Cobb B, McKenzie C, Riley ET. Implementation of programmed intermittent epidural bolus for the maintenance of labor analgesia. Anesth Analg. 2016;123:965–71.
14. Klumpner TT, Lange EMS, Ahmed HS, Fitzgerald PC, Wong CA, Toledo P. An in vitro evaluation of the pressure generated during programmed intermittent epidural bolus injection at varying infusion delivery speeds. J Clin Anesth. 2016;34:632–7.
15. Dinges E, Heier J, Bollag L. It's not easy being green, or is it? Alkaline battery versus a/C power for programmed intermittent epidural bolus pumps. Int J Obstet Anesth Elsevier. 2018;33:100–1.

Ultrasound-guided versus low dose computed tomography scanning guidance for lumbar facet joint injections: same accuracy and efficiency

Ling Ye[1], Chuanbing Wen[2*†] and Hui Liu[1*†]

Abstract

Background: The purpose of this study was to investigate the feasibility, accuracy and efficiency of the facet joint injections in the lumbar spine by ultrasound guided versus lose dose computed tomography (CT) guidance.

Methods: First the examination on the joint space of the facet joints of the lumbar spine was obtained by the ultrasound in 10 patients. Second forty patients were randomized assigned into two groups: ultrasound group and low dose CT group. Comparison was made in the clinical efficiency between the ultrasound-guided group and CT group. The feasibility, accuracy and efficiency of the ultrasound-guided lumbar facet joint injections were also evaluated.

Results: A total of 88 lumbar facet joints from L_1 to S_1 were clearly visualized in the 10 patients. Both the ultrasound and the CT measurements showed the same average depth and lateral distance to the reference point ($P > 0.05$). And 86.5% of the facet joint injections (64/74) were correctly performed under the ultrasound guidance in the first time. The exact placement of the needle tips was evaluated by CT. After the lumbar facet joint injections, the clinical efficiency was almost the same in the ultrasound-guided group as in the CT group.

Conclusions: The lumbar facet joint space can be accurately demonstrated by ultrasound. The ultrasound-guided facet joint injection in the lumbar spine obtained almost the same satisfactory feasibility, accuracy and clinical efficiency compared with low dose CT. Ultrasound technique could provide the real-time monitoring.

Keywords: Ultrasound, Computed tomography, Accuracy, Efficiency, Lumbar facet joint injection

* Correspondence: chunbingwen@163.com; huaxiliuhui@163.com
†Chuanbing Wen and Hui Liu contributed equally to this work.
[2]Department of Pain Management, Sichuan Academy of Medical Sciences & Sichuan Provincial People's Hospital, Chengdu, Sichuan Province 610072, People's Republic of China
[1]Department of Pain management, West China Hospital, Sichuan University, Chengdu, Sichuan Province 610041, People's Republic of China

Background

The facet joint-related pain is very common, and it has been identified as a common source of the low back pain [1–3]. However, we cannot diagnose it solely based on physical examination [4] or radiographic imaging [5]. Facet joint block is a commonly used method for relieve the low back pain, and for diagnosis and treatment of the facet joint-related pain [6]. Facet joint blocks are usually performed with the help of the fluoroscopic guidance or the computed tomography (CT) scanning guidance for a precise localization of the needle tips and avoidance of complications [7–9]. But the two techniques are inevitably associated with significant radiation doses for both the patient and the pain physicians [10].

Ultrasound is not associated with an exposure to radiation, and equipment is not too expensive, which is portable and can be used as a real-time monitoring image guide tool. Ultrasonography has been applied for guidance in nerve blocks [11–15]. Ultrasound can exactly indicate the injection sites and monitor the needle insertion and the spread of local anesthetics in real time. The success and validity of the lumbar facet joint injections may depend on the accurate insertion of the needle tip. Inaccurate positioning of a needle tip may result in an inadvertent spread of the local anesthetic into the intervertebral foramen, the epidural space, or even the subarachnoid space, which can cause some serious complications [16, 17].

The present study was designed to evaluate the feasibility and accuracy of the ultrasound-guided lumbar facet joint injections, which were compared with CT. The pain relief was also assessed.

Materials and methods

The study was approved by the institutional ethics committee of West China Hospital, Sichuan University (Chengdu, China). Informed consents were obtained from all the participants. All the procedures were performed by the same group of doctors.

The first part - the CT analysis study

Ten adult patients with low back pain who were required CT scan (5 women, 5 men) were enrolled between Jan 3, 2016 to March 3, 2016 in West China Hospital, Sichuan University, Chengdu. All the patients met the following inclusion criteria: 18–80 years old. The patients were excluded as following: the body mass index (BMI) ≥ 25 kg/m^2; spinal deformities including congenital scoliosis and kyphosis, secondary deformities such as ankylosing spondylitis, spinal tuberculosis, neuromuscular scoliosis, Scheumann disease and osteoporosis.

All the demographic data were recorded. The patients were placed in a prone position, with the abdomen supported by the pillows to compensate for the lumbar lordosis. Ultrasound examinations were performed by one ultrasound investigator experienced in the musculoskeletal ultrasound examination, and a standard ultrasound device (Philips, HDI 3500 or 5000) was used, which used a broadband curved array transducer working at 3–5 MHz and a broadband linear array working at 12–15 MHz. To identify the spinal levels, the posterior parasagittal sonograms were obtained at levels L1 to S1 (Fig. 1) [18–20].

To get the ultrasound view, first the transducer was placed on the long axis of the facet column, which appears like a camel's hump. Then the transducer was rotated 90°to get the short axis view. The lumbar facet joints were delineated with the help of the transverse sonograms at each level. The transducer was first placed in the midline for scanning the short axis view of the lumbar spine. Then the transducer is relocated more cranially until spinous process was seen in the middle of the view. The lateral border comprises bilateral inferior articular process, superior articular process and transverse process. The sonogram of each plane was measured by the ultrasound measuring device. The lateral distance (A) was defined as the horizontal distance from the middle of the tip of the spinous process to the reference point; the depth (B) was defined as the vertical distance from the middle point between the tips of the spinous processes to the reference point; the oblique line (C) indicates the distance from the middle point between the tips of the spinous processes to the reference point. The above three distances were measured to assess the position of the facet joint space in the transverse sonograms. The distances A, B and C of each sonogram were evaluated by a spiral CT (low dose, 100 kV, 35 mAs) on the same plane with the same approach, reformatted to 1-mm axial slices (Fig. 2). All the values are presented as means ± SD.

The second part – The clinical study

Forty adult patients (20 women, 20 men) were consecutively enrolled between April 1, 2016 to Dec20, 2016 in

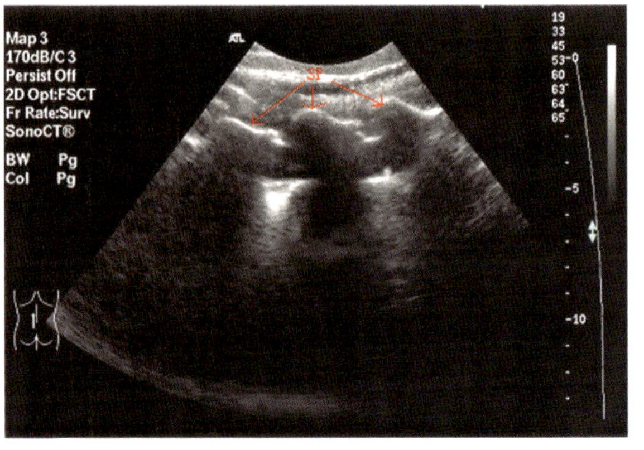

Fig. 1 The spinous processes of the lumbar spine demonstrated in a posterior paravertebral parasagittal sonogram. Arrow: spinous process (SP)

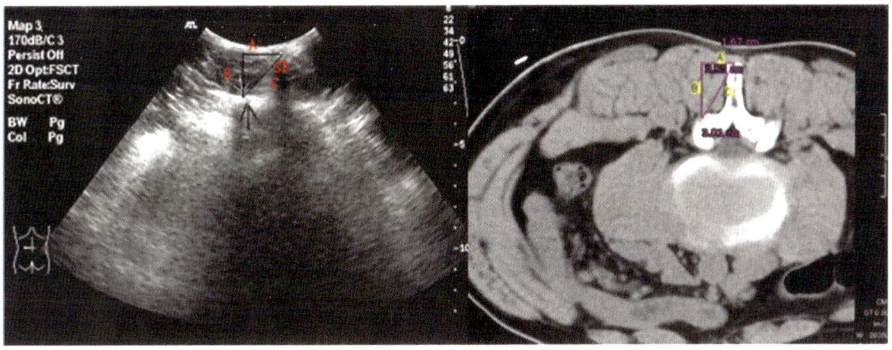

Fig. 2 The lateral distance (**a**) defined as the horizontal distance from the middle point between the tips of the spinous processes to the reference point, the depth (**b**) defined as the vertical distance from the middle of the tip of the spinous process to the reference point, and the oblique line (**c**) defined as the distance from the middle point between the tips of the spinous processes to the reference point

West China Hospital, Sichuan University, Chengdu (Fig. 3). The inclusion criteria were as following: 18–80 years old; having undergone CT or MRI of their lumbar spine, with the visible lumbar facet joint spaces. The patients were excluded as following: any potential contraindications, such as a spinal tumor, spinal deformities, spinal instability, discitis, and fracture; local or systemic infection or spinal infections; allergy to steroids or anesthetics; previous surgery; uncorrectable coagulopathy; pregnant; BMI ≥ 25 kg/m2. Based on the computer-generated randomization table, the patients were randomized assigned to two groups: patients in the group 1 were scheduled for the ultrasound-guided infiltrations (the US group), patients in the group 2 were scheduled for the lose dose CT guidance (the CT group, low dose, 100 kV, 35 mAs).

The US group

The patients were placed in a prone position with the abdomen supported by the pillows. One doctor

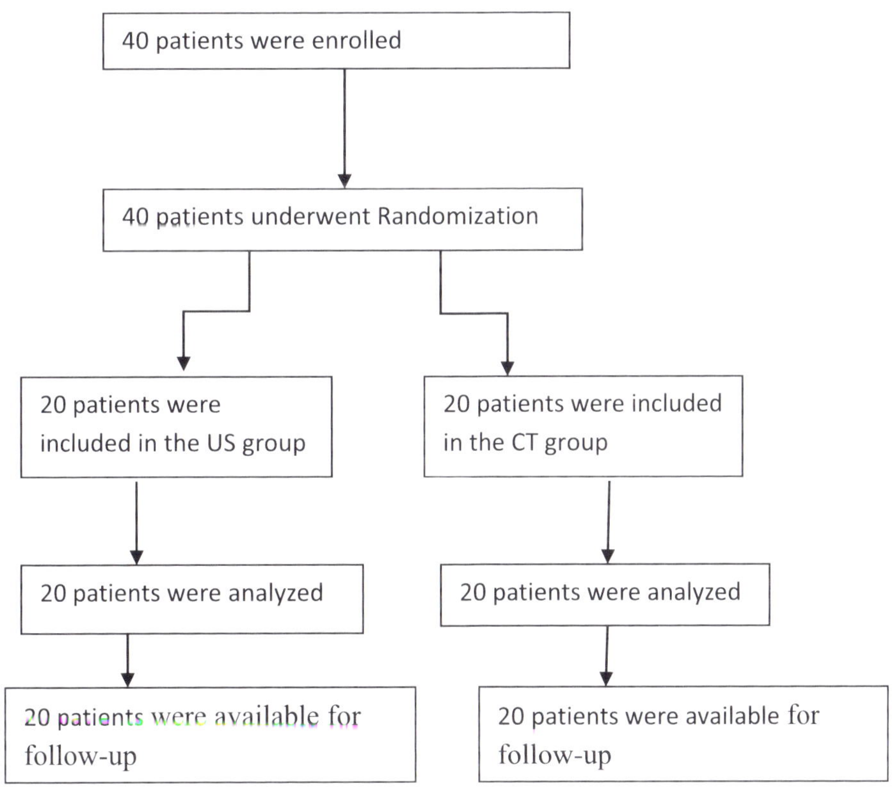

Fig. 3 Patient flow chart: randomization, treatment, and inclusion in analysis

experienced in the musculoskeletal ultrasound performed the ultrasound-guided facet joints injection in the lumbar spine in the US group (20 patients). This ultrasound-guided approach to the facet joint blocks was as the same as that in the first part. The skin was routinely sterilized. A spinal needle (20 gauge, 90 mm) was inserted into the ideal target position. When the needle tip was properly placed, 2 ml of a mixture that contained 0.5 ml of 2% lidocaine, 0.4 mg of compound betamethasone was injected into the facet joint space.

The CT group

The patients were placed in the same position as in the US group. The facet joint space was identified as did in the first part study described above. The needle tip was verified under the CT monitoring (Fig. 4) [18–20]. Then, the same drug was injected in the facet joint space as that in the US group.

Measurements

In both the groups, the visual analog scale (VAS) score regarding the low back pain before the facet joint injections were recorded. VAS and the remission rate (VAS < 3) of half an hour, one day, two days, 6 weeks after the procedures were recorded. The accuracy rate of the ultrasound procedure was defined as the percentage of the facet joint space surveyed by ultrasound. The levels of the facet joint injections were recorded in the two groups. The achievement rate in the US group was also recorded.

Statistical analysis

On the basis of our pilot study data, A sample size of 18 allowed the detection of a 20% difference in the proportion with an α 0.05 (two-tailed) and a β of 0.20, power of 0.8. To account for attrition, a sample size of 20 was selected for each group.

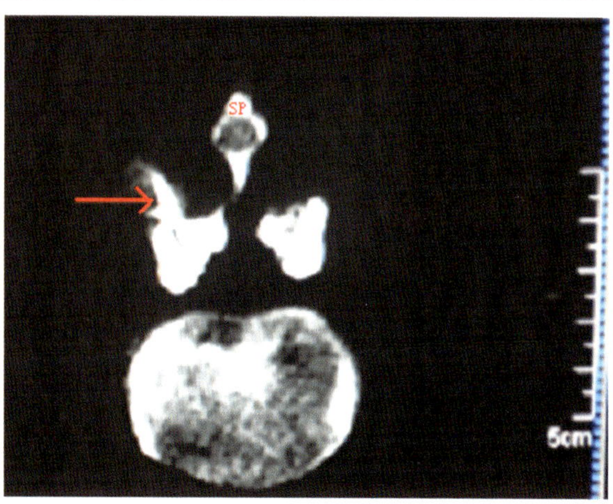

Fig. 4 The needle tip verified under the CT monitoring. SP: Spinous process; arrow: needle

Statistical analysis was performed with SAS and spss17.0. The features of the patients in the two parts were presented as medians (ranges). The distances are expressed as means ± SD (ranges), and they were analyzed for normality by means of the multivariant matched-pairs t test the A, B and C values in the volunteer study. P values less than 0.05 were considered statistically significant.

Results

The first part - The CT analysis study

In all the patients (5 women, 5 men; median age, 56.2 ± 14.8 kg; height, 159.1 ± 6.56 cm; weight, 56.6 ± 4.11 kg; BMI, 22.37 ± 1.21), there were 88 facet joints that were entirely visible, accounting for 88%. Ultrasound and CT showed the same mean values of distances A, B and C($P > 0.05$) (Table 1). In three patients, 12 facet joints could not be identified for providing a lumbar approach to the facet joint by ultrasound, but they could be identified by CT.

The second part - The clinical study

All the patients in the two groups suffered from chronic low back pain, with visual analogue scale (VAS) > 3(0–10) (the US group:7.00 ± 0.88; the CT group: 6.25 ± 2.31; $P > 0.05$) before the blocking procedure. There was no significant difference between the two groups (Table 2). An obvious paravertebral lumbar tenderness was found by ultrasound in the 20 patients, involving 74 facet joints

Table 1 A, B, C values of ultrasound and CT in the same spine level

Ultrasound			CT	
	Left(cm)	right(cm)	left(cm)	right(cm)
AL1/2	1.56 ± 0.19	1.54 ± 0.25	1.55 ± 0.21	1.51 ± 0.23
BL1/2	2.17 ± 0.22	2.16 ± 0.28	2.17 ± 0.21	2.17 ± 0.32
CL1/2	2.67 ± 0.26	2.66 ± 0.26	2.68 ± 0.25	2.65 ± 0.31
AL2/3	1.54 ± 0.22	1.58 ± 0.28	1.51 ± 0.21	1.56 ± 0.26
BL2/3	2.35 ± 0.25	2.39 ± 0.24	2.39 ± 0.26	2.41 ± 0.23
CL2/3	2.84 ± 0.26	2.87 ± 0.26	2.85 ± 0.24	2.88 ± 0.24
AL3/4	1.77 ± 0.32	1.79 ± 0.28	1.76 ± 0.32	1.82 ± 0.30
BL3/4	2.46 ± 0.23	2.46 ± 0.24	2.49 ± 0.23	2.47 ± 0.22
CL3/4	3.05 ± 0.23	3.05 ± 0.23	3.06 ± 0.23	3.08 ± 0.22
AL4/5	1.97 ± 0.32	2.03 ± 0.32	1.97 ± 0.32	2.03 ± 0.32
BL4/5	2.27 ± 0.37	2.29 ± 0.35	2.28 ± 0.42	2.30 ± 0.33
CL4/5	3.06 ± 0.23	3.07 ± 0.33	3.08 ± 0.24	3.08 ± 0.31
AL5S1	2.12 ± 0.35	2.15 ± 0.29	2.11 ± 0.37	2.16 ± 0.31
BL5S1	2.21 ± 0.33	2.25 ± 0.23	2.22 ± 0.35	2.26 ± 0.27
CL5S1	3.08 ± 0.26	3.09 ± 0.31	3.09 ± 0.26	3.15 ± 0.34

Table 2 Demographic data of the two groups

	US group	CT group	P
F/M	9/11	12/8	
Years	55 ± 12.4	54.5 ± 14.4	$P > 0.05$
Disease course (mon)	52.6 ± 11.2	42.6 ± 5.2	$P > 0.05$
BMI	24.3 ± 0.80	24.7 ± 2.19	$P > 0.05$
VAS	7.00 ± 0.88	6.25 ± 2.31	$P > 0.05$

F female, *M* male, *BMI* body mass index, *VAS* visual analog scale

associated with the injection, which were confirmed by the CT scan. 86.5% of the needles (64/74) could be successfully guided by ultrasound into the right facet joint space in the first time. In some patients, adaptation was necessary for the needling during the ultrasound guidance. Under CT, only 10 of the 74 needles had to be slightly corrected in position. No signs of the nerve root block, and no other neurological symptoms were observed. Half an hour after the injections, 14 patients had a reduction in the pain, with a remission rate ≥ 50% in the US group, and 12 patients, in the CT group.

In the US group, 30 min, 1 day, 2 days and 6 weeks after the procedures, there were 16, 18, 18 and 18 patients who had a decrease (≥3) in the VAS score respectively, and there were 14, 16, 16 and 16 patients had a reduction in the pain severity respectively, with a remission rate ≥ 50%, respectively; the follow-up after 6 weeks revealed a 73% pain remission rate (Table 2). Only 2 patients reported pain aggravation 30 min after procedure and then relived after 1 day.

In the CT group, 30 min, 1 day, 2 days and 6 weeks after the puncture procedures, there were 15, 16, 16 and 16 patients who had a decrease (≥3) in the VAS score respectively, and 14, 16, 16 and 16 patients who had a reduction in the pain severity respectively, with a remission rate ≥ 50%, respectively; the follow-up after 6 weeks revealed a 57% pain remission rate (Table 3). There were 4 patients reported pain aggravation 30 min after procedure and then relived after 1 day.

Discussion

In the present study, the lumbar facet joint space can be accurately demonstrated by the ultrasound. The feasibility, accuracy and clinical efficiency of the ultrasound-guided approach for the lumbar facet joint injections were very satisfactory for the patients with low back pain.

The facet joints are often affected by the mechanical derangements or the degenerative alterations; thus, the reflex muscular spasm or the referred pain can be easily developed [21]. The facet syndrome has been defined as a lumbosacral pain with or without a sciatic pain, particularly associated with a twisting or rotary strain of the lumbosacral region. The pain can be unilateral or bilateral and is typically enhanced by hyperextension of the lumbar spine or the locally applied pressure on the facet joints. No specific anatomic or radiologic findings have been confirmed to be correlated with the clinical diagnosis of the facet syndrome. Consequently, the primarily-diagnostic facet joint blocks are required in many patients, using a fluoroscopy device or a CT scan or in the blind manner based on the indication by the X-ray examination.

The advantages of the ultrasound guidance include (but not limited to) an increased success rate, decreased complications caused by the needle malpositioning, a faster effect of the blocks, and a reduced amount of the local anesthetics [21–27]. Besides, no exposure to radiation for the patient and the doctor is an important advantage, which makes the ultrasound guidance applicable for the pregnant patient. As we know, fluoroscopy has a complication rate of 5–10%, and CT has a complication rate about 0.5%. The previous researches revealed some life-threatening complications caused by the fluoroscopy-guided infiltrations, such as pleural perforation and pneumothorax [7]. The ultrasound guidance is useful in facilitating peripheral and neuraxial blocks and offers the direct visualization of the target, adjacent structures, and local anesthetic spread [7, 28].

Kullmer, et al. described the ultrasound use for the facet joint infiltration of the lumbar spine only for the periarticular region, but they could not ensure the precise application of the intraarticular local anesthetic without the fluoroscopy monitoring or the use of the contrast media [25]. The facet joint blocks are mainly used for diagnosis and the needle placement, and a small volume of the local anesthetic is necessary to minimize the rate of the false-positive block or complication. Theoretically, the facet joint infiltration in the periarticular region may cause a false-positive result because of the aberrant local anesthetic spread (epidural, nerve root, multifidus muscle). The direct intraarticular injection is considered indispensable for treatment of the facet joint-related pain. 27 The recent researches presented the new methodology of the ultrasound-guided lumbar facet nerve block and lumbar facet joint infiltration in the cadavers or the patients in the first part [29–31].

The present study showed that the ultrasound could identify the lumbar facet joint space exactly in the

Table 3 Patients of remission rate ≥ 50% and VAS after procedures

	Remission rate		VAS	
	US group	CT group	US group	CT group
30 min	14	14	2.95 ± 0.18	2.98 ± 0.21
1 day	16	16	2.76 ± 0.14	2.98 ± 0.18
2 days	16	16	2.81 ± 0.20	2.83 ± 0.17
6 weeks	16	16	2.86 ± 0.15	2.84 ± 0.15

Effect of Shenmai injection on cognitive function after cardiopulmonary bypass in cardiac surgical patients: a randomized controlled trial

Lei Chen[1†], Liangrong Wang[1†], Qian Zhuo[2], Qiong Zhang[1], Feifei Chen[1], Liling Li[1] and Lina Lin[1*]

Abstract

Background: Postoperative cognitive dysfunction (POCD) is a common complication after cardiac surgery that influences the clinical outcomes and quality of life of patients. This study aimed to evaluate the effects of Shenmai injection (SMI) on POCD of patients who underwent cardiac valve replacement under cardiopulmonary bypass (CPB).

Methods: This prospective, randomized, controlled trial was conducted from September 2014 to January 2017. Eighty-eight patients receiving cardiac valve replacement under CPB were randomized into the control (C) or the SMI (S) group. SMI (0.6 mL/kg) was administered intravenously from the time of anesthesia induction to the beginning of CPB. Cognitive function was assessed at 3 days before surgery and 3 days, 7 days, and 1 month after surgery using the Beijing version of the Montreal Cognitive Assessment (MoCA-BJ) score. The serum levels of neuroglobin (Ngb), hypoxia-inducible factor-1α (HIF-1α), and neuron-specific enolase (NSE) were measured at 30 min after induction (T_0), immediately after the endonasal temperature rewarmed to 36 °C (T_1), and 1 h (T_2), 6 h (T_3), 24 h (T_4), 48 h (T_5), and 72 h (T_6) after CPB.

Results: Compared with the baseline values at T_0, the serum Ngb levels in group C were significantly decreased at T_{1-2} and then increased at T_{3-6}, while the levels in group S were decreased at T_{1-2} and increased at T_{4-6}, compared to group C ($p < 0.05$). The serum HIF-1α levels at T_{1-4} and the serum NSE levels at T_{1-6} were significantly increased in both groups ($p < 0.05$). The serum levels of Ngb at T_3, HIF-1α at T_{1-3}, and NSE at $T_{3-4,6}$ were lower in group S, compared to group C ($p < 0.01$). The MoCA-BJ scores were decreased at 3 and 7 days after surgery in both groups, and the MoCA-BJ scores in group S were higher than those in group C at 3 and 7 days after surgery ($p < 0.01$).

Conclusion: Cognitive function is impaired postoperatively in patients who have undergone cardiac valve replacement under CPB. In addition, treatment with the traditional Chinese medicine SMI decreases the serum levels of Ngb, HIF-1α, and NSE as well as attenuates cognitive dysfunction.

Keywords: Cardiopulmonary bypass, Cognitive dysfunction, Shenmai injection, Cerebral protection

* Correspondence: luckstone009@163.com
†Lei Chen and Liangrong Wang contributed equally to this work.
[1]Department of Anesthesiology, The First Affiliated Hospital of Wenzhou Medical University, Wenzhou, Zhejiang Province, China
Full list of author information is available at the end of the article

Background

Postoperative cognitive dysfunction (POCD) is considered as a common complication of cardiovascular surgery and causes several adverse effects, such as a delayed long-term recovery, a reduced quality of life, and an increased mortality rate [1, 2]. Cerebral embolization, systemic inflammatory response, and low cerebral oxygenation to cerebral hypoperfusion are usually implicated as potential factors for short-term POCD after cardiac surgery [3, 4]. In addition, oxygenation and upregulation of neuroglobin (Ngb) and hypoxia-inducible factor-1α (HIF-1α) expression have been considered as a protective mechanism responding to ischemic injury to neurons, while neuron-specific enolase (NSE) is a marker of neuronal damage. Therefore, the circulating levels of Ngb, HIF-1α, and NSE have been used as indicators for cerebral injury [5, 6]. However, whether circulating Ngb, HIF-1α, and NSE levels could serve as early indicators for cognitive dysfunction after cardiac surgery has not been reported.

With the increasing understanding of the mechanisms involved, various treatments have been introduced over the last decade. Shenmai injection (SMI), a Chinese traditional medicine mainly consisting of the two herbal components Radix ginseng Rubra and Radix ophiopogonis, is extensively used in China as an organ protector [7]. Our previous studies [7–10] have demonstrated the protective effects of SMI against oxidative injury and the inflammatory response, showing its potential as a therapeutic agent for the prevention of lung injury after cardiopulmonary bypass (CPB). However, reports concerning the effects of SMI on cognitive function in patients undergoing cardiac valve replacement under CPB are not available.

Therefore, this prospective, randomized, controlled trial was designed to evaluate the predictive effects of serum Ngb, HIF-1α, and NSE on POCD after CPB as well as the protective effect provided by SMI administration in patients undergoing cardiac valve replacement under CPB. The Beijing version of the Montreal Cognitive Assessment (MoCA-BJ; range, 0–30) was analyzed for assessing the cognitive function; and blood gas parameters of the jugular veins as well as Ngb, HIF-1α, and NSE expression levels were used to evaluate cerebral injury.

Methods

Study design and patients

This prospective, randomized, controlled trial was conducted from September 2014 to January 2017 at the First Affiliated Hospital of Wenzhou Medical University. This trial was registered with Clinicaltrials.gov as ChiCTR-TRC-14004373 on March 11, 2014. After approval by the hospital's Clinical Research Ethics Committee and written informed consent from the patients, 90 patients receiving cardiac valve replacement under CPB were screened. This study was reported according to the CONSORT Extension for Chinese Herbal Medicine Formulas 2017: Recommendations, Explanation, and Elaboration checklist [11].

Inclusion criteria included American Society of Anesthesiologists physical status II–III, aged 40–69 years old, body mass index of 18–29 kg/m^2, left ventricular ejection fraction ≥0.3, and preoperative MoCA-BJ score ≥ 26. Patients were excluded from this study if they had a diagnosis of diabetes mellitus, hypertension, peripheral vascular disease, pulmonary disease, neurological disease, mental disorder, renal insufficiency, liver dysfunction, infective endocarditis, or previous coronary heart disease before screening. In addition, patients who received SMI treatment within 6 months were also excluded.

Surgical interventions

At 30 min before surgery, 0.2 mg/kg morphine and 0.3 mg/kg scopolamine were given intramuscularly. After a standard monitor was attached, a peripheral venous access was secured. Before induction, a 20-G arterial catheter was cannulated, and the sensor/transducer (FloTrac) was connected to record the waveform. Anesthesia was induced intravenously with 0.01 mg/kg midazolam, 0.6 μg/kg sufentanil, 0.3 mg/kg etomidate, and 0.15 mg/kg vecuronium bromide, and then tracheal intubation was facilitated. The patients received intermittent positive-pressure ventilation with a tidal volume of 8–10 mL/kg and a respiratory rate of 10 beats per min to maintain the end-tidal carbon dioxide pressure at approximately 35 mmHg. Continuous administration of sevoflurane and propofol combined with intermittent injection of sufentanil and vecuronium were used to maintain the depth of anesthesia, which was monitored by the bispectral index. After anesthesia, the right internal jugular vein was reversely cannulated to the bulbar level for continuous blood sampling.

All patients received standard CPB management. CPB was instituted with a membrane oxygenator. The body temperature was maintained under mild hypothermia (32–33 °C), and α-stat was used for acid-base management. The pump flow was maintained at a rate of 2.0–2.5 $L/min/m^2$ using a nonpulsatile flow, and a blood cardioplegic solution was used. During the perioperative period including CPB, the mean arterial blood pressure was maintained at 55–80 mmHg using norepinephrine or vasopressin. Milrinone was used if the left ventricular ejection fraction was less than 30% after CPB, as measured by transesophageal echocardiography, in case of right ventricular dysfunction or pulmonary hypertension. A blood transfusion was needed if the hematocrit level fell below 21% during CPB or below 25% during the remaining perioperative period. Fresh frozen plasma was transfused when the international normalized ratio was greater than 1.5 with excessive bleeding greater than 200 mL/h for two consecutive hours in the postoperative period. Platelet concentrates were transfused when the platelet count was less than 50,000/mm^3 with excessive bleeding greater than 200 mL/h for two consecutive hours in the postoperative period. All patients were transferred to the Coronary Care Unit (CCU) after surgery and received standard management according to institutional guidelines by the CCU staff.

SMI administration

SMI composed of Radix ginseng Rubra and Radix Ophiopogonis was a product of Sanjiu Pharmaceutical Co. Ltd. (Yaan, China; batch No. Z51021845, provided as 1 g of crude drug in an ampoule of 10 mL). In group S, SMI at a dose of 0.6 mL/kg, dissolved in 250 mL of normal saline, was administered intravenously from the time of anesthesia induction to the beginning of CPB at a rate of 10 mL/min. The control patients were given an equal volume of normal saline instead.

Outcome measures

The durations of aortic cross clamping, CPB, and anesthesia maintenance were recorded, respectively. The hemodynamic parameters, including the mean arterial blood pressure and heart rate, as well as the blood gas parameters of the jugular veins, which included the jugular venous oxygen saturation (S_JvO_2), jugular venous oxygen partial pressure (P_JvO_2), hemoglobin, hematocrit, and lactic acid (Lacjv) of the jugular venous blood samples, were collected at 30 min after induction (T_0), immediately after the endonasal temperature rewarmed to 36 °C (T_1), the end of cardiac surgery (T_2), and 6 h (T_3), 24 h (T_4), 48 h (T_5), and 72 h (T_6) after CPB, respectively. The MoCA-BJ scores were evaluated at 3 days before surgery as well as 3 days, 7 days, and 1 month after surgery.

The remaining blood sample was centrifuged to separate the serum, which was then stored at − 20 °C for subsequent analyses of Ngb, HIF-1α, and NSE. Indicators were determined using commercially available enzyme-linked immunosorbent assay kits (Westang Biotechnology Co. Ltd., Shanghai, China), according to the manufacturer's instructions. The levels of these indicators were measured by investigators unaware of the group allocation and the blood gas results.

Sample size calculation and randomization

The sample size was planned and calculated according to comparison of the MoCA-BJ on the third and seventh day postsurgery. With a power of 66% and a significance level of 5%, a total of 17 patients would be required in each group to make a difference of − 3.4 in the MoCA-BJ on the third day postsurgery, with a dropout rate of 10%. With a power of 31% and a significance level of 5%, a total of 28 patients would be required in each group to make a difference of − 1.7 in the MoCA-BJ on the seventh day postsurgery, with a dropout rate of 10%. Thus, enrollment of 88 patients was planned to minimize statistical errors.

Patients were randomized using a sealed envelope system. Eighty-eight patients were randomized to either the SMI (group S, 44 cases) or the control (group C, 44 cases) group. The medical staff collecting and analyzing the MoCA-BJ scores was blinded to the treatment allocation.

Statistical analysis

Data were tested for normal distribution using the Kolmogorov–Smirnov test. Continuous, normally distributed data were expressed as the mean ± standard deviation. Categorical data were expressed as numbers. Data on the block level were expressed as a median (range) and analyzed with the Mann–Whitney test. For comparison of demographic and operative data, categorical data were compared with the χ^2 test and quantitative data were compared with the Student's t-test. For comparison of outcomes within the same group at different time points, data were analyzed by repeated-measures analysis of variance using the Bonferroni method. For comparison of outcomes between different groups at the same time point, the paired t-test was conducted. A P value < 0.05 was considered significant. Analysis was performed using SPSS software, version 17.0 for Windows.

Results

Patient enrollment and characteristics

The study flow diagram is shown in Fig. 1. A total of 80 patients completed the study. No significant differences between the two groups were found in terms of the clinical characteristics, including gender, age, body mass index, surgical procedure type, duration of aortic cross clamping, CPB, and anesthesia maintenance ($p > 0.05$) (Table 1).

Hemodynamic parameters

In comparison to T_0, the mean arterial blood pressure was decreased at T_1 ($p < 0.001$) and increased at $T_{4,6}$ ($p = 0.005$ and $p = 0.041$) in group C, while it was decreased at $T_{1,3}$ ($p < 0.001$ and $p = 0.021$) and increased at $T_{4–6}$ ($p = 0.002$, $p = 0.002$, and $p = 0.006$) in group S. The heart rate was significantly decreased at T_1 and increased at $T_{2–6}$ in both groups ($p < 0.001$). There were no differences in hemodynamic variables (mean arterial blood pressure and heart rate) at any time points ($p > 0.05$) between these two groups (Table 2).

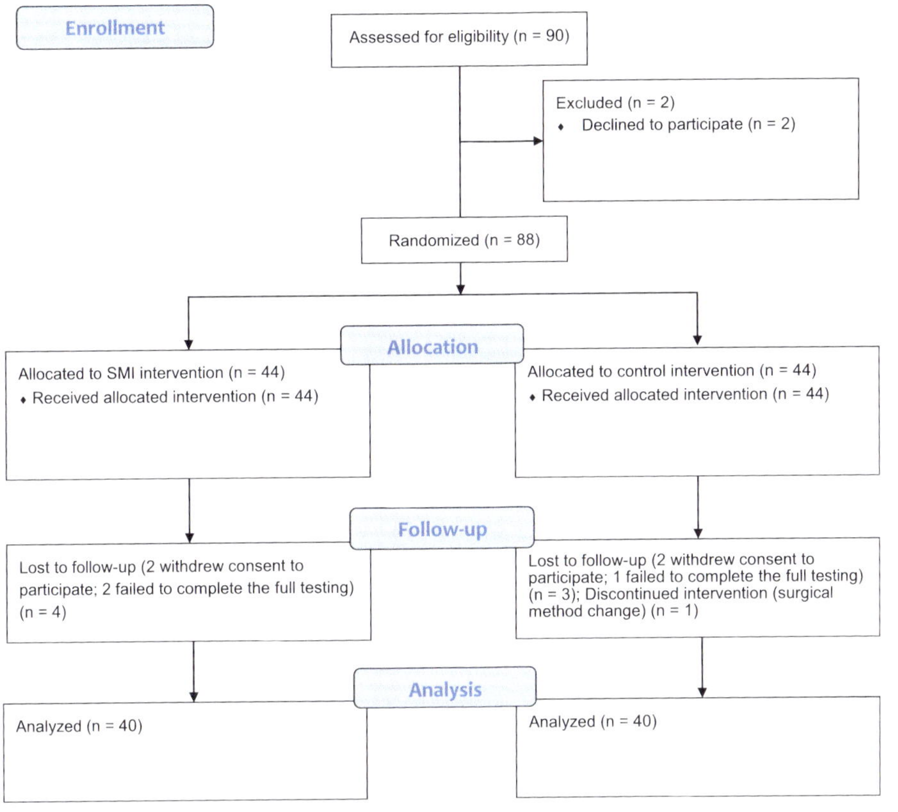

Fig. 1 CONSORT 2010 Flow Diagram

Blood gas analysis

Table 3 shows the blood gas parameters. Compared to the baseline values at T_0, the levels of S_jvO_2 and P_jvO_2 were increased significantly at T_2 ($p = 0.001$ and $p < 0.001$) in group C and T_{1-2} ($p < 0.001$) in group S; the values were much higher in group S at T_{1-3} than in group C ($p < 0.001$) (Fig. 2). The levels of Lacjv were increased at T_{1-4} (group C: $p < 0.001$, $p < 0.001$, $p < 0.001$, and $p = 0.003$ and group S: $p < 0.001$, $p < 0.001$, $p < 0.001$, and $p = 0.002$) and decreased at T_6 (group C: $p = 0.003$; group S: $p = 0.001$) in both groups, compared with T_0; however the level at T_4 in group S was lower than that in group C ($p < 0.001$) (Fig. 2). The levels of hemoglobin and hematocrit were lower at T_{1-6} than at T_0 ($p < 0.001$), but no differences were found between the two groups ($p > 0.05$).

Table 1 Clinical Characteristics of Patients ($n = 40$ in Each Group)

	Group C	Group S
Gender (M/F)	23/17	22/18
Age (yr)	55 ± 10	58 ± 9
Body mass index (kg/m2)	23.0 ± 2.8	24.2 ± 2.4
Valve replacement(n)		
single valve replacement	24	26
double valve replacement	16	14
Duration of ACC (min)	89 ± 21	86 ± 20
Duration ofCPB(min)	116 ± 22	111 ± 24
Duration of anesthesiamaintenance (min)	247 ± 33	239 ± 29

ACC aortic cross clamp, *CPB* cardiopulmonary bypass
Data are presented as mean ± SD, or numbers

Concentrations of Ngb, HIF-1α, and NSE

Table 4 shows the serum levels of Ngb, HIF-1α, and NSE in both groups. Compared with T_0, the levels of serum Ngb in group C were significantly decreased at T_{1-2} ($p < 0.001$ and $p = 0.004$) and significantly increased at T_{3-6} ($p < 0.001$), with two peaks at T_3 and T_6, respectively; while the levels in group S were significantly decreased at T_{1-2} ($p < 0.001$) and significantly increased at T_{4-6} ($p = 0.023$, $p < 0.001$ and $p < 0.001$), with the highest levels at T_6. The levels of serum HIF-1α were increased at T_{1-4} and had peaks at T_2 in both groups (group C: $p < 0.001$, $p < 0.001$, $p < 0.001$, and $p = 0.001$; group S: $p = 0.001$, $p < 0.001$, $p < 0.001$, and $p = 0.023$). The serum NSE levels in both groups were significantly increased at T_{1-6} ($p < 0.001$). The serum levels of Ngb at T_3 ($p < 0.001$), HIF-1α at T_{1-3} ($p < 0.001$), and NSE at $T_{3-4,6}$ ($p < 0.001$, $p = 0.002$, and $p < 0.001$) were lower in group S than in group C (Fig. 3).

Table 2 MAP and HR (n = 40 in Each Group)

	Group	T_0	T_1	T_2	T_3	T_4	T_5	T_6
MAP	C	73 ± 10	60 ± 6*	71 ± 9	71 ± 8	83 ± 8*	80 ± 9	80 ± 9†
(mm Hg)	S	74 ± 7	62 ± 6*	71 ± 8	69 ± 5†	81 ± 9*	83 ± 9*	80 ± 6*
HR	C	64 ± 13	0*	86 ± 10*	91 ± 11*	81 ± 9*	85 ± 7*	80 ± 11*
(bpm/min)	S	62 ± 10	0*	88 ± 10*	93 ± 9*	83 ± 11*	85 ± 7*	81 ± 10*

T_0, 30 min after the induction; T_1, immediately after temperature rewarmed to 36 °C; T_2, end of cardiac surgery; T_{3-6}, 6 h, 24 h, 48 h, 72 h after CPB
Data are expressed as mean ± SD
* $p < 0.01$ vs. $\mathbf{T_0}$.† $p < 0.05$ vs. $\mathbf{T_0}$

MoCA-BJ analysis

Compared to preoperative values at 3 days before surgery, the MoCA-BJ scores were decreased at 3 and 7 days after surgery in both groups (group C: $p < 0.001$; group S: $p < 0.001$, $p = 0.001$). The MoCA-BJ scores of group S were higher than those in group C at 3 and 7 days after surgery ($p < 0.001$) (Fig. 4). The scores of Clock, Naming, Memory, Serial 7, and Sentence rep in group C ($p = 0.025$, $p < 0.001$, $p < 0.001$, $p < 0.001$ and $p = 0.015$) and the score of Memory in group S ($p = 0.012$) were lower than the preoperative baseline values at 3 days after surgery. Compared to group C, the scores of Cube, Memory, Serial 7, and Sentence rep were elevated at 3 days after surgery in group S ($p = 0.005$, $p = 0.005$, $p = 0.008$, and $p < 0.001$) (Fig. 5).

Discussion

Recent technological advances have contributed to an increasingly lower rate of clinically evident complications, but POCD remains an important clinical problem associated with cardiac surgery [12, 13]. Its manifestations may include impairment in visuospatial and executive functions, naming, attention, language, delayed recall (memory), and orientation [14]. Presently, the MoCA and the Mini-Mental State Examination (MMSE) are the most commonly used neuropsychological tests for POCD. As a simple cognitive screening tool, the MoCA-BJ was used in this study to balance the influences of various ages and education levels; [15] and its sensitivity and specificity are better than those of the MMSE [16, 17]. As shown in this study, the total MoCA-BJ scores were significantly lower at 3 and 7 days after surgery in patients receiving cardiac surgery in group C, and the scores basically recovered to baseline values at 1 month after surgery, suggesting that the patients suffered from POCD in the early but not the late stage after cardiac surgery. The results also showed that several cognitive domains, especially memory, were badly impaired; these results were identical to previous ones [18, 19]. For example, Yu et al. [16] have reported that among all the cognitive subdomains, delayed recall (Memory) was shown to be the best index to differentiate POCD from the normal controls. Similarly, Jones et al. [20] have reported that the severity of heart/circulation problems independently contributed to a worse delayed recall (Memory) performance. Our results showed that the Memory scores were lower than the baseline values at 3 days after surgery in both groups, but the scores in group S were improved after SMI administration. In addition, changes in the Clock, Naming, Serial 7, and Sentence rep scores were similar as the delayed recall evaluation, which were all lower than the preoperative baselines values.

Table 3 Blood Gas Parameters (n = 40 in Each Group)

	Group	T_0	T_1	T_2	T_3	T_4	T_5	T_6
SJ vO2	C	58.2 ± 12.6	48.4 ± 4.7*	64.3 ± 8.0*	54.7 ± 8.9	54.8 ± 5.4	50.7 ± 6.1*	53.3 ± 8.7
(%)	S	57.7 ± 8.8	70.5 ± 12.0*‡	75.8 ± 7.4*‡	59.9 ± 4.6‡	56.1 ± 3.8	52.1 ± 6.0*	50.8 ± 4.4*
PJ vO2	C	33.8 ± 8.1	29.5 ± 2.8*	40.1 ± 6.0*	32.1 ± 5.1	31.0 ± 2.5†	28.3 ± 3.0*	29.7 ± 4.2†
(mmHg)	S	34.1 ± 3.9	45.7 ± 11.8*‡	50.4 ± 8.0*‡	34.6 ± 4.0‡	30.5 ± 2.1*	28.8 ± 3.1*	28.6 ± 2.5*
Lacjv	C	1.1 ± 0.5	1.7 ± 0.7*	1.9 ± 1.0*	2.1 ± 1.0*	2.0 ± 0.8*	1.0 ± 0.3	0.8 ± 0.3*
(mmol/L)	S	1.1 ± 0.5	1.7 ± 0.7*	1.9 ± 0.8*	1.9 ± 0.8*	1.4 ± 0.6*‡	1.0 ± 0.3	0.8 ± 0.3*
Hb	C	12.8 ± 1.4	8.1 ± 0.9*	9.5 ± 1.1*	10.5 ± 1.3*	11.1 ± 1.3*	9.9 ± 1.1*	9.8 ± 1.1*
(g/dL)	S	13.0 ± 1.1	8.1 ± 0.7*	9.6 ± 1.0*	10.3 ± 0.9*	11.3 ± 0.9*	10.1 ± 1.3*	10.2 ± 1.4*
HCT	C	37.8 ± 4.1	24.0 ± 2.8*	28.0 ± 3.1*	30.9 ± 3.2*	32.5 ± 3.9*	29.2 ± 3.3*	28.7 ± 3.1*
(%)	S	38.1 ± 3.3	24.0 ± 1.9*	28.3 ± 3.0*	30.4 ± 2.6*	33.2 ± 2.7*	29.7 ± 3.9*	30.1 ± 4.0*

T_0, 30 min after the induction; T_1, immediately after temperature rewarmed to 36 °C; T_2, end of cardiac surgery; T_{3-6}, 6 h, 24 h, 48 h, 72 h after CPB
Data are expressed as mean ± SD
* $p < 0.01$ vs. $\mathbf{T_0}$.† $p < 0.05$ vs. $\mathbf{T_0}$.‡ $p < 0.01$ vs. group C

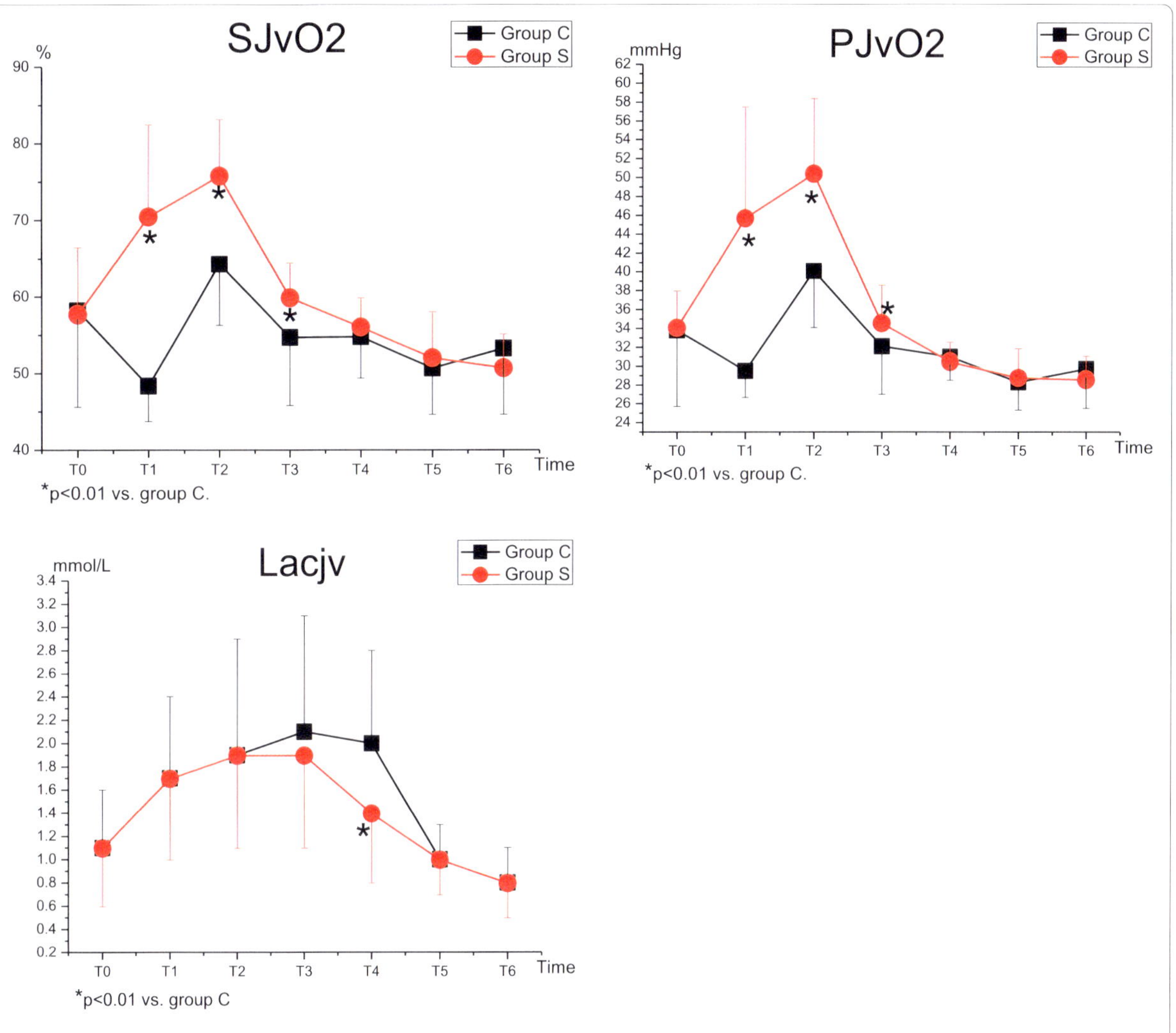

*p<0.01 vs. group C.

Fig. 2 Blood Gas Parameters

Table 4 Serum Levels of Ngb, HIF-1α and NSE(n = 40 in Each Group)

	Group	T_0	T_1	T_2	T_3	T_4	T_5	T_6
Ngb	C	1.23 ± 0.42	0.53 ± 0.19*	0.93 ± 0.43*	2.83 ± 1.14*	1.89 ± 0.77*	1.92 ± 0.83*	2.33 ± 0.74*
(ng/mL)	S	1.35 ± 0.39	0.61 ± 0.23*	0.93 ± 0.32*	1.20 ± 0.61‡	1.62 ± 0.59†	1.94 ± 0.80*	2.35 ± 0.83*
HIF-1α	C	2.01 ± 0.55	4.54 ± 1.38*	10.98 ± 2.55*	6.56 ± 2.06*	2.48 ± 0.99*	2.04 ± 0.62	2.33 ± 1.12
(ng/mL)	S	1.93 ± 0.68	2.37 ± 1.04*‡	9.11 ± 1.49*‡	4.69 ± 2.01*‡	2.36 ± 1.30†	2.15 ± 0.90	1.98 ± 0.77
NSE	C	5.05 ± 1.21	18.47 ± 5.72*	34.93 ± 12.33*	40.77 ± 15.73*	14.25 ± 5.67*	9.54 ± 3.50*	12.27 ± 5.76*
(ng/mL)	S	5.28 ± 1.35	17.67 ± 5.51*	33.82 ± 12.78*	27.96 ± 6.53*‡	10.51 ± 4.94*‡	8.25 ± 3.61*	6.44 ± 1.35*‡

T_0, 30 min after the induction; T_1, immediately after temperature rewarmed to 36 °C; T_2, end of cardiac surgery; T_{3-6}, 6 h, 24 h, 48 h, 72 h after CPB
Data are expressed as mean ± SD
* $p < 0.01$ vs. T_0.† $p < 0.05$ vs. T_0.‡ $p < 0.01$ vs. group C

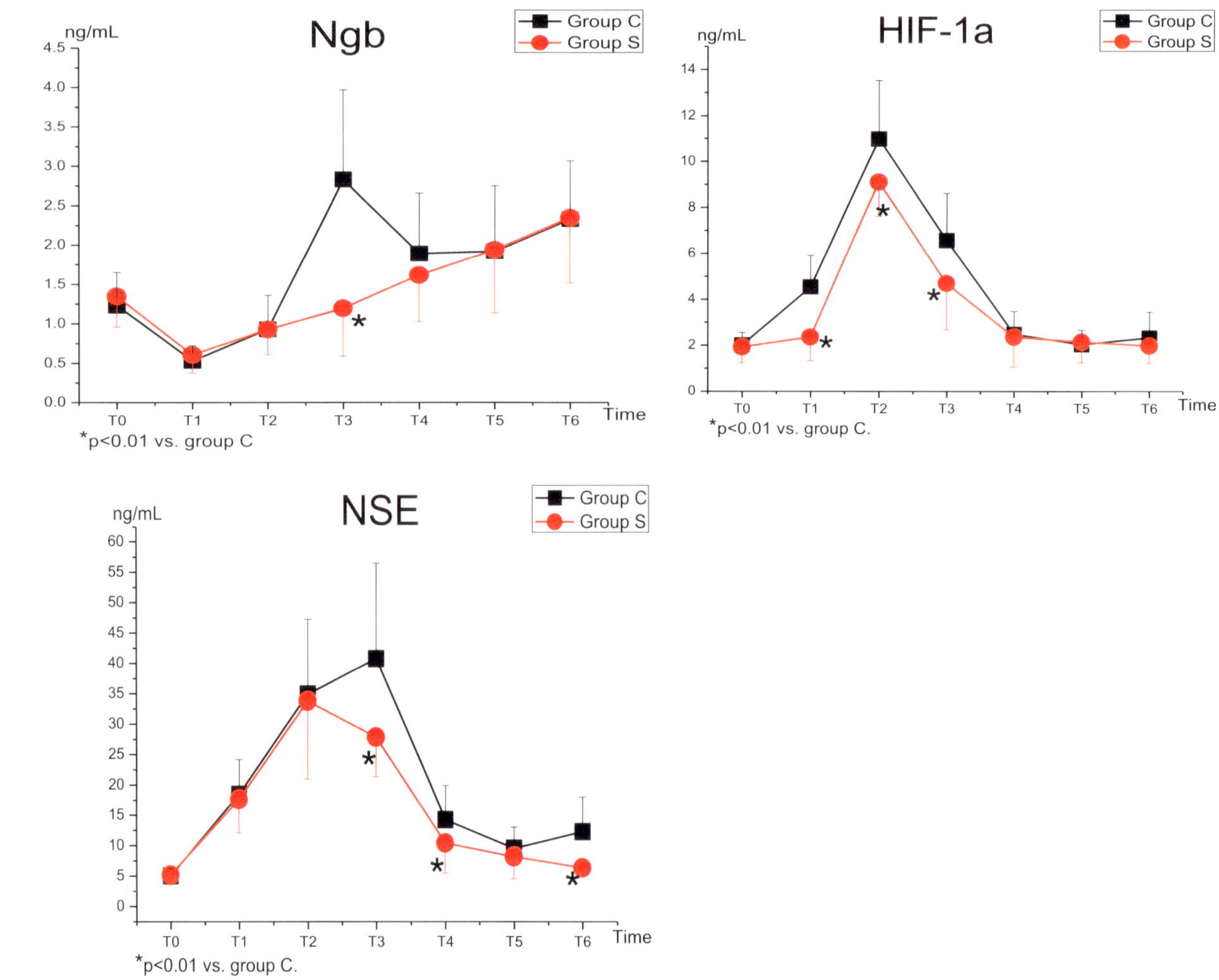

*p<0.01 vs. group C.

Fig. 3 Serum Levels of Ngb, HIF-1α and NSE

Though the cognitive damages after cardiac surgery have been well described, the exact mechanisms involved have not been elucidated. Zheng et al. [21] have reported an association between decreased regional cerebral oxygen saturation ($rScO_2$), desaturation, and POCD in adult patients receiving cardiac surgery. The blood flow of the internal jugular vein bulbar is mainly from the cerebral hemisphere, and the levels of S_JvO_2 and P_JvO_2 can indirectly reflect $rScO_2$ [22, 23]. As shown in our study, compared to the baseline values, the levels of S_JvO2 and P_JvO2 were significantly decreased and the levels of Lacjv were increased in patients undergoing CPB, suggesting that cerebral anoxia may at least partly contribute to POCD.

Ngb, a novel neuroprotective protein, affords protection against hypoxia/ischemia and oxidative stress-induced injury in the nervous system. Ngb overexpression enhances cell survival under conditions of anoxia or oxygen and glucose deprivation [24], and it protects neurons against cerebral ischemia-reperfusion injury [25]. Previous data have implied that the upregulated expression of Ngb could be an endogenous compensatory or protective mechanism in response to sublethal hypoxic/ischemic insults to brain neurons, and Barzo et al. [26] have reported that a predominantly vasogenic edema formation occurred immediately after brain injury and a more widespread and slower cytotoxic edema formation resulted later, which may lead to two peaks of Ngb expression following brain injury. Furthermore, recent studies have found that the Ngb levels are increased in early and moderately advanced Alzheimer's disease subjects [27]. These findings may explain the results uncovered in our study.

HIF-1α has emerged as a critical oxygen-sensitive transcription factor that orchestrates the body's protective response to hypoxia and can protect organs against acute ischemic injury [28]. Moreover, it has been

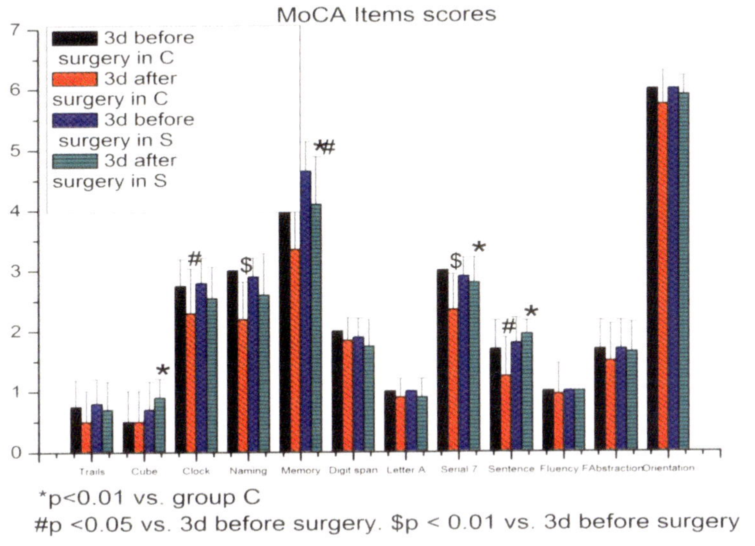

Fig. 5 MoCA-BJ Items scores

recently documented that the expression of HIF-1α under hypoxia has protective effects on astrocytes, thus playing an important role in cerebral protection [29]. Its protective effects also have been proven in a model of cultured cortical neurons exposed to moderate hypoxia [30, 31]. As shown in our study, the serum HIF-1α level began to increase before the Ngb level. The role of HIF-1α in the regulation of oxygen homeostasis in tissue may be correlated with Ngb expression [32]. Additionally, a recent study has demonstrated that HIF-1α contributes to the upregulation of Ngb expression under hypoxic conditions in mice [33]. However, further studies are necessary to elucidate the exact mechanisms of HIF-1α in Ngb regulation under hypoxic and other pathological conditions.

NSE, which was originally described by Moore and McGregor in 1965, [34] has been considered as a traditional marker to assess neuronal damage; [35] however, clinical trials have shown controversial results regarding the correlation between cognitive dysfunction and the circulating NSE level. Some studies have found a correlation between the NSE level and the clinical outcome of neurocognitive dysfunction, [36–38] but others have failed to do so [39, 40]. In our study, the serum NSE levels were significantly increased after CPB. Therefore, NSE may be an indicative parameter for POCD.

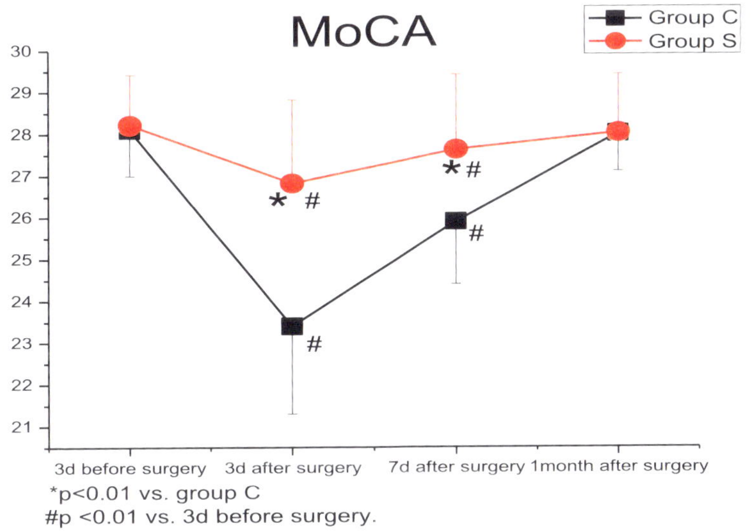

Fig. 4 Total MoCA-BJ scores

SMI, a traditional Chinese herbal medicine, is widely used in mainland China for the treatment of cardio/cerebrovascular disorders and as an adjunct therapy to tumor chemotherapy [41]. The active component of SMI is radix ginseng rubra, which contains Ginsenoside Rg3 and Ginsenoside Rb1. The protective effects of Ginsenoside Rb1 have been well proven in various models of cerebral ischemia-reperfusion injury [42, 43]. Its possible mechanism of the protective effect on the central nervous system involves calcium channel blockade, estrogen-like action, and antiperoxidation, which may inhibit cerebral nerve cell apoptosis and ameliorate mitochondrial dysfunction, etc [44]. Hence, we hypothesized that treatment with SMI might present beneficial effects against reperfusion injury and improve cognitive function after cardiac valve replacement under CPB. As shown in our study, even though the MoCA-BJ score in group S was decreased at 3 days after surgery but was still improved as compared to group C at the early stage after CPB, SMI treatment increased the levels of S_jvO_2 and P_jvO_2 as well as decreased the serum Ngb, HIF-1α, and NSE levels at different time points. These data implied that SMI may attenuate cerebral anoxia and neuronal damage, subsequently improving cognitive function and reducing the incidence of POCD.

Several limitations of this study should be noted. First, enrollment of patients did not consider the traditional Chinese medicine syndromes, and the lack of traditional Chinese medicine syndrome diagnosis during patient enrolment was another potential source of selection bias. Second, whether SMI exerts protective effects by improving cerebral oxygenation directly or by other implied mechanisms should be investigated in future studies. Finally, the optimal dosage of SMI and its main effective ingredient were not determined in the current study. Our future studies will address these issues.

Conclusions

In conclusion, cognitive function is impaired postoperatively in patients undergoing cardiac surgery with CPB. The novel biomarkers Ngb, HIF-1α, and NSE could serve as early indicators for POCD. Treatment with SMI, a traditional Chinese medicine, decreases the levels of serum Ngb, HIF-1α, and NSE, thus improving cognitive function.

Abbreviations

CCU: Coronary Care Unit; CPB: Cardiopulmonary bypass; HIF-1α: Hypoxia-inducible factor-1α; MoCA-BJ: Beijing version of the Montreal Cognitive Assessment; Ngb: Neuroglobin; NSE: Neuron-specific enolase; POCD: Postoperative cognitive dysfunction; $rScO_2$: Regional cerebral oxygen saturation; SMI: Shenmai Injection

Funding

The present study was granted by Wenzhou Municipal Science and Technology Bureau (No. H20100010).

Authors' contributions

LNL and LRW designed this study and wrote the manuscript. CL and LLL performed the experiments. QZ1 collected all data. QZ2 and FFC assisted with data analysis. All the authors approved the final version of the manuscript. CL and LRW were co-first authors and contributed equally to this study.

Competing interests

The authors declare that they have no competing interests.

Author details

[1]Department of Anesthesiology, The First Affiliated Hospital of Wenzhou Medical University, Wenzhou, Zhejiang Province, China. [2]Wenzhou People's Hospital, Wenzhou, Zhejiang Province, China.

References

1. Tonkovic D, Marinic DK, Baronica R, Oberhofer D, Pavlovic DB, Peric M. Postoperative mental disorders in cardiovascular surgery. Acta Med Croatica. 2012;66:67–72.
2. Hartholt KA, van der Cammen TJ, Klimek M. Postoperative cognitive dysfunction in geriatric patients. Z Gerontol Geriatr. 2012;45:411–6. https://doi.org/10.1007/s00391-012-0326-2.
3. Djaiani G, Katznelson R, Fedorko L, Rao V, Green R, Carroll J, Katski J. Early benefit of preserved cognitive function is not sustained at one-year after cardiac surgery: a longitudinal follow-up of the randomized controlled trial. Can J Anaesth. 2012;59:449–55. https://doi.org/10.1007/s12630-012-9675-y.
4. Papadopoulos G, Karanikolas M, Liarmakopoulou A, Papathanakos G, Korre M, Beris A. Cerebral oximetry and cognitive dysfunction in elderly patients undergoing surgery for hip fractures: a prospective observational study. Open Orthop J. 2012;6:400–5. https://doi.org/10.2174/1874325001206010400.
5. Hota KB, Hota SK, Srivastava RB, Singh SB. Neuroglobin regulates hypoxic response of neuronal cells through Hif-1alpha- and Nrf2-mediated mechanism. J Cereb Blood Flow Metab. 2012 Jun;32(6):1046–60. https://doi.org/10.1038/jcbfm.2012.21.
6. Yildirim AO, Eroglu M, Kaldirim U, Eyi YE, Simsek K, Durusu M, Yamanel L, Arziman I, Tuncer SK, Toygar M, Balkan A, Cayci T, Demirbas S, Oter S, Bilgi C. Serum neuron-specific enolase and S-100beta levels as prognostic follow-up markers for oxygen administered carbon monoxide intoxication cases. Indian J Biochem Biophys. 2015;52:29–33.
7. Wang L, Wang W, Zhao X, Jin L, Bai Y, Yao H, Zhuo Q, Lin L. Effect of Shenmai injection, a traditional Chinese medicine, on pulmonary dysfunction after tourniquet-induced limb ischemia-reperfusion. J Trauma. 2011;71:893–7. https://doi.org/10.1097/TA.0b013e318205e279.
8. Lin L, Wang L, Chen F, Hu M, Miao J, Wang J. Effect and significance of Shenmai injection on value of vascular endothelial active factors of heart valve replacement patients. Zhongguo Zhong Yao Za Zhi. 2009;34:1155–8.
9. Lin LN, Zhang SG, Wang WT, Xi JH, Qiu XX, Dai YY. Effect of Shenmai injection on expression and activity of heme oxygenase-1 in reperfusion injury after pulmonary ischemia in rabbits. Zhongguo Zhong yao za zhi. 2008;33:296–9.
10. Chen FF, Lin LN, Miao JX. Protective effect of Shenmai injection on lung injury induced by cardiac pulmonary bypass. Zhongguo Zhong Xi Yi Jie He Za Zhi. 2009;29:414–7.
11. Cheng CW, Wu TX, Shang HC, Li YP, Altman DG, Moher D, Bian ZX, Group C-CF. CONSORT extension for Chinese herbal medicine formulas 2017: recommendations, explanation, and elaboration (traditional Chinese version). Ann Intern Med. 2017;167:W7–W20. https://doi.org/10.7326/IsTranslatedFrom_M17-2977_1.

12. Schwarz N, Schonburg M, Kastaun S, Gerriets T, Kaps M. Cognitive deterioration after cardiosurgery. Nervenarzt. 2011;82(190):192–7. https://doi.org/10.1007/s00115-010-3116-3.
13. Lombard FW, Mathew JP. Neurocognitive dysfunction following cardiac surgery. Semin Cardiothorac Vasc Anesth. 2010;14:102–10. https://doi.org/10.1177/1089253210371519.
14. Nie K, Zhang Y, Wang L, Zhao J, Huang Z, Gan R, Li S, Wang L. A pilot study of psychometric properties of the Beijing version of Montreal cognitive assessment in patients with idiopathic Parkinson's disease in China. J Clin Neurosci. 2012;19:1497–500. https://doi.org/10.1016/j.jocn.2011.11.039.
15. Nasreddine ZS. Montreal Cognitive Assessment. https://www.mocatest.org/. 2003/2012-10-4.
16. Yu J, Li J, Huang X. The Beijing version of the Montreal cognitive assessment as a brief screening tool for mild cognitive impairment: a community-based study. BMC Psychiatry. 2012;12:156. https://doi.org/10.1186/1471-244X-12-156.
17. Tan JP, Li N, Gao J, Wang LN, Zhao YM, Yu BC, Du W, Zhang WJ, Cui LQ, Wang QS, Li JJ, Yang JS, Yu JM, Xia XN, Zhou PY. Optimal cutoff scores for dementia and mild cognitive impairment of the Montreal cognitive assessment among elderly and oldest-old Chinese population. J Alzheimers Dis. 2015;43:1403–12. https://doi.org/10.3233/JAD-141278.
18. Burkhart CS, Steiner LA. Can postoperative cognitive dysfunction be avoided? Hosp Pract (1995). 2012;40:214–23. https://doi.org/10.3810/hp.2012.02.962.
19. An LN, Yue Y, Guo WZ, Miao YL, Mi WD, Zhang H, Lei ZL, Han SJ, Dong L. Surgical trauma induces iron accumulation and oxidative stress in a rodent model of postoperative cognitive dysfunction. Biol Trace Elem Res. 2013; 151:277–83. https://doi.org/10.1007/s12011-012-9564-9.
20. Jones JD, Malaty I, Price CC, Okun MS, Bowers D. Health comorbidities and cognition in 1948 patients with idiopathic Parkinson's disease. Parkinsonism Relat Disord. 2012;18:1073–8. https://doi.org/10.1016/j.parkreldis.2012.06.004.
21. Zheng F, Sheinberg R, Yee MS, Ono M, Zheng Y, Hogue CW. Cerebral near-infrared spectroscopy monitoring and neurologic outcomes in adult cardiac surgery patients: a systematic review. Anesth Analg. 2013;116:663–76. https://doi.org/10.1213/ANE.0b013e318277a255.
22. Walther T, Dhein S, Ullmann C, Schneider K, Bilz T, Rastan A, Garbade J, Falk V, Emrich FC, Muth P, Mohr FW, Kostelka M. Cerebral protection during controlled hypoperfusion in a piglet model: comparison of moderate (25°C) versus deep (18°C) hypothermia at various flow rates using intraoperative measurements and ex vivo investigation. Thorac Cardiovasc Surg. 2013;61: 546–52. https://doi.org/10.1055/s-0032-1324710.
23. Sari A, Yamashita S, Ohosita S, Ogasahara H, Yamada K, Yonei A, Yokota K. Cerebrovascular reactivity to CO2 in patients with hepatic or septic encephalopathy. Resuscitation. 1990;19:125–34.
24. Fordel E, Thijs L, Martinet W, Schrijvers D, Moens L, Dewilde S. Anoxia or oxygen and glucose deprivation in SH-SY5Y cells: a step closer to the unraveling of neuroglobin and cytoglobin functions. Gene. 2007;398:114–22.
25. Li SQ, Li WB, Zhang M, Wu YZ, Hu YY. The role of neuroglobin in the neuroprotection of limb ischemic preconditioning in rats. Mol Neurobiol. 2013;47:197–208. https://doi.org/10.1007/s12035-012-8373-7.
26. Barzo P, Marmarou A, Fatouros P, Hayasaki K, Corwin F. Biphasic pathophysiological response of vasogenic and cellular edema in traumatic brain swelling. Acta Neurochir Suppl. 1997;70:119–22.
27. Sun F, Mao X, Xie L, Greenberg DA, Jin K. Neuroglobin protein is upregulated in Alzheimer's disease. J Alzheimers Dis. 2013;36:659–63. https://doi.org/10.3233/JAD-130323.
28. Ong SG, Hausenloy DJ. Hypoxia-inducible factor as a therapeutic target for cardioprotection. Pharmacol Ther. 2012;136:69–81. https://doi.org/10.1016/j.pharmthera.2012.07.005.
29. Badawi Y, Ramamoorthy P, Shi H. Hypoxia-inducible factor 1 protects hypoxic astrocytes against glutamate toxicity. ASN Neuro. 2012;4:231–41. https://doi.org/10.1042/AN20120006.
30. Li D, Bai T, Brorson JR. Adaptation to moderate hypoxia protects cortical neurons against ischemia-reperfusion injury and excitotoxicity independently of HIF-1alpha. Exp Neurol. 2011;230:302–10. https://doi.org/10.1016/j.expneurol.2011.05.009.
31. Shao G, Gao CY, Lu GW. Alterations of hypoxia-inducible factor-1 alpha in the hippocampus of mice acutely and repeatedly exposed to hypoxia. Neurosignals. 2005;14:255–61.
32. Di Giulio C, Zara S, Cataldi A, Porzionato A, Pokorski M, De Caro R. Human carotid body HIF and NGB expression during human development and aging. Adv Exp Med Biol 2012;758:265–271. doi: https://doi.org/10.1007/978-94-007-4584-1_36.
33. Liu N, Yu Z, Xiang S, Zhao S, Tjarnlund-Wolf A, Xing C, Zhang J, Wang X. Transcriptional regulation mechanisms of hypoxia-induced neuroglobin gene expression. Biochem J. 2012;443:153–64. https://doi.org/10.1042/BJ20111856.
34. Moore BW, McGregor D. Chromatographic and electrophoretic fractionation of soluble proteins of brain and liver. J Biol Chem. 1965;240:1647–53.
35. Giacoppo S, Bramanti P, Barresi M, Celi D, Foti Cuzzola V, Palella E, Marino S. Predictive biomarkers of recovery in traumatic brain injury. Neurocrit Care. 2012;16:470–7. https://doi.org/10.1007/s12028-012-9707-z.
36. Zhang B, Huang Y, Su Z, Wang S, Wang S, Wang J, Wang A, Lai X. Neurological, functional, and biomechanical characteristics after high-velocity behind armor blunt trauma of the spine. J Trauma. 2011;71:1680–8. https://doi.org/10.1097/TA.0b013e318231bce7.
37. Prohl J, Rother J, Kluge S, de Heer G, Liepert J, Bodenburg S, Pawlik K, Kreymann G. Prediction of short-term and long-term outcomes after cardiac arrest: a prospective multivariate approach combining biochemical, clinical, electrophysiological, and neuropsychological investigations. Crit Care Med. 2007;35:1230–7.
38. Ramlawi B, Rudolph JL, Mieno S, Khabbaz K, Sodha NR, Boodhwani M, Levkoff SE, Marcantonio ER, Sellke FW. Serologic markers of brain injury and cognitive function after cardiopulmonary bypass. Ann Surg. 2006;244:593–601.
39. Reinsfelt B, Ricksten SE, Zetterberg H, Blennow K, Freden-Lindqvist J, Westerlind A. Cerebrospinal fluid markers of brain injury, inflammation, and blood-brain barrier dysfunction in cardiac surgery. Ann Thorac Surg. 2012; 94:549–55. https://doi.org/10.1016/j.athoracsur.2012.04.044.
40. McDonagh DL, Mathew JP, White WD, Phillips-Bute B, Laskowitz DT, Podgoreanu MV, Newman MF, Neurologic Outcome Research G. Cognitive function after major noncardiac surgery, apolipoprotein E4 genotype, and biomarkers of brain injury. Anesthesiology. 2010;112:852–9. https://doi.org/10.1097/ALN.0b013e3181d31fd7.
41. Lu LY, Zheng GQ, Wang Y. An overview of systematic reviews of shenmai injection for healthcare. Evid Based Complement Alternat Med. 2014;2014: 840650. https://doi.org/10.1155/2014/840650.
42. Zhu J, Jiang Y, Wu L, Lu T, Xu G, Liu X. Suppression of local inflammation contributes to the neuroprotective effect of ginsenoside Rb1 in rats with cerebral ischemia. Neuroscience. 2012;202:342–51. https://doi.org/10.1016/j.neuroscience.2011.11.070.
43. Yang CX, Liu JX, Sun ZL, Gao XQ, Deng L, Yuan QL. Effects of Ginsenoside RB1 on neural cell apoptosis and expressions of Bcl-2 and Bax in rats following subjected to cerebral ischemia-reperfusion. Sichuan da xue xue bao Yi xue ban. 2008;39:214–7.
44. Wang WX, Wang W, Chen KJ. Protective effect and mechanism of ginsenosides on central nerve system of animals. Zhongguo Zhong Xi Yi Jie He Za Zhi. 2005;25:89–93.

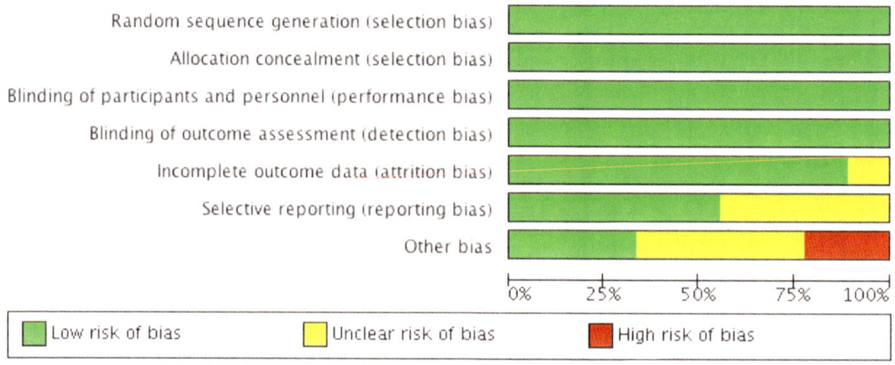

Fig. 1 Cochrane risk of bias assessment for mortality outcome

Sub-group analysis

According to Goligher's study [10], we defined positive oxygenation response to PEEP as $\Delta PaO_2/FiO_2 > 0$ mmHg when compared mean PaO_2/FiO_2 at baseline (lower PEEP) and after PEEP increased to a higher PEEP level in the high PEEP group. However, in the low PEEP group, oxygenation response to PEEP was unavailable because the baseline PEEP did not increase to a high level during the study period. We analysed the sub-groups according to whether patients in the high PEEP group had positive oxygenation response to PEEP to determine whether high PEEP could improve outcomes in patients who respond to increased PEEP by improved oxygenation. In addition, the PEEP value in the low PEEP group and the severity of ARDS also affected whether high PEEP reduced mortality. Therefore, we also performed sub-group analysis to determine whether PEEP greater than 10 cmH_2O in the low PEEP group or baseline PaO_2/FiO_2 equal to or less than 150 mmHg could have some effect on mortality between the high and low PEEP groups.

Summary measures

The meta-analysis was performed according to the Cochrane Collaboration guidelines. All statistical analyses were performed with Review Manager, version 5.3 (the Nordic Cochrane Centre, Copenhagen, Denmark), the Cochrane Collaboration's software for preparing and maintaining Cochrane systematic reviews. The pooled-effects estimates for binary variables are expressed as risk ratios with 95% CIs, whereas continuous variables are expressed as weighted mean differences with 95% CIs.

Synthesis of results

We tested the difference in the estimated value of the treatment effect between the experimental and control groups with a 2-sided z-test. Statistical significance was defined as $P < 0.05$. We predefined heterogeneity as low, moderate, and high with I^2 statistics greater than 25, 50, and 75%, respectively [11]. A meta-analysis with a random-effects model was applied with I^2 statistics greater than 50%. For other I^2 values, a fixed-effects model was selected. Funnel plot were used to analyse publication bias.

Results

Study selection

Our initial electronic and manual search identified 8124 studies. Ultimately, nine RCTs fulfilled the inclusion criteria and were included in the cumulative meta-analysis (Fig. 2). The characteristics of the included studies are

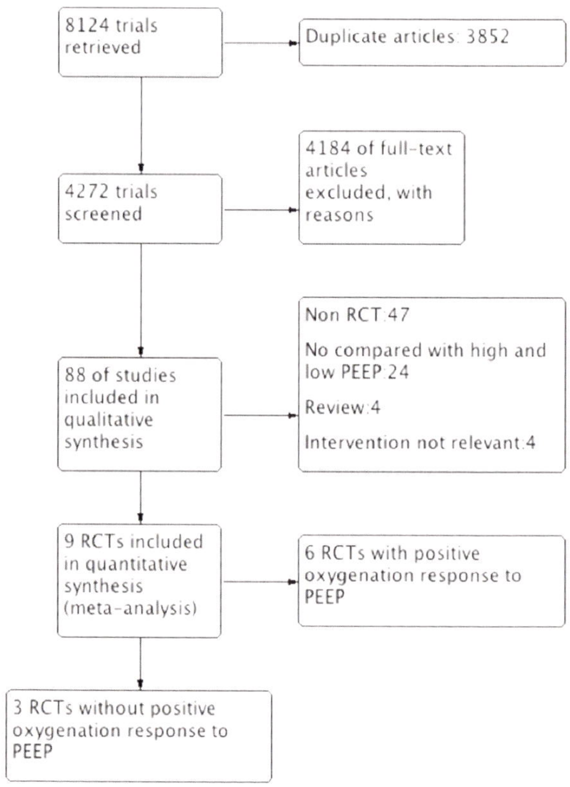

Fig. 2 Study flow diagram

Table 1 Characteristics of the included patients

Trial	Jadad score	Inclusion criteria	method of PEEP selection	Number of Patients (HP/LP)	Age (HP/LP)	PEEP (cmH_2O) (HP/LP)	Gender (HP vs. LP) [male/female]	PaO_2/FIO_2 (mmHg) (HP/LP)
Amato/1998 [12]	3	Lung injury score ≥ 2.5	HP[a]:LIP[c] + 2 cmH_2O LP[b]:FiO_2-PEEP	29/ 24	36/33	13.2 ± 0.4/9.3 ± 0.5	–	112/134
Ranieri/1999 [13]	3	PaO_2:FIO_2 ≤ 200 mmHg	HP[a]:LIP[c] + 2 cm H2O LP[b]:FiO_2-PEEP	18/19	51/49	14.8 ± 2.7/6.5 ± 1.7	7/11 vs. 10/19	149/142
Brower/2004 [3]	4	PaO_2:FIO_2 ≤ 300 mmHg	HP[a]:FiO_2-PEEP (ARDSnet) LP[b]:FiO_2-PEEP (PEEP more than 12 cmH_2O)	276/273	54/49	14.7 ± 3.5/8.9 ± 3.5	145/128 vs.157/119	151/165
Villar/2006 [14]	3	PaO_2:FIO_2 ≤ 200 mmHg	HP[a]:LIP[c] + 2 cmH_2O LP[b]:FiO_2-PEEP	50/45	48/52	14.1 ± 2.8/9.0 ± 2.7	23/27 vs.27/18	111/109
Meade/2008 [5]	4	PaO_2:FIO_2 ≤ 250 mmHg	FiO_2-PEEP	475/508	54.5/56.9	15.6 ± 3.9/10.1 ± 3.0	282/193 vs. 307/201	144.8/144.6
Mercat/2008 [15]	4	PaO_2:FIO_2 ≤ 300 mmHg	HP[a]:Pplat LP[b]: FiO_2-PEEP	385/382	60/60	14.6 ± 3.2/7.1 ± 1.8	260/125 vs. 256/126	144/143
Talmor/2008 [16]	3	PaO_2:FIO_2 ≤ 200 mmHg	HP[a]:Transpulmonary pressure LP[b]:FiO_2-PEEP	30/31	54.5/51.2	17 ± 6.0/10 ± 4.0	19/11 vs. 17/14	91/107
Huh/2009 [17]	3	PaO_2:FIO_2 ≤ 200 mmHg	HP[a]:saturation decrease more than 2% and drop of static compliance LP[b]:FiO_2-PEEP	30/27	55/62		18/12 vs. 17/10	115/110
ART/2017 [8]	3	PaO_2:FIO_2 ≤ 200 mmHg	HP[a]: Maximum alveolar recruitment by compliance + 2 cmH_2O LP[b]: FiO_2-PEEP	501/509	51.3/56	16.8 ± 3.8/13.0 ± 0.3	313/188 vs. 318/191	119.5/117.2

[a]*HP* High PEEP group, [b]*LP* Low PEEP group, [c]*LIP* lower inflection point

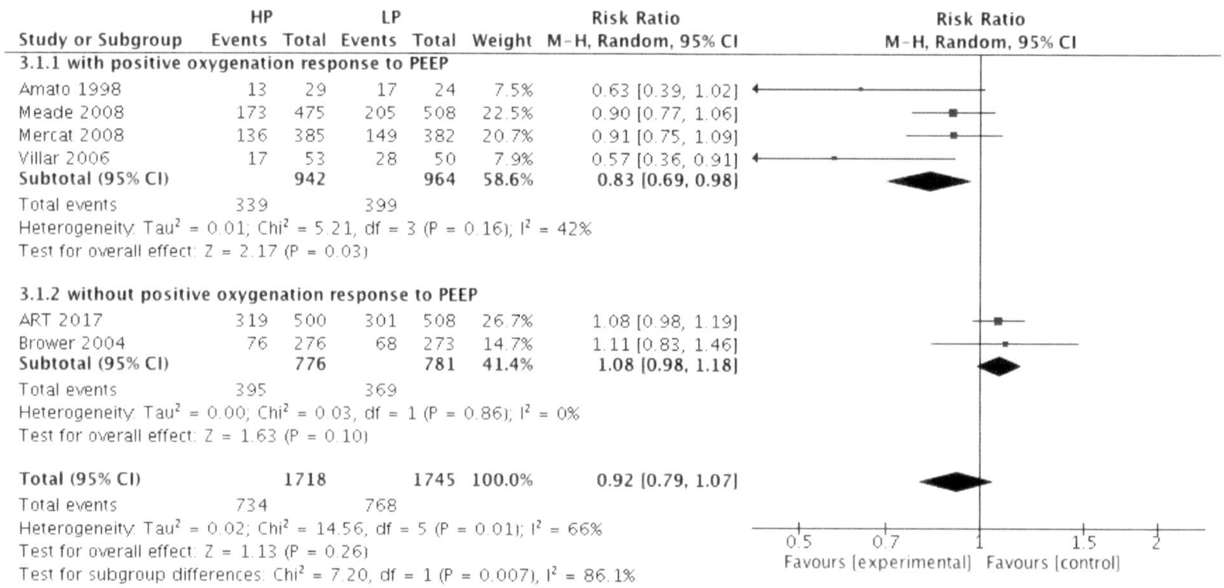

Fig. 3 Effect of high PEEP on hospital mortality in ARDS patients with or without positive oxygenation response to PEEP

shown in Table 1. A total of 3612 patients, including 1794 patients in the high PEEP group and 1818 patients in the low PEEP group, were included in our meta-analysis.

Effect of high PEEP on hospital mortality in ARDS patients

There was no difference in hospital mortality between the high PEEP and low PEEP groups (RR = 0.92; 95% CI, 0.79 to 1.07; *P* = 0.26) (Fig. 3). In ARDS with positive oxygenation response to PEEP (from 4 RCTs), hospital mortality was lower in the high PEEP group than the low PEEP group (RR = 0.83; 95% CI, 0.69 to 0.98; *P* = 0.03) (Fig. 3). However, hospital mortality was comparable between groups in patients without positive oxygenation response to PEEP (RR = 1.08; 95% CI, 0.98 to 1.18; *P* = 0.1) (Fig. 3).

For ARDS patients in the low PEEP group who received a PEEP level lower than 10 cmH_2O (from 4 RCTs), hospital mortality was no different in the high and low PEEP groups (RR = 0.83; 95% CI, 0.64 to 1.08; *P* = 0.16) (Fig. 4). There was no significant difference in

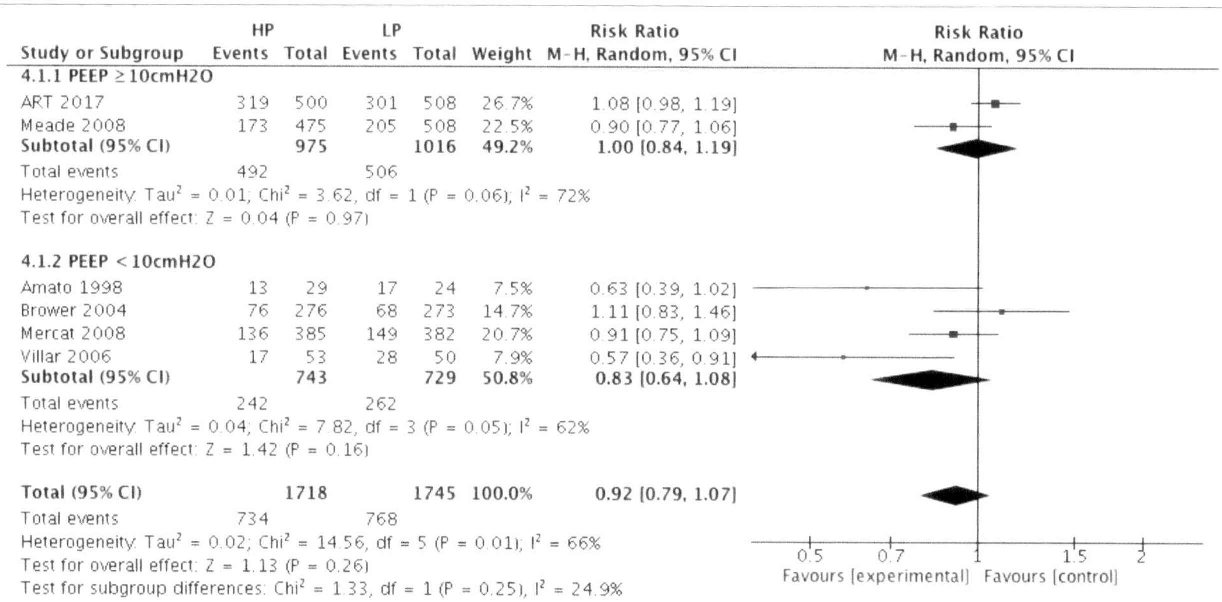

Fig. 4 Effect of high PEEP on hospital mortality while the PEEP level of patients in low PEEP group was different

Study or Subgroup	HP Events	HP Total	LP Events	LP Total	Weight	Risk Ratio M-H, Random, 95% CI
5.1.1 PaO2/FiO2 > 150mmHg						
Brower 2004	76	276	68	273	14.7%	1.11 [0.83, 1.46]
Subtotal (95% CI)		**276**		**273**	**14.7%**	**1.11 [0.83, 1.46]**
Total events	76		68			
Heterogeneity: Not applicable						
Test for overall effect: Z = 0.70 (P = 0.48)						
5.1.2 PaO2/FiO2 ≤ 150mmHg						
Amato 1998	13	29	17	24	7.5%	0.63 [0.39, 1.02]
ART 2017	319	500	301	508	26.7%	1.08 [0.98, 1.19]
Meade 2008	173	475	205	508	22.5%	0.90 [0.77, 1.06]
Mercat 2008	136	385	149	382	20.7%	0.91 [0.75, 1.09]
Villar 2006	17	53	28	50	7.9%	0.57 [0.36, 0.91]
Subtotal (95% CI)		**1442**		**1472**	**85.3%**	**0.88 [0.74, 1.05]**
Total events	658		700			
Heterogeneity: Tau^2 = 0.02; Chi^2 = 14.05, df = 4 (P = 0.007); I^2 = 72%						
Test for overall effect: Z = 1.43 (P = 0.15)						
Total (95% CI)		**1718**		**1745**	**100.0%**	**0.92 [0.79, 1.07]**
Total events	734		768			
Heterogeneity: Tau^2 = 0.02; Chi^2 = 14.56, df = 5 (P = 0.01); I^2 = 66%						
Test for overall effect: Z = 1.13 (P = 0.26)						
Test for subgroup differences: Chi^2 = 1.82, df = 1 (P = 0.18), I^2 = 45.2%						

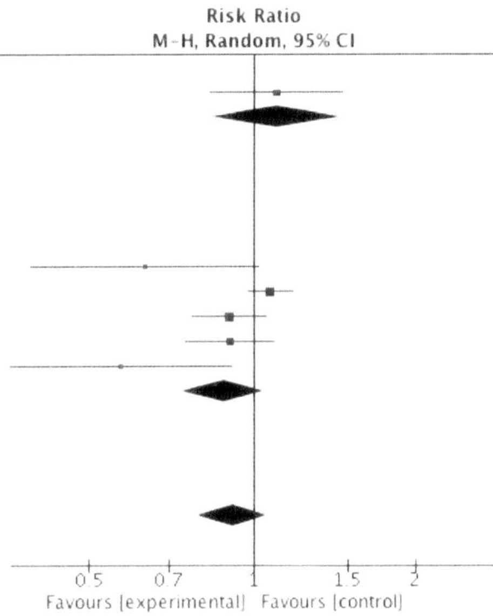

Fig. 5 Effect of high PEEP on hospital mortality of moderate and severe ARDS patients between high and low PEEP groups

hospital mortality between high and low PEEP groups (RR = 1.0; 95% CI, 0.84 to 1.19; P = 0.97) for ARDS patients in the low PEEP group who received a PEEP level equal or higher than 10 cmH_2O (Fig. 4). For ARDS patients with baseline $PaO_2/FiO_2 \leq 150$ mmHg (from 5 RCTs), there was no significant difference in hospital mortality between high and low PEEP groups (RR = 0.88; 95% CI, 0.74 to 1.05; P = 0.15) (Fig. 5).

Effect of high PEEP on 28-day mortality in ARDS patients

Twenty-eight-day mortality was reported in seven RCTs and was similar in the high and low PEEP groups (RR = 0.88; 95% CI,0.72 to 1.07; P = 0.19) (Fig. 6). In ARDS patients with positive oxygenation response to PEEP (5 RCTs), 28-day mortality was lower in the high PEEP group than the low PEEP group (RR = 0.83; 95% CI, 0.67 to 1.01; P = 0.07) (Fig. 6).

Study or Subgroup	HP Events	HP Total	LP Events	LP Total	Weight	Risk Ratio M-H, Random, 95% CI
6.1.1 with positive oxygenation response to PEEP						
Amato 1998	11	29	17	24	9.7%	0.54 [0.31, 0.91]
Huh 2009	12	30	9	27	6.6%	1.20 [0.60, 2.39]
Meade 2008	135	475	164	508	23.7%	0.88 [0.73, 1.06]
Mercat 2008	107	385	119	382	22.1%	0.89 [0.72, 1.11]
Talmor 2008	5	30	12	31	4.1%	0.43 [0.17, 1.07]
Subtotal (95% CI)		**949**		**972**	**66.2%**	**0.83 [0.67, 1.01]**
Total events	270		321			
Heterogeneity: Tau^2 = 0.02; Chi^2 = 6.30, df = 4 (P = 0.18); I^2 = 37%						
Test for overall effect: Z = 1.83 (P = 0.07)						
6.1.2 without positive oxygenation response to PEEP						
ART 2017	277	501	251	509	27.3%	1.12 [1.00, 1.26]
Ranieri 1999	7	18	11	19	6.5%	0.67 [0.34, 1.35]
Subtotal (95% CI)		**519**		**528**	**33.8%**	**0.98 [0.63, 1.53]**
Total events	284		262			
Heterogeneity: Tau^2 = 0.07; Chi^2 = 2.03, df = 1 (P = 0.15); I^2 = 51%						
Test for overall effect: Z = 0.10 (P = 0.92)						
Total (95% CI)		**1468**		**1500**	**100.0%**	**0.88 [0.72, 1.07]**
Total events	554		583			
Heterogeneity: Tau^2 = 0.03; Chi^2 = 16.65, df = 6 (P = 0.01); I^2 = 64%						
Test for overall effect: Z = 1.30 (P = 0.19)						
Test for subgroup differences: Chi^2 = 0.46, df = 1 (P = 0.50), I^2 = 0%						

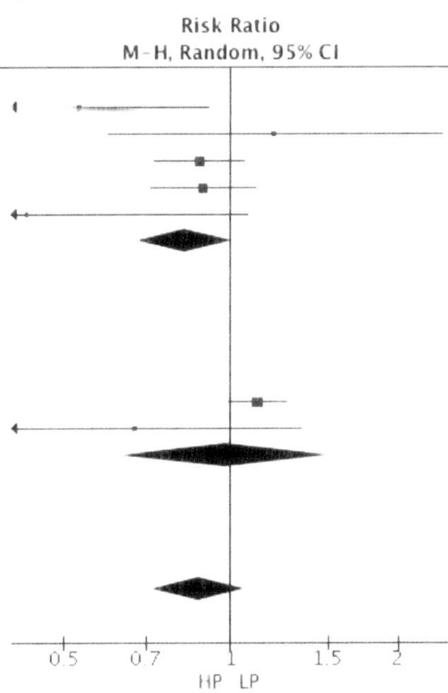

Fig. 6 Effect of high PEEP on 28-day mortality in ARDS patients

Study or Subgroup	PR Events	PR Total	PN Events	PN Total	Weight	Risk Ratio M-H, Random, 95% CI
7.1.1 PEEP ≥10cmH2O						
ART 2017	277	501	251	509	27.3%	1.12 [1.00, 1.26]
Meade 2008	135	475	164	508	23.7%	0.88 [0.73, 1.06]
Talmor 2008	5	30	12	31	4.1%	0.43 [0.17, 1.07]
Subtotal (95% CI)		**1006**		**1048**	**55.1%**	**0.93 [0.70, 1.24]**
Total events	417		427			
Heterogeneity: Tau² = 0.04; Chi² = 8.33, df = 2 (P = 0.02); I² = 76%						
Test for overall effect: Z = 0.47 (P = 0.64)						
7.1.2 PEEP <10cmH2O						
Amato 1998	11	29	17	24	9.7%	0.54 [0.31, 0.91]
Huh 2009	12	30	9	27	6.6%	1.20 [0.60, 2.39]
Mercat 2008	107	385	119	382	22.1%	0.89 [0.72, 1.11]
Ranieri 1999	7	18	11	19	6.5%	0.67 [0.34, 1.35]
Subtotal (95% CI)		**462**		**452**	**44.9%**	**0.80 [0.60, 1.07]**
Total events	137		156			
Heterogeneity: Tau² = 0.03; Chi² = 4.50, df = 3 (P = 0.21); I² = 33%						
Test for overall effect: Z = 1.48 (P = 0.14)						
Total (95% CI)		**1468**		**1500**	**100.0%**	**0.88 [0.72, 1.07]**
Total events	554		583			
Heterogeneity: Tau² = 0.03; Chi² = 16.65, df = 6 (P = 0.01); I² = 64%						
Test for overall effect: Z = 1.30 (P = 0.19)						
Test for subgroup differences: Chi² = 0.53, df = 1 (P = 0.47), I² = 0%						

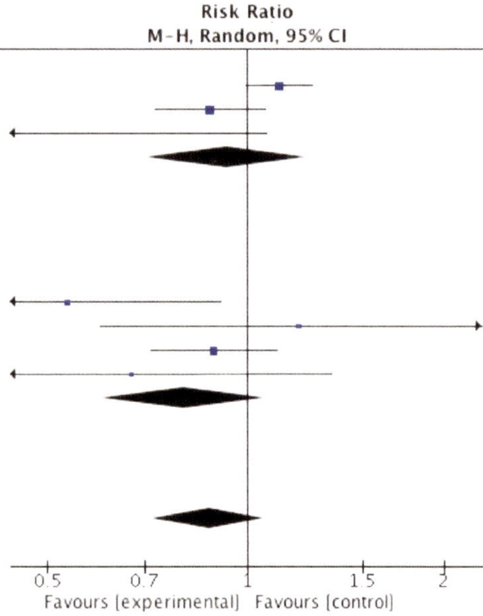

Fig. 7 Effect of high PEEP on 28-day mortality while the PEEP level of patients in low PEEP group was different

There was no difference in 28-day mortality between the high and low PEEP groups, regardless of the PEEP level used in the low PEEP group (For PEEP less than 10 cmH_2O, RR = 0.80; 95% CI, 0.60 to 1.07; $P = 0.14$) (For PEEP equal and more than10 cmH_2O, RR = 0.93; 95% CI, 0.70 to 1.24; $P = 0.64$) (Fig. 7).

Effect of high PEEP on ICU mortality in ARDS patients

ICU mortality was reported in five RCTs. A high PEEP strategy did not decrease the ICU mortality compared to the low PEEP strategy (RR = 0.83; 95% CI, 0.65 to 1.07; $P = 0.15$) (Fig. 8). In ARDS with positive oxygenation response to PEEP (4 RCTs), ICU mortality was lower in the high PEEP group than the low PEEP group (RR = 0.74; 95% CI, 0.56 to 0.98; $P = 0.04$) (Fig. 8). However, ICU mortality was not different between the high and low PEEP groups among ARDS patients without a positive oxygenation response to PEEP.

For ARDS patients in the low PEEP group who received a PEEP level lower than 10 cmH_2O (from 3 RCTs), ICU mortality was lower in the high PEEP group

Study or Subgroup	HP Events	HP Total	LP Events	LP Total	Weight	Risk Ratio M-H, Random, 95% CI
8.1.1 with positive oxygenation response to PEEP						
Amato 1998	11	29	17	24	13.2%	0.54 [0.31, 0.91]
Huh 2009	14	30	13	27	12.7%	0.97 [0.56, 1.68]
Meade 2008	145	475	178	508	28.2%	0.87 [0.73, 1.04]
Villar 2006	16	53	27	50	14.7%	0.56 [0.34, 0.91]
Subtotal (95% CI)		**587**		**609**	**68.8%**	**0.74 [0.56, 0.98]**
Total events	186		235			
Heterogeneity: Tau² = 0.04; Chi² = 5.64, df = 3 (P = 0.13); I² = 47%						
Test for overall effect: Z = 2.10 (P = 0.04)						
8.1.2 without positive oxygenation response to PEEP						
ART 2017	303	500	284	509	31.2%	1.09 [0.98, 1.21]
Subtotal (95% CI)		**500**		**509**	**31.2%**	**1.09 [0.98, 1.21]**
Total events	303		284			
Heterogeneity: Not applicable						
Test for overall effect: Z = 1.55 (P = 0.12)						
Total (95% CI)		**1087**		**1118**	**100.0%**	**0.83 [0.65, 1.07]**
Total events	489		519			
Heterogeneity: Tau² = 0.05; Chi² = 15.82, df = 4 (P = 0.003); I² = 75%						
Test for overall effect: Z = 1.46 (P = 0.15)						
Test for subgroup differences: Chi² = 6.32, df = 1 (P = 0.01), I² = 84.2%						

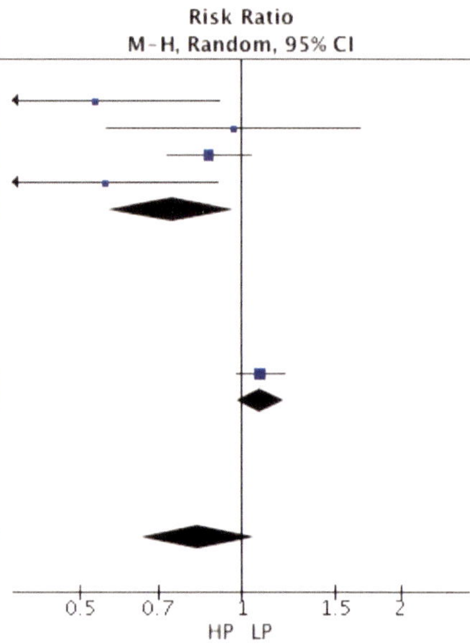

Fig. 8 Effect of high PEEP on ICU mortality in ARDS patients

Study or Subgroup	HP Events	HP Total	LP Events	LP Total	Weight	Risk Ratio M-H, Random, 95% CI
9.1.1 PEEP≥10cmH2O						
ART 2017	303	500	284	509	31.2%	1.09 [0.98, 1.21]
Meade 2008	145	475	178	508	28.2%	0.87 [0.73, 1.04]
Subtotal (95% CI)		**975**		**1017**	**59.4%**	**0.98 [0.79, 1.23]**
Total events	448		462			
Heterogeneity: Tau² = 0.02; Chi² = 4.54, df = 1 (P = 0.03); I² = 78%						
Test for overall effect: Z = 0.14 (P = 0.89)						
9.1.2 PEEP<10cmH2O						
Amato 1998	11	29	17	24	13.2%	0.54 [0.31, 0.91]
Huh 2009	14	30	13	27	12.7%	0.97 [0.56, 1.68]
Villar 2006	16	53	27	50	14.7%	0.56 [0.34, 0.91]
Subtotal (95% CI)		**112**		**101**	**40.6%**	**0.65 [0.45, 0.94]**
Total events	41		57			
Heterogeneity: Tau² = 0.03; Chi² = 2.93, df = 2 (P = 0.23); I² = 32%						
Test for overall effect: Z = 2.29 (P = 0.02)						
Total (95% CI)		**1087**		**1118**	**100.0%**	**0.83 [0.65, 1.07]**
Total events	489		519			
Heterogeneity: Tau² = 0.05; Chi² = 15.82, df = 4 (P = 0.003); I² = 75%						
Test for overall effect: Z = 1.46 (P = 0.15)						
Test for subgroup differences: Chi² = 3.56, df = 1 (P = 0.06), I² = 71.9%						

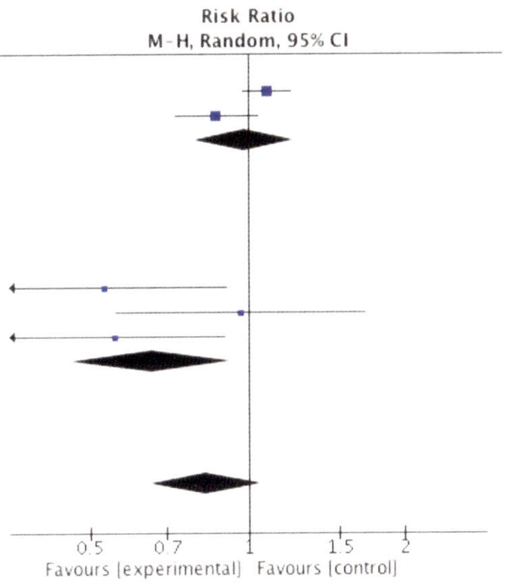

Fig. 9 Effect of high PEEP on ICU mortality while the PEEP level of patients in low PEEP group was different

than the low PEEP group (RR = 0.65; 95% CI, 0.45 to 0.94; $P = 0.02$) (Fig. 9). In contrast, there was no significant difference in ICU mortality between the high and low PEEP groups if the PEEP level was equal and more than 10 cmH_2O in the low PEEP group (RR = 0.98; 95% CI, 0.79 to 1.23; $P = 0.89$) (Fig. 9).

Effect of high PEEP on clinically objectified barotrauma in ARDS patients

Seven RCTs reported data on clinically objectified barotrauma, including 1746 patients in the high PEEP group and 1768 patients in the low PEEP group. A meta-analysis with a random-effects model showed that the incidence of clinically objectified barotrauma in the high and low PEEP groups were 9.97% (174/1746) and 6.8% (120/1768), respectively. High PEEP did not increase the incidence of clinically objectified barotrauma (RR = 1.24; 95% CI, 0.74 to 2.09, $P = 0.41$) (Fig. 10). However, in ARDS patients without positive oxygenation response to PEEP, high PEEP increased the incidence of clinically objectified barotrauma (RR = 2.50; 95% CI, 1.64 to 3.79, $P < 0.0001$) (Fig. 10).

Study or Subgroup	HP Events	HP Total	LP Events	LP Total	Weight	Risk Ratio M-H, Random, 95% CI
10.1.1 with positive oxygenation response to PEEP						
Amato 1998	2	29	10	24	8.6%	0.17 [0.04, 0.68]
Huh 2009	3	30	3	27	7.9%	0.90 [0.20, 4.09]
Meade 2008	53	475	46	508	21.4%	1.23 [0.85, 1.79]
Mercat 2008	26	385	22	382	18.9%	1.17 [0.68, 2.03]
Villar 2006	2	50	4	45	7.0%	0.45 [0.09, 2.34]
Subtotal (95% CI)		**969**		**986**	**63.7%**	**0.85 [0.48, 1.49]**
Total events	86		85			
Heterogeneity: Tau² = 0.18; Chi² = 8.48, df = 4 (P = 0.08); I² = 53%						
Test for overall effect: Z = 0.58 (P = 0.57)						
10.1.2 without positive oxygenation response to PEEP						
ART 2017	28	501	8	509	15.6%	3.56 [1.64, 7.73]
Brower 2004	60	276	27	273	20.7%	2.20 [1.44, 3.35]
Subtotal (95% CI)		**777**		**782**	**36.3%**	**2.50 [1.64, 3.79]**
Total events	88		35			
Heterogeneity: Tau² = 0.02; Chi² = 1.15, df = 1 (P = 0.28); I² = 13%						
Test for overall effect: Z = 4.29 (P < 0.0001)						
Total (95% CI)		**1746**		**1768**	**100.0%**	**1.24 [0.74, 2.09]**
Total events	174		120			
Heterogeneity: Tau² = 0.29; Chi² = 21.46, df = 6 (P = 0.002); I² = 72%						
Test for overall effect: Z = 0.83 (P = 0.41)						
Test for subgroup differences: Chi² = 9.16, df = 1 (P = 0.002), I² = 89.1%						

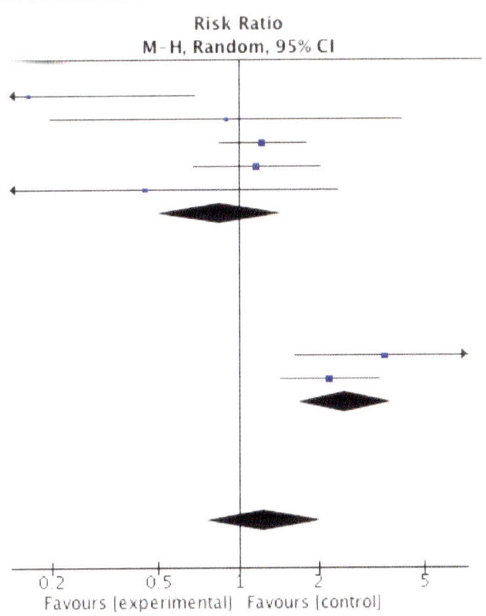

Fig. 10 Effect of high PEEP on clinically objectified barotrauma in ARDS patients

Discussion

Our meta-analysis showed that high PEEP did not improve outcomes in patients with ARDS. However, subgroup analysis showed that it may decrease hospital mortality as well as ICU and 28-d mortality in ARDS patients with clinically positive oxygenation response to PEEP. In addition, in ARDS patients without positive oxygenation response to PEEP, high PEEP increased the incidence of clinically objectified barotrauma. The results were different from Goligher's study [18], which found that recruitment manoeuvres in combination with higher PEEP could reduce mortality in ARDS patients.

Evidence from previous studies showed that high PEEP does not decrease mortality in patients with ARDS [7, 8, 19, 20], which is in line with our results. However, several issues must be considered when interpreting this result. First, there was a large variation in the PEEP level between the different studies. For example, Huh et al. [17] set a high PEEP of 10 cmH_2O, while the high PEEP was 16.3 cmH_2O in Amato's study [12]. Similarly, the PEEP level varied from 6.5 to 13 cmH_2O in the low PEEP groups among the included studies. Therefore, the different PEEP levels may have led to the different results. Subgroup results showed that the PEEP level in the low PEEP group greatly impacted the effect of PEEP on ICU mortality. Second, patient characteristics also impacted the effect of PEEP. Among these studies, the severity of ARDS in patients varied widely. For example, baseline PaO_2/FiO_2 ranged from 110.8 ± 6.3 to 165 ± 77 mmHg. Oxygenation response to PEEP was also significantly associated with the severity of ARDS. The potential lung with response to PEEP was considerably stronger in more severe ARDS patients than in less severe individuals. A previous meta-analysis showed that a high PEEP reduced mortality in patients with ARDS but not ALI [8] However, in the present study, there was no difference of hospital mortality between groups of ARDS patients with a baseline PaO_2/FiO_2 less than 150 mmHg.

The purpose of PEEP is to recruit collapsed alveoli in a gravity-dependent lung but not to induce the alveoli to overdistend in the non-dependent lung. Patients with ARDS exhibit significant dependent atelectasis due to increased lung weight resulting from interstitial and alveolar edema. Both higher PEEP and recruitment manoeuvres can reduce atelectasis and increase end-expiratory lung volume. Physically, we need higher pressure to open alveoli and only need a relative lower PEEP to keep the lung open. Therefore, it was noted that higher PEEP should follow the recruitment manoeuvres. Goligher et al. showed that combine with recruitment manoeuvres and higher PEEP could reduce mortality of patients with ARDS [18]. The results were also demonstrated in the study by Constantin et al. [21]. However, the study by Goligher et al. [10] indicated that the percentage of potentially respond to PEEP was extremely variable. Our results demonstrated the hypothesis that only patients who respond to increased PEEP by improved oxygenation benefitted more from higher PEEP. PEEP could have different effects on clinical outcomes based on the nature of the clinical response to PEEP itself. In ARDS patients with clinically positive oxygenation response to PEEP, the main effect of a high PEEP might be recruiting the collapsed lung, which may reduce ventilation-induced lung injury (VILI). In contrast, a high PEEP might result in alveolar overdistension, which induces lung injury in ARDS patients without positive oxygenation response to PEEP. These reasons could help to explain why our subgroup analysis showed that high PEEP reduced mortality in ARDS patients with clinically positive oxygenation response to PEEP.

The severity of ARDS can be used to titrate PEEP. There are many methods for PEEP titration, such as oxygenation, stress index and transpulmonary pressure. Chiumello et al. found that oxygenation-guided PEEP provided PEEP levels related to oxygenation response to PEEP in the lung that progressively increased from mild to moderate and severe ARDS [19]. In assessing the oxygenation response to PEEP at 5 cmH_2O PEEP based on the Berlin definition [6, 22], a simple Friday-night ventilation strategy can be used in patients with ARDS [23]. Therefore, while we only included studies in which the PEEP level was lower than 10 cmH_2O in the low PEEP group, decreased ICU mortality was found in the high PEEP group.

There are many methods that can be used with ARDS patients at present. To date, prolonged sessions of prone positioning has not only been shown to be efficient at significantly increasing oxygenation and decreasing driving pressure in severe ARDS in the APRONET study [24], but the PROSEVA trial also showed that prone positioning was associated with improved patient survival [25]. However, the LUNG SAFE study showed that the rate of prone positioning was low because of selection bias or the clinician's perception [26]. On the other hand, neuromuscular blockers could be used in severe ARDS, but they are controversial. Many previous studies found that the mortality of ARDS treated with neuromuscular blockers was not decreased. However, neuromuscular blockers could exert beneficial effects in patients with moderate ARDS, at least in part, by limiting expiratory efforts as shown in Guervilly's study [27]. In our study, there were 3 RCTs that included prone position or neuromuscular blockers. Unfortunately, due to the lack of prognostic data, statistical analysis was not possible.

We did not find a significant difference in clinically objectified barotrauma between high PEEP and low PEEP groups. Lung-protective strategies were used in all of the included studies, which decreased the incidence of clinically objectified barotrauma [28, 29]. In addition, most patients in these studies had moderate or severe ARDS, which indicates that more lung area was responsive to increased PEEP. However, in ARDS patients without positive oxygenation response to PEEP, high PEEP increased the incidence of clinically objectified barotrauma. It was shown in a recent study that an exceedingly high pressure was used to recruit the lung, especially in ARDS patients without positive oxygenation response to PEEP, and mortality may increase [8].

Some limitations of our analysis should be noted. First, we were unable to obtain patient-level data despite asking for these data from the authors of the included studies. The lung oxygenation response to PEEP was evaluated based on the mean PaO_2/FiO_2 values reported in each study but not the individual patient data. That finding means most of the patients in the study with positive oxygenation response to increased PEEP were in their respective groups.

Second, the definition of positive oxygenation response to PEEP based on Goligher's study is not highly precise [10]. We also did not assess other factors that may affect the oxygenation response to PEEP. These factors may have affected the accuracy of our results. In this meta-analysis, we only included the data from the included studies. In addition, we did not used the data on SpO_2, $PaCO_2$ and respiratory compliance at the two different PEEP levels. We only used the PaO_2/FiO_2 data at higher and lower PEEP levels. Therefore, we defined the groups as positive oxygenation response to PEEP if the mean PaO_2/FiO_2 was higher in the high PEEP group than at baseline. Based on this definition, we found that patients with clinically positive oxygenation response to PEEP benefitted from high PEEP.

Third, the methods of PEEP titration were different between the included studies, which may have induced bias in our study. Oxygenation response to PEEP should be considered during PEEP titration in patients with ARDS. However, no clinical trial has shown that oxygenation response to PEEP using assessment–guided PEEP titration could improve the outcomes in patients with ARDS, which indicates further studies are needed.

Conclusion

In this study, high PEEP did not improve outcomes in patients with ARDS as a whole. However, subgroup analysis showed that high PEEP decreased hospital and ICU mortality in ARDS patients with a clinically objective positive oxygenation response to PEEP.

Abbreviations

ALI: Acute lung injury; ARDS: Acute respiratory distress syndrome; ARF: Acute respiratory failure; ICU: Intensive care unit; PEEP: Positive end-expiratory pressure; RCT: Randomized controlled trials; VILI: Ventilation-induced lung injury

Acknowledgements

Not available.

Funding

This work was supported by the National Natural Science Foundation of China under grant No. 81670074, the Jiangsu Provincial Medical Youth Talent grant No. QNRC2016807, and the Third Level Talents of the "333 High Level Talents Training Project" in the fifth phase in Jiangsu (LGY2016051).

Authors' contributions

LQG, LL conceived the study, participated in the design, collected the data, performed statistical analyses, and drafted the manuscript. HBQ and YY participated in the design, and helped to draft the manuscript. JFX, YZH and CP helped to perform statistical analyses and to revise it critically for important intellectual content. All authors read and approved the final manuscript.

Competing interests

The authors declare that they have no competing interests.

References

1. Esteban A, Ferguson ND, Meade MO, Frutos-Vivar F, Apezteguia C, Brochard L, VENTILA Group, et al. Evolution of mechanical ventilation in response to clinical research. Am J Respir Crit Care Med. 2008;177:170–7.
2. Gattinoni L, Caironi P, Cressoni M, et al. Lung recruitment in patients with the acute respiratory distress syndrome. N Engl J Med. 2006;354:1775–86.
3. Brower RG, Lanken PN, Mac Intyre N, et al. Higher versus lower positive end expiratory pressures in patients with the acute respiratory distress syndrome. N Engl J Med. 2004;351:327–36.
4. Gattinoni L, Caironi P. Refining ventilatory treatment for acute lung injury and acute respiratory distress syndrome. JAMA. 2008;299(6):691–3.
5. Meade MO, Cook DJ, Guyatt GH, et al. Lung open ventilation study investigators. Ventilation strategy using low tidal volumes, recruitment maneuvers, and high positive end-expiratory pressure for acute lung injury and acute respiratory distress syndrome: a randomized controlled trial. JAMA. 2008;299:637–45.
6. Borges JB, Okamoto VN, Matos GFJ, Caramez MPR, Arantes PR, Barrios F, et al. Reversibility of lung collapse and hypoxemia in early acute respiratory distress syndrome. Am J Respir Crit Care Med. 2006;174:268–78.
7. Putensen C, Theuerkauf N, Zinserling J, et al. Meta-analysis: ventilation strategies and outcomes of the acute respiratory distress syndrome and acute lung injury. Ann Intern Med. 2009;151:566–76.
8. Cavalcanti AB, Suzumura ÉA, Laranjeira LN, et al. Effect of lung recruitment and titrated positive end-expiratory pressure (PEEP) vs low PEEP on mortality in patients with acute respiratory distress syndrome: a randomized clinical trial. JAMA. 2017;318(14):1335–45.
9. Briel M, Meade M, Mercat A, et al. Higher vs lower positive end-expiratory pressure in patients with acute lung injury and acute respiratory distress syndrome systematic review and Meta-analysis. JAMA. 2010;303(9):865–73.

10. Goligher EC, Kavanagh BP, Rubenfeld GD, et al. Oxygenation response to PEEP predicts mortality in ARDS: a secondary analysis of the LOVS and ExPress trials. Am J Respir Crit Care Med. 2014;190(1):70–6.
11. Higgins JP, Thompson SG, Deeks JJ, Altman DG. Measuring inconsistency in meta-analyses. BMJ. 2003;327:557–60.
12. Amato MSP, Barbas CSV, Medeiros DM, et al. Effect of a protective-ventilation strategy on mortality in the acute respiratory distress syndrome. N Engl J Med. 1998;338:347–54.
13. Ranieri VM, Suter PM, Tortorella C, et al. Effect of mechanical ventilation on inflammatory mediators in patients with acute respiratory distress syndrome: a randomized controlled trial. JAMA. 1999;282:54–61.
14. Villar J, Kacmarek RM, Pérez-Méndez L, et al. A high positive end-expiratory pressure, low tidal volume ventilatory strategy improves outcome in persistent acute respiratory distress syndrome: A randomized, controlled trial*. Crit Care Med. 2006;34:1311–8.
15. Mercat A, Richard JC, Vielle B, et al. Expiratory pressure (Express) study group. Positive end-expiratory pressure setting in adults with acute lung injury and acute respiratory distress syndrome: a randomized controlled trial. JAMA. 2008;299:646–55.
16. Talmor D, Sarge T, Malhotra A, et al. Mechanical ventilation guided by esophageal pressure in acute lung injury. N Engl J Med. 2008;359:2095–104.
17. Huh JW, Jung H, Sook Choi H, et al. Efficacy of positive end-expiratory pressure titration after the alveolar recruitment manoeuvre in patients with acute respiratory distress syndrome. Crit Care. 2009;13:R22.
18. Goligher EC, Hodgson CL, Adhikari NKJ, et al. Lung recruitment maneuvers for adult patients with acute respiratory distress syndrome. A systematic review and Meta-analysis. Ann Am Thorac Soc. 2017;14(Supplement_4): S304–11.
19. Chiumello D, Cressoni M, Carlesso E, et al. Bedside selection of positive end-expiratory pressure in mild, moderate, and severe acute respiratory distress syndrome. Crit Care Med. 2014;42(2):252–64.
20. Dasenbrook EC, Needham DM, Brower RG, et al. Higher PEEP in patients with acute lung injury: a systematic review and Meta-analysis. Respir Care. 2011;56(5):568–75.
21. Constantin JM, Jaber S, Futier E, et al. Respiratory effects of different recruitment maneuvers in acute respiratory distress syndrome. Critical Care. 2008;12:R50.
22. Ranieri VM, Rubenfeld GD, Thompson BT, et al. Acute respiratory distress syndrome: the Berlin definition. JAMA. 2012;307:2526–33.
23. Gattinoni L, Carlesso E, Brazzi L, et al. Friday night ventilation: a safety starting tool kit for mechanically ventilated patients. Minerva Anestesiol. 2014;80(9):1046–57.
24. Guérin C, Beuret P, Constantin JM, et al. A prospective international observational prevalence study on prone positioning of ARDS patients: the APRONET (ARDS prone position network) study. Intensive Care Med. 2017; 44(1):22–37.
25. Guérin C, Reignier J, Richard JC, et al. Prone positioning in severe acute respiratory distress syndrome. N Engl J Med. 2013;368(23):2159–68.
26. Bellani G, Laffey JG, Pham T, et al. Epidemiology, patterns of care, and mortality for patients with acute respiratory distress syndrome in intensive care units in 50 countries. JAMA. 2016;315(8):788–800.
27. Guervilly C, Bisbal M, Forel JM, et al. Effects of neuromuscular blockers on transpulmonary pressures in moderate to severe acute respiratory distress syndrome. Intensive Care Med. 2016;43(3):408–18.
28. Remblay LN, Slutsky AS. Ventilator-induced lung injury: from the bench to the bedside. Intensive Care Med. 2006;32(1):24–33.
29. Tagami T, Sawabe M, Kushimoto S, et al. Quantitative diagnosis of diffuse alveolar damage using extravascular lung water. Crit Care Med. 2013;41(9):2144–50.

24

Preoperative anxiety and associated factors among adult surgical patients in Debre Markos and Felege Hiwot referral hospitals, Northwest Ethiopia

Henok Mulugeta[1*], Mulatu Ayana[2], Mezinew Sintayehu[1], Getenet Dessie[3] and Tesfu Zewdu[4]

Abstract

Background: Anxiety during the preoperative period is the most common problem with a number of postoperative complications such as an increase in postoperative pain, delay of healing and prolong the hospital stay. Further, patients with a high level of preoperative anxiety require higher doses of anesthetic agents and recover poorly. Despite its serious health complications, its magnitude and associated factors have been poorly explored in Ethiopia particularly in the selected study areas.

Objective: To assess preoperative anxiety and associated factors among adult surgical patients in Debre Markos and Felege Hiwot Referral Hospitals, Northwest Ethiopia.

Method: An institution based cross-sectional study was conducted on 353 patients scheduled for surgery using a systematic random sampling technique. The data were collected using the state version of the state-trait anxiety inventory scale. All collected data were entered into Epi-Data version 3.1 and analysis was done by using SPSS version 20 software. Binary logistic regression was performed to assess the effect of independent variables on the dependent variable. A p-value ≤ 0.05 was considered as statistically significant.

Results: Overall, 61% (95%CI (55.5–65.7)) patients had significant high level of preoperative anxiety. The most common reported factor responsible for preoperative anxiety was fear of complications 187(52.4%). There was a statistically significant high level of pre-operative anxiety among female patients [AOR 2.19 (95%CI (1.29–3.71))] and patients who lack preoperative information [AOR 2.03(95%CI (1.22–3.39))].

Conclusion: The prevalence of preoperative anxiety was high. The level of preoperative anxiety significantly associated with sex, preoperative information provision, and previous surgical experience. Preoperative psychosocial assessment should be incorporated into a routine nursing practice and every patient should be provided with preoperative information before surgery.

Keywords: Anxiety, Major surgery, Preoperative anxiety, Ethiopia

* Correspondence: mulugetahenok68@gmail.com
[1]Department of Nursing, College of Health Science, Debre Markos University, P.O. Box 269, Debre Markos, Ethiopia
Full list of author information is available at the end of the article

Background

Anxiety is defined as a feeling of unease, worry, fear, tension, and apprehension. It is a response to external or internal stimuli that can have behavioral, emotional, cognitive, and physical symptoms [1]. Perioperative period is one of the worrying events for most surgical patients. It often triggers emotional, cognitive and physiological responses. The goal of perioperative nursing care is to provide better environments and quality of life of a patient before, during and after operation [2].

Preoperative anxiety is a challenging problem in the preoperative care of patients. A common low level of anxiety is an expected reaction to the unpredictable and potentially life-threatening circumstances, especially for a patient's first surgical experience. However, higher and extended level of preoperative anxiety results in a delay in wound healing as well as requires larger doses of anesthetics and recover poorly. Most patients in the preoperative phase experience anxiety and it is commonly considered as a usual patient response [3–5].

Preoperative anxiety has a number of postoperative complications on the patient, and one of these complications is pain. Pain is the common complaint of post-operative patients which is mostly occur due to preoperative anxiety as a common factor. Pre-operative anxiety has been found to lead to a number of problems such as nausea, vomiting, cardiovascular disturbances such as tachycardia and hypertension, and increased the risk of infection. Studies also showed that a large proportion of surgical patients experience considerable preoperative anxiety and this reported to affect 60–80% of surgical patients [6–8].

The degree to which each patient manifests anxiety depends on many factors such as the patient's susceptibility to preoperative anxiety, age, gender, past experiences with the surgery, educational status, type and extent of the proposed surgery, current health status, and socioeconomic status. Identifying risk factors helps the nurse to provide psychological support during the preoperative visit so that stress can be reduced. Some group of patients, for example, females, younger patients, patients who have no previous history of surgical operation experience have an increased level of preoperative anxiety [9–12].

A study done in Canada, Saudi Arabia, and Sri Lanka showed that the overall prevalence of preoperative anxiety was 89%, 55%, and 76.7%, respectively [11, 13, 14]. Similarly, a study conducted in Austria reported that the overall preoperative anxiety was 45.3% among admitted surgical patients [15]. Moreover, the result of a study done in a tertiary hospital in Nigeria and a pilot study in Niger showed that 51.0% and 90% of surgical patients had significant preoperative anxiety respectively [16, 17].

In Ethiopia, a limited study has been conducted on preoperative anxiety among surgical patients. In a recent study conducted in South Western Ethiopia, 70.3% of preoperative patients had significant preoperative anxiety [18]. The magnitude of preoperative anxiety among adult surgical patients in the Ethiopian population is not well-known yet. Therefore, the objective of this study was to assess the prevalence of preoperative anxiety and associated factors among adult surgical patients in Debre Markos and Felege Hiwot Referral Hospitals.

Methods

Study design and setting

An institution based cross-sectional study design was conducted in Debre Markos and Felege Hiwot referral hospitals from February 01 to April 30, 2017, on 353 patients scheduled for surgery. Debre Markos Referral Hospital is one of the referral hospitals in the Amhara region which is found in Debre Markos town. Debre Markos town, found in the northwest of Addis Ababa, is the capital city of East Gojjam zone, which is found from 265 km from Bahirdar, the capital city of Amhara national Regional state and 300 km from Addis Ababa, the capital city of Ethiopia. Felege-Hiwot referral hospital is found in Bahir Dar. Bahir Dar is found 558 km far away from the capital city of Ethiopia, Addis Ababa.

Eligibility criteria

Inclusion criteria: All adult elective major surgical Patients age > =18 years.

Exclusion criteria: Patients have known psychiatric illness and those who were on any type of anxiolytic medications. Critically ill patients who were not sufficiently alert to be able to respond to questions.

Sample size and sampling technique

The sample size was determined by using a single proportion for a finite population with assumptions of 95% confidence level, marginal error (d) of 5% and the prevalence (P) of 70.3% [18]. So, this proportion was used to determine the sample size.

$$n = \frac{(Z\alpha/2)^2 P(1-P)}{D^2}$$

Where: n = the desired sample size

Za/2 = standard normal score (at 95% confidence level)

Where: Z = 1.96

P = prevalence (70.3%)

D = degree of accuracy desired (5%)

$$n=\frac{(1.96)^2(0.703)(1-0.703)}{(0.05)^2}$$

$=321+$ **Non-responsive rate**$(10\%)=353$ **major surgical patients**

Samples were selected from the two referral hospitals (Debre Markos referral hospital and Felege Hiwot referral hospital) in Northwest Ethiopia. Then the total number of adult elective major surgical patient admission from February to April 2016 (last year) was taken to estimate the current admission and the total sample size from each hospital calculated by using a proportion to size allocation formula. Then a systematic random sampling technique was employed to approach the study participants. The sampling fraction (Kth) was calculated by dividing N/n (753/353 = 2). Accordingly, every other patient was selected to participate in the study until the required sample size was achieved.

Variables

Dependent Variable: Preoperative anxiety (High/low).

Independent Variables: Socio-demographic characteristics, previous surgical experience, previous hospitalization, preoperative information, awareness of the disease and awareness of the type of surgical procedure.

Operational definitions and definition of terms

Adult: a person who is greater than 18 years old.

Surgery/ Operation: a procedure that involves cutting a patient's tissues [18].

Anxiety: is a vague feeling of dread or apprehension [1].

Level of anxiety: - expressed by a score of S- STAI as high-level anxiety and low-level anxiety [16].

High-level anxiety: - Patient who score S- STAI > 44 [16].

Low-level anxiety: - Patient who score S- STAI ≤44 [16].

Major surgery: any surgical operation that is performed in the major operating room using spinal or general anesthesia. Example: Cholecystectomy, hemorrhoidectomy, hernia repair, thyroidectomy, orthopedic surgeries, appendectomy, prostatectomy, colon surgeries.

Data collection and instruments

The data were collected using validated and standardized preoperative anxiety measuring tool that is State Version (Y-1) of State-Trait Anxiety Inventory Scale (S-STAI), which is adapted from other studies [16, 18], with some modification to increase the comparability of the finding. The questions and statements were grouped and arranged according to the particular objectives that can address based on experts' comments. The STAI Form Y is the absolute instrument for measuring preoperative anxiety in adults. The questionnaire was prepared in English and it was translated into the local language, Amharic and back to English for consistency.

State-Trait Anxiety Inventory Scale (S-STAI) is a self-report measure that has two subscales. First, the State Anxiety Scale (S-Anxiety) evaluates the current state of anxiety, asking how respondents feel "right now," using items that measure subjective feelings of apprehension, tension, nervousness, worry, and activation/arousal of the autonomic nervous system. The Trait Anxiety Scale (T-Anxiety) evaluates relatively stable aspects of "anxiety proneness," including general states of calmness, confidence, and security. Reliability and validity of the STAI are well reported (Cronbach's alpha = 0.86) and measurement of state anxiety is recommended in the perioperative period.

The STAI has 40 items, 20 items allocated to each of the S-Anxiety and T-Anxiety subscales. Responses for the S-Anxiety scale assess the intensity of current feelings "at this moment": 1) not at all, 2) somewhat, 3) moderately so, and 4) very much so. Responses for the T-Anxiety scale assess the frequency of feelings "in general": 1) almost never, 2) sometimes, 3) often, and 4) almost always. In the state portion of STAI (Y-1), ten statements express anxiety (item number 3, 4, 6, 7, 9, 12, 13, 14, 17 and 18) while the remaining 10 statements (item number 1, 2, 5, 8, 10, 11, 15, 16, 19 and 20) represent the relaxed and pleasant state of patient [19].

A rating of 4 indicates the presence of high level of anxiety for ten S-Anxiety items and a high rating indicates the absence of anxiety for the remaining ten S-Anxiety items. The scoring weights for the anxiety-absent items are reversed. The scores of STAI range from a minimum of 20 to a maximum score of 80. The score of more than 44 on STAI was taken as significant anxiety and patient was categorized as high anxiety (STAI score > 44) while low anxiety (STAI score ≤ 44). The selection of this value was based on previously published researches [16, 18–22].

The data were collected through interview using structured questionnaire by trained four BSc nurses and the data collection took only 20 min to complete for one patient. Two Supervisors were closely supervised the process of data collection.

Data quality control

To assure the quality of data training about the questionnaire was given to data collectors for one day prior to data collection, a pretest was done on 10% of the sampled population. Collected data were checked for its completeness and clarity on daily basis and corrections were made accordingly. Follow up and supervision was also conducted by supervisors during data collection.

Data processing and analysis

The collected data were entered into Epi-Data version 3.1 and exported to SPSS version 20 for data cleaning and analysis. Descriptive analysis was performed to describe the number and percentage of socio-demographic characteristics of the sample and other variables. The binary logistic regression model was fitted to estimate the effect size of independent variables on the dependent variable. Odds ratio with its 95% confidence interval was used to estimate the strength of association. First, a bivariate analysis was computed to test the association between each independent variable with the dependent variable. In bivariable analysis, all independent variables with a p-value of less than 0.2 were included for further analysis in the multivariable regression model. Then to control for possible confounders multivariable backward logistic regression was performed to explore the risk of "high anxiety" associated with the patient characteristics. A p-value of 0.05 or below was considered to declare statistically significant association or effect. The results were presented in text, tables, and graphs based on the types of data.

Results

Socio- demographic characteristics

A total of 353 elective major surgical patients participated in the study with a response rate of 100%. One hundred Eighty-two (51.6%) of the participants were males and the majority (61.2%) belong to the age of 18–39 years with a median age of 40 (IQR = 28.5–50) years. The result of this study showed that 135(64.6%), 73(20.7%), 24(6.8%), 19(5.4%), and 9(5%) were married, single, widowed, divorced, and separated respectively. The ethnic and religious composition of the patients showed that322 (91.2%) were Amhara and 307 (87%) were Orthodox Christians. Among all respondents, 188(53.3%) did not attend formal education. The occupational status of the participants showed that 124(35.1%) were farmers, 49(13.9%) were merchants, 49(13.9%) were housewives, 65(18.4%) were private workers, 35(9.9%) were a governmental employee and 31(8.8%) were students. Out of the total respondents, 208(59%) came from rural areas. Socio-demographic characteristics summarized in Table 1.

Table 1 Socio demographic characteristics of surgical patients in the referral hospitals

Variables	Response	Frequency (n)	Percentage (%)
Age (in Years)	18–39	168	47.6
	40–49	88	24.9
	50–59	44	12.5
	≥ 60	53	15
Sex	Male	182	51.6
	Female	171	48.4
Educational status	Not attended formal education	188	53.3
	Primary education (1–8)	74	21
	Secondary education (9–12)	49	13.9
	College and above	42	11.9
Religion	Orthodox	307	87
	Muslim	26	7.4
	Protestant	17	4.8
	Catholic	3	0.8
Ethnicity	Amhara	322	91.2
	Oromo	18	5.1
	Tigre	13	3.7
Residence	Urban	208	59
	Rural	145	41
Income (in ETB)	≤ 1000	121	34.3
	1001–2500	96	27.2
	2501–3999	56	15.9
	≥ 4000	80	22.7
Family size	≤ 3	91	25.8
	4–6	184	52.1
	>6	78	22.1

Previous health status history of the patient

Among all respondents, 144(40.8%) had a history of previous hospitalization and 61(17.3%) had previous surgical operation experience. Past health status condition of surgical patients was presented in Table 2.

Current health status history of the study participants

Majority of the total study participants 229(64.9%) know their diagnosis and 191(54.1%) had knowledge of the type of surgery to be performed. Respondents were asked whether they had got preoperative information or not. Among those, 179(51%) of them were not provided with appropriate preoperative information about the surgical operation and preoperative anxiety. Current health status history of the study participants was summarized in Table 3.

Among those who had got preoperative information, 140(39.7%) respondents got information only about operative procedures, while 17 respondents got information

Table 2 Past health status condition of surgical patients the referral hospitals

Variables	Responses	Frequency	Percentage
Previous hospitalization	Yes	144	40.8
	No	209	59.2
Previous surgical operation	Yes	61	17.3
	No	292	82.7
Time of the previous operation (in years)	≤ 1 year	10	2.8
	2–5 years	30	8.5
	≥ 6 years	7	2
Time of the previous operation (in months)	≤ 5	9	2.5
	> 5	5	1.4
Frequency of the previous operation performed	Once	50	14.2
	Twice	10	2.8
	Thrice or more	1	0.3
Any previous surgery complications	Yes	9	2.5
	No	52	14.7
Preoperative information during the previous surgery	Yes	22	6.2
	No	24	6.8
	I don't remember	15	4.2

about operative procedures expected recovery, anesthesia and surgery complications (Fig. 1).

Prevalence of preoperative anxiety

The prevalence of preoperative anxiety (state anxiety) was assessed using the state version of the State-Trait Anxiety Inventory scale (STAI). Overall 61% (95%CI (55.5–65.7)) of surgical patients in this study had significant high level of preoperative anxiety (having S-STAI scores above 44). The median score for state-anxiety (S-STAI) was 49 with IQR of 38.5–56.5. Concerning the state anxiety items, 141(39.9%) of patients scored moderately calm with a median score of 2 with IQR of 2–3. STAI state (Y-1) anxiety score of surgical patients was presented in Table 4.

Table 3 Awareness of study participants on their current health status and Preoperative information provision

Variables	Responses	Frequency	Percentage
Know the disease (diagnosis)	Yes	229	64.9
	No	124	35.1
Know the type of surgery to be performed	Yes	191	54.1
	No	162	45.9
Presence of pain on admission	Yes	122	34.6
	No	231	65.4
Preoperative information provision	Yes	174	49
	No	179	51
Satisfaction with information provided	Yes	129	36.5
	No	45	12.7

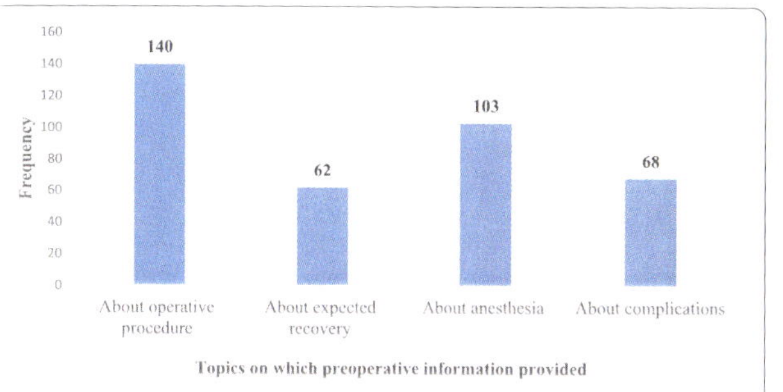

Fig. 1 Preoperative information topics for surgical patients in the referral hospitals

Reported factors responsible for preoperative anxiety among surgical patients

There are various responsible factors for preoperative anxiety in patients undergoing a surgical operation. In this study, among the factors responsible for preoperative anxiety, the most common reported factors responsible for preoperative anxiety were fear of complications 187(52.4%), concern about family 178(50.4%), fear of postoperative pain 177(50.1%) and fear of death 170(48.2%). Reported factors responsible for preoperative anxiety among surgical patients were presented in Table 5.

Statistical analysis of factors associated with preoperative anxiety

In bivariable analysis, the factors with a p-value of less than 0.20 were sex, age, marital status, educational level, occupation, residence, family size, preoperative information, and previous surgical experience. However, those variables such as awareness of the diagnosis, awareness of the type of surgery to be performed and previous hospitalization did not show any significant association up to P-value of 0.2 so that subsequently were not included in the final model.

Multivariable backward logistic regression analysis showed that a model with the five independent variables: sex, educational level, preoperative information provision, and previous surgical experience, family size was significantly associated with preoperative anxiety. The odds of having preoperative anxiety was 2.19 (95%CI (1.29–3.71)) times higher among females as compared to males (Table 6).

Discussion

The overall prevalence of preoperative anxiety in this study was 61% (95%CI (55.5–65.7)) as suggested by STAI score of more than 44 which showed that most of the

Table 4 STAI state (Y-1) anxiety score of surgical patients in referral hospitals

S. No	Variables	Not at all N (%)	Somewhat N (%)	Moderately N (%)	Very much N (%)
1	I feel calm[a]	36 (10.2)	155 (43.9)	141 (39.9)	21 (5.9)
2	I feel secure[a]	45 (12.7)	150 (42.5)	131 (37.1)	27 (7.6)
3	I feel tense	113 (32)	150 (42.5)	67 (19)	23 (6.5)
4	I am strained	47 (13.3)	189 (53.5)	93 (26.3)	24 (6.8)
5	I feel at ease[a]	70 (19.8)	165 (46.7)	103 (29.2)	15 (4.2)
6	I feel upset	178 (50.4)	95 (26.9)	67 (19)	13 (3.7)
7	I am presently worrying…	86 (24.4)	168 (47.6)	84 (23.8)	15 (4.2)
8	I feel satisfied[a]	57 (16.1)	187 (53)	93 (26.3)	16 (4.5)
9	I feel frightened	75 (21.2)	185 (52.4)	75 (21.2)	18 (5.1)
10	I feel comfortable[a]	74 (21)	169 (47.9)	105 (29.7)	5 (1.4)
11	I feel self-confident[a]	22 (6.2)	138 (39.1)	137 (38.8)	56 (15.9)
12	I feel nervous	122 (34.6)	152 (43.1)	64 (18.1)	15 (4.2)
13	I feel jittery	122 (34.6)	172 (48.7)	48 (13.6)	11 (3.1)
14	I feel indecisive	146 (41.4)	157 (44.5)	44 (12.5)	6 (1.7)
15	I am relaxed[a]	110 (31.2)	143 (40.5)	93 (26.3)	7 (2)
16	I feel content[a]	113 (32)	151 (42.8)	74 (21)	15 (4.2)
17	I am worried	44 (12.5)	201 (56.9)	73 (20.7)	35 (9.9)
18	I feel confused	138 (39.1)	137 (38.8)	56 (15.9)	22 (6.2)
19	I feel steady[a]	83 (23.5)	140 (39.7)	114 (32.3)	16 (4.5)
20	I feel pleasant[a]	104 (29.5)	153 (43.3)	75 (21.1)	21 (5.9)

Note: [a] Positive questions which are reverse coded

patients awaiting elective surgery experienced a high level of preoperative anxiety. This result was similar to the previous study conducted among Pakistan surgical patients using a similar tool in which the overall prevalence of preoperative anxiety was 62%(STAI score of more than 44) [22]. In parallel, similar results were seen from another study conducted in Indian surgical patients using a different tool, where the overall prevalence of preoperative anxiety was 58.9% [23].

The result of this study found to be higher than another study conducted in Austria, Saudi Arabia and Nigeria where the overall prevalence of preoperative

Table 5 Factors responsible for preoperative anxiety among surgical patients in the referral hospitals

Variables	Responses		State anxiety score Median (IQR)
	Frequency (N)	Percent (%)	
Fear of complications	185	52.4	50 (39–58)
Concern about family	178	50.4	49 (37–56)
Postoperative pain	177	50.1	49 (40–56)
Fear of death	170	48.2	51 (41–59)
Change of environment	160	45.3	57 (41–61)
Results of operation	150	42.5	49 (39–56)
Harm from doctor/nurse mistake	107	30.3	53 (46–59)
Fear of unknown	104	29.5	50 (40–59)
Fear of physical disability	96	27.2	53 (47–61)
Waiting for operation	65	18.4	48 (39–54)
Financial loss	62	17.6	53 (49–61)
Nil per mouth	60	17	50 (39–60)
Awareness during surgery	60	17	52 (39–60)

Note: Proportion (%) cannot be 100% because it is based on multiple response questions

Table 6 Bivariable and Multivariable logistic regression analysis of factors associated with preoperative anxiety

VARIABLES	Level of anxiety		COR (95%CI)	AOR (95%CI)
	High (%)	Low (%)		
Sex				
Male	83 (38.8)	99 (71.2)	1	1
Female	131 (61.2)	40 (28.8)	3.91 (2.47–6.18)	2.19 (1.29–3.71)
Educational level				
Not attended formal Edu.	126 (58.9)	62 (44.6)	8.64 (3.77–19.77)	7.06 (2.88–17.29)
Primary education (1–8)	54 (25.2)	20 (14.4)	11.48 (4.55–28.95)	7.07 (2.63–19.02)
Secondary education (9–12)	26 (12.1)	23 (16.5)	4.80 (1.85–12.46)	5.04 (1.81–13.99)
College and above	8 (3.7)	34 (24.5)	1	1
Preoperative information				
Yes	87 (40.7)	87 (62.6)	1	1
No	127 (59.3)	52 (37.4)	2.44 (1.58–3.79)	2.03 (1.22–3.39)
Previous surgical experience				
Yes	19 (8.9)	42 (30.2)	1	1
No	195 (91.1)	97 (69.9)	4.44 (2.45–8.05)	3.05 (1.57–5.95)
Family size				
< =3	66 (30.8)	25 (18)	2.15 (1.13–4.08)	3.21 (1.50–6.90)
4–6	105 (49.1)	79 (56.8)	1.08 (0.64–1.84)	1.23 (0.67–2.27)
>6	43 (20.1)	35 (25.2)	1	1

anxiety among admitted surgical patients was 45.3% and 55% and 51% respectively [14–16]. This might be due to the fact that most of the study participants in this study were poor and lower-class patients with poor educational status so that they had no access to information regarding anesthesia and the surgical procedure they were about to undergo.

The prevalence of preoperative anxiety in this study is lower than other similar studies conducted in Canada, Seri Lanka and Niger where the overall prevalence was 89%, 76.7%, 90% respectively [11, 13, 17]. The possible reason for the lower proportion of anxiety in this study might be due to strong family and social support implemented in our society. In addition, the difference could be due to methodological issues and measurement tool used to quantify the level of preoperative anxiety. Furthermore, the prevalence of anxiety in this study is lower than other similar study conducted among surgical patients in Jimma University Specialized Teaching Hospital, South Western Ethiopia [18]. This might be due to a difference in socio-demographic characteristics of the study participants.

There are various factors responsible for preoperative anxiety in patients undergoing a surgical operation. In this study, the most common responsible factor for preoperative anxiety was fear of complications. This was in line with a research done in Nigeria [16]. Concern about family and fear of postoperative pain in this study were the second and third most common responsible factors respectively. This was inconsistent with another study where concern about family and fear of postoperative pain were ranked the first and the second common responsible factors for preoperative anxiety respectively [24]. A study done in check republic demonstrated that their patient's most common cause of preoperative anxiety was fear of postoperative pain while in this study it was ranked third [25]. Similarly, fear of death in this study was the fourth top responsible factor, but it was the most common cause of anxiety in another study [18].

The socio-demographic characteristics that were significantly associated with preoperative anxiety were sex and educational level. The findings of this study showed that female patients had a statistically significant higher level of preoperative anxiety than males. These associations have also been demonstrated by previous similar studies [13, 17, 23–27]. The difference could be because women are sensitive to fearful events and differences in hormone fluctuations. In addition, females more easily express their anxiety than men, and separation from the family affects women more. However, one study showed no association between sex and preoperative anxiety [28].

In this study history of previous surgical experience was a significant factor for preoperative anxiety. Patients with a history of previous surgical experience were less anxious than patients coming for surgery for the first time. This was in line with other similar studies [13, 25]. This could be because of less fear of surgery or less misunderstandings about anesthesia and surgery. Contrary to this, a number of studies showed that a history of previous surgical experience and level of preoperative anxiety were not significantly associated [18, 22–24].

Another finding of this study was the level of education were significantly associated with the level of anxiety. In this study, the level of anxiety decreases with increasing level of education. This was consistent with another similar study [29]. This could be because increase level of education helps patients in preparing and reducing anxiety preoperatively. In addition, a larger proportion of anxious patients with lower education level may be because of their poor awareness related to anesthesia and surgery. Contrary to this, the results of other similar studies revealed that the level of preoperative anxiety appeared to increase with increasing level of education [18, 22, 27].

The findings of this study showed that patients who had information regarding the surgical procedure and anesthesia had a lower state-anxiety score. A marked decrease was observed in the state anxiety score of patients who had preoperative information. This was in line with many other studies [7, 18, 28, 30].

Limitation of the study

Although this has provided valuable information regarding the prevalence of preoperative anxiety and associated factors among surgical patients, there were some limitations that could be addressed in future research. First, this study did not measure patients' anxiety level before admission. Second, Comparison of the level of anxiety preoperatively and postoperatively among respondents was not done. Lastly, the Pediatric group was excluded.

Conclusion

In this study, the prevalence of preoperative anxiety was high. The level of preoperative anxiety significantly associated with sex, educational level, preoperative information provision, and previous surgical experience. In addition, Fear of complications, concern about family and fear of postoperative pain were the most common factors responsible for preoperative anxiety. Preoperative psychosocial assessment should be incorporated into a routine preoperative nursing practice and adequate, and appropriate preoperative information should be provided for surgical patients before surgery.

Abbreviations

AOR: Adjusted Odds Ratio; APAIS: Amsterdam Preoperative Anxiety and Information Scale; CI: Confidence Interval; COR: Crude Odds Ratio; HADS: Hospital Anxiety and Depression Scale; IQR: Interquartile Range; JUSH: Jimma University Specialized Hospital; SPSS: Statistical Package for Social Sciences; STAI: State-Trait Anxiety Inventory; VAS: Visual Analog Scale

Acknowledgments

The authors would like to thank the participants of the study for their cooperation and Debre Markos and Felege Hiwot referral hospital staffs for their support.

Funding

Not applicable.

Authors' contributions

HM, MA and GD have contributed to the design, data collection, data analysis, interpretation and manuscript development. TZ and MS have contributed to data collection, interpretation, and revision of the final manuscript. All authors read and approved the final manuscript.

Competing interests

The authors declare that they have no competing interests.

Author details

[1]Department of Nursing, College of Health Science, Debre Markos University, P.O. Box 269, Debre Markos, Ethiopia. [2]Department of Public Health, College of Health Science, Debre Markos University, P.O. Box 269, Debre Markos, Ethiopia. [3]Department of Nursing, School of Health Science, College of Medicine and Health Science, Bahir Dar University, P.O. Box 79, Bahir Dar, Ethiopia. [4]Department of Nursing, College of Health Science, Assosa University, P.O. Box 18, Assosa, Ethiopia.

References

1. Videbeck S, Videbeck S. Psychiatric-mental health nursing. 5th edition. Lippincott Williams & Wilkins; 2013.
2. Sigdel S. Perioperative anxiety. Clin Trials Patent. 2015;1(1):2.
3. Boker A, Brownell L, Donen N. The Amsterdam preoperative anxiety and information scale provides a simple and reliable measure of preoperative anxiety. Can J Anesth. 2002;49(8):792–8.
4. Stirling L, Raab G, Alder EM, Robertson F. Randomized trial of essential oils to reduce perioperative patient anxiety: feasibility study. J Adv Nurs. 2007; 60(5):494–501.
5. Vileikyte L. Stress and wound healing. Clin Dermatol. 2007;25(1):49–55.
6. Bailey L. Strategies for decreasing patient anxiety in the perioperative setting. AORN J. 2010;92(4):445–60.
7. Jlala HA, French J, Foxall GL, Hardman JG, Bedforth NM. Effect of preoperative multimedia information on perioperative anxiety in patients undergoing procedures under regional anaesthesia. Br J Anaesth. 2010; 104(3):369–74.
8. Pokharel K, Bhattarai B, Tripathi M, Khatiwada S, Subedi A. Nepalese patients' anxiety and concerns before surgery. J Clin Anesth. 2011;23(5):372–8.

9. Frazier SK, Moser DK, Daley LK, McKinley S, Riegel B, Garvin BJ, An K. Critical care nurses' beliefs about and reported management of anxiety. Am J Crit Care. 2003;12(1):19–27.
10. Haugen AS, Eide GE, Olsen MV, Haukeland B, Remme ÅR, Wahl AK. Anxiety in the operating theatre: a study of frequency and environmental impact in patients having local, plexus or regional anaesthesia. J Clin Nurs. 2009; 18(16):2301–10.
11. Perks A, Chakravarti S, Manninen P. Preoperative anxiety in neurosurgical patients. J Neurosurg Anesthesiol. 2009;21(2):127–30.
12. Pritchard MJ. Identifying and assessing anxiety in pre-operative patients. Nurs Stand. 2009;23(51):35–40.
13. Matthias AT, Samarasekera DN. Preoperative anxiety in surgical patients-experience of a single unit. Acta Anaesthesiol Taiwanica. 2012;50(1):3–6.
14. Uddin I, Kurkuman A, Jamil T. Pre-operative anxiety in patients admitted for elective surgery in king Saud hospital, Unaizah, Al-Qassim, Kingdom of Saudi Arabia. Pak J Med Sci. 2002;18(4):306–10.
15. Wetsch WA, Pircher I, Lederer W, Kinzl J, Traweger C, Heinz-Erian P, Benzer A. Preoperative stress and anxiety in day-care patients and inpatients undergoing fast-track surgery. Br J Anaesth. 2009;103(2):199–205.
16. Akinsulore A, Owojuyigbe AM, Faponle AF, Fatoye FO. Assessment of preoperative and postoperative anxiety among elective major surgery patients in a tertiary hospital in Nigeria. Middle East J Anaesthesiol. 2015; 23(2):235–40.
17. Ebirim L, Tobin M. Factors responsible for pre-operative anxiety in elective surgical patients at a university teaching hospital: A pilot study. Int J Anesth. 2010;29(2):1–6.
18. Nigussie S, Belachew T, Wolancho W. Predictors of preoperative anxiety among surgical patients in Jimma University specialized teaching hospital, South Western Ethiopia. BMC Surg. 2014;14(1):1.
19. Spielberger CD: Manual for the state-trait anxiety inventory STAI (form Y) ("self-evaluation questionnaire"). 1983.
20. Carr E, Brockbank K, Allen S, Strike P. Patterns and frequency of anxiety in women undergoing gynaecological surgery. J Clin Nurs. 2006;15(3):341-52.
21. Millar K, Jelicic M, Bonke B, Asbury A. Assessment of preoperative anxiety: comparison of measures in patients awaiting surgery for breast cancer. Br J Anaesth. 1995;74(2):180–3.
22. Jafar MF, Khan FA. Frequency of preoperative anxiety in Pakistani surgical patients. J Pak Med Assoc. 2009;59(6):359.
23. Saini S, Dayal M. Preoperative Anxiety in Indian Surgical Patients-Experience of a Single Unit. Indian J Appl Res. 2016;6(9):476-9.
24. Jawaid M, Mushtaq A, Mukhtar S, Khan Z. Preoperative anxiety before elective surgery. Neurosciences. 2007;12(2):145–8.
25. Homzová P, Zeleníková R. Measuring preoperative anxiety in patients undergoing elective surgery in Czech republic. Education. 2015;38:11.
26. Aalouane R, Rammouz I, Tahiri-Alaoui D, Elrhazi K, Boujraf S. Determining factors of anxiety in patients at the preoperative stage. Neurosciences (Riyadh). 2011;16(2):146–9.
27. Yilmaz M, Sezer H, Gürler H, Bekar M. Predictors of preoperative anxiety in surgical inpatients. J Clin Nurs. 2012;21(7–8):956–64.
28. Kiyohara LY, Kayano LK, Oliveira LM, Yamamoto MU, Inagaki MM, Ogawa NY, Gonzales PESM, Mandelbaum R, Okubo ST, Watanuki T. Surgery information reduces anxiety in the pre-operative period. Revista do Hospital das Clínicas. 2004;59(2):51–6.
29. Prathapan S, Wanigabandu LU, Lamahewage N, De Silva D, Serasinghe V, Dadigamuwa N, Sannasuriya M, Rajakaruna M. Anxiety of patients undergoing general anaesthesia and their myths and beliefs. Sri Lankan J Anaesthesiol. 2013;22(1):11–14.
30. Aasa A, Hovback M, Bertero CM. The importance of preoperative information for patient participation in colorectal surgery care. J Clin Nurs. 2013;22(11–12):1604–12.

25

Prediction of hemodynamic fluctuations after induction of general anesthesia using propofol in non-cardiac surgery: a retrospective cohort study

Sho Kawasaki[1,2], Chikako Kiyohara[2*], Shoji Tokunaga[3] and Sumio Hoka[1]

Abstract

Background: Although propofol is a common anesthetic agent for the induction of general anesthesia, hemodynamic fluctuations are occasionally prominent during induction/intubation. The aims of this study were to determine the influential factors on enhanced hemodynamic fluctuation and to establish a prediction formula to quickly determine the dose of propofol to protect against hemodynamic fluctuations.

Methods: This retrospective cohort study patients ($n = 2097$) were 18 years or older. They underwent general anesthesia induction using propofol and orotracheal intubation for non-cardiac surgery at Kyushu University Hospital during April 2015 to March 2016. Preoperative patient clinical information was collected from anesthesia preoperative evaluation records. Intraoperative data were obtained from computerized anesthesia records. If patients' post-induction mean arterial blood pressure (MAP) decreased or increased 30% or more from their pre-induction MAP, they were determined to have enhanced hemodynamic fluctuations. Unconditional logistic regression was used to assess the adjusted odds ratios (ORs) and 95% confidence intervals (CIs). Structural equation modeling (SEM) was conducted to simultaneously examine the direct and indirect effect (path coefficient = r) of potential variables.

Results: In the SEM analysis, age was significantly associated with enhanced hemodynamic fluctuations (adjusted odds ratio = 1.008, 95% CI = 1.001–1.015, $P = 0.03$). Age (path coefficient (r) = − 0.0113, 95% CI = − 0.0126–0.010, $P < 0.001$), American Society of Anesthesiologists physical status (ASA-PS) ($r = -0.0788$, 95% CI = − 0.1431–0.0145, $P = 0.02$), sex ($r = 0.057$, 95% CI = 0.0149–0.9906, $P = 0.01$), and fentanyl dose ($r = 0.1087$, 95% CI = 0.0707–0.1467, $P < 0.001$) influenced the dose of propofol in induction. The prediction formula of "Propofol dose (mg) = [2.374 − 0.0113 × age (year) − 0.0788 (if ASA-PS 3 or 4) + 0.057 (if female) + 0.1087 × fentanyl dose (μg/kg)] × body weight (kg)" was derived.

Conclusions: Age was associated with hemodynamic fluctuations in induction. Although the prediction formula is considered to be acceptable, future studies validating whether it can decrease patients' risk of enhanced hemodynamic fluctuations in clinical situations are necessary.

Keywords: Propofol, Anesthesia induction, Hemodynamics, Prediction formula

* Correspondence: chikako@phealth.med.kyushu-u.ac.jp
[2]Department of Preventive Medicine, Graduate School of Medical Sciences, Kyushu University, Maidashi 3-1-1, Higashi-ku, Fukuoka, Fukuoka, Japan
Full list of author information is available at the end of the article

Background

Propofol is a common anesthetic agent for the induction of general anesthesia. Rapid infusion of propofol often causes hypotension [1–5]. Intraoperative hypotension may lead to negative outcomes such as myocardial injury, stroke, acute kidney injury, and death [6–10]. Conversely, laryngoscopy and tracheal intubation often cause hypertension [11–15]. Hypertension associated with intubation may cause negative outcomes such as myocardial infarction, heart failure, pulmonary edema, and cerebral and subarachnoid hemorrhage [16–18]. Thus, preventing hemodynamic fluctuations, or stabilizing hemodynamics, would avoid some harmful complications. The recommended dose of propofol in induction of general anesthesia is 2–2.5 mg/kg.

The American Society of Anesthesiologists physical status (ASA-PS) scale is a widely used grading system to measure the preoperative health of surgical patients. The ASA-PS scale is a subjective assessment of a patient's overall health that is based on 6 categories (1 [healthy and no complications] to 6 [brain death]). Elderly patients and/or patients with ASA-PS scores of 3 or higher (having moderate to severe comorbidities) require a reduction in dose of propofol due to adverse prognosis [19–21]. However, the relationship between characteristics of patients and anesthesia induction dose of propofol has not yet been fully evaluated.

Since reliable guidelines for determining the propofol dose in anesthesia induction do not exist, this determination has been entrusted to each anesthesiologist. Although anesthetic devices and drugs have undergone improvements, intraoperative hemodynamic fluctuations continue to occur [22]. Structural equation modeling (SEM) is a multivariate statistical tool for evaluating complex relations in several research fields. SEM is a useful method for evaluating simultaneous causal associations among factors, which allows factors to be both dependent and independent. By explicitly accounting for the underlying roles of the factors of enhanced hemodynamic fluctuations, SEM can provide more insight and a better understanding of how risk factors influence the outcome.

The aims of this study were to identify the predictors of hemodynamic fluctuations after induction of general anesthesia and to develop a prediction formula, using SEM analysis, to calculate the appropriate propofol dose in induction.

Materials and methods

Patient population and ethics

Our retrospective cohort study protocol was approved by the Institutional Review Board (IRB) of Kyushu University Hospital in March 2018 (IRB# 29–630). The IRB waived the need for written informed consent from participants. Because all patients received usual care and were not subjected to research activities, written informed consent was not obtained. This article adheres to the applicable Strengthening the Reporting of Observational Studies in Epidemiology (STROBE) guidelines.

Patients who were 18 years old or older (range: 18 to 96 years old) and underwent general anesthesia induction using propofol subsequently with tracheal intubation for non-cardiac surgery were included in this study. All patients ($n = 2760$) underwent inpatient anesthesia and surgery at the Kyushu University Hospital in Fukuoka, Japan, during the period April 2015 to March 2016. Patients who were missing important covariates regarding intubation or hemodynamic data were excluded ($n = 56$). Patients who did not receive oral intubation or who underwent repeated attempts at intubation were also excluded ($n = 607$). A total of 2097 participants were included in this analysis.

Validation study of the prediction formula

In another part of the study, the prediction formula was then applied to 1974 patients, who were admitted to the same hospital during the period April 2016 to March 2017 in order to validate the derived prediction formula. A sample size of 1974 patients was expected to yield sufficient subjects to validate the prediction formula. This separate cohort was comparable in confounders to the study cohort.

Clinical data

Preoperative patient clinical information was collected from anesthesia preoperative evaluation records (NIHON KOHDEN Corp, Tokyo, Japan). The records consisted of demographic data, laboratory data, and medical history. Intraoperative data were obtained from computerized anesthesia records (NIHON KOHDEN Corp.). These data from the patient monitoring system and anesthesia machine were automatically stored in anesthesia records, whereas drug dose and anesthesia techniques were registered manually. No patients received anesthetic premedication. In the operation room, the patients were placed on the operating table in the supine position. Baseline data, such as electrocardiography, non-invasive blood pressure, and pulse oximetry, were obtained from the records of standard monitors. An invasive arterial catheter was inserted after induction of general anesthesia if necessary. Heart rate was continuously recorded, and non-invasive arterial blood pressure was recorded every 2.5 min. Basically, arterial blood pressure was recorded continuously after insertion of the invasive arterial catheter. Induction of general anesthesia was elicited by propofol, fentanyl, remifentanil, rocuronium, and inhalation anesthetics (sevoflurane or desflurane in oxygen). Propofol was administered according to the instruction manual. Selection of induction drugs and doses depended on the anesthesiologist's clinical judgment based on the patients' medical conditions. Laryngoscopy and orotracheal intubation were performed by an attending anesthesiologist (residents or specialists).

Definition of main outcome

Baseline arterial blood pressure (pre-induction) was defined as the first measurement in the operating room under awake conditions. While, arterial blood pressure after induction (post-induction) was measured within 3 min after tracheal intubation. In case of insertion of an invasive arterial catheter, arterial blood pressure 1 min after tracheal intubation was measured. Several definitions of hemodynamic fluctuations have been previously published. However, Bijker et al. reviewed the major journals and concluded that hypotension is best defined as 20–30% reduction of mean arterial blood pressure (MAP) [22]. In addition, Goldman et al. reported that postoperative cardiac death was significantly associated with a 33% or greater fall in intraoperative systolic blood pressure (SBP) from baseline for more than 10 min [23]. Moreover, Bijker et al. reported that a decrease in MAP of more than 30% from baseline was associated with the occurrence of a postoperative stroke (odds ratio [OR] = 1.013 for every minute of hypotension, 99% confidence interval [CI] = 1.000–1.025) [7]. Based on the results mentioned above, if a patient's post-induction MAP decreased or increased 30% or more from their pre-induction MAP, they were determined to have enhanced hemodynamic fluctuations before and after anesthesia induction.

Statistical analysis

Differences in patient characteristics between the fluctuation status categories were compared using the Student t-test for normally distributed continuous variables and the Mann-Whitney U test for not-normally distributed continuous variables. Categorical variables were compared using the Pearson chi-squared test or the Fisher exact test where appropriate. Variables with a *P* value of less than 0.20 in univariate analyses or clinical relevance were entered into the multivariate logistic regression model. Multivariate logistic regression analysis was used to adjust for potential confounding variables and to identify the association of independent variables with hemodynamic fluctuations. Similarly, variables with a *P* value of less than 0.20 in multivariate analysis or clinical relevance were entered into SEM. SEM could be performed to simultaneously examine the direct and indirect effect of potential variables. A path coefficient indicates the direct effect of a variable assumed to be a cause on another variable assumed to be an effect [24]. As path coefficients are estimated from correlations, they should be standardized. In our study, SEM was used to reveal the propofol-mediated effect of potential variables to hemodynamic fluctuations and the effect of potential variables to propofol dose in anesthesia induction. The potential variables are often highly intercorrelated (multicollinearity). Multicollinearity was assessed using variance inflation factor (VIF) [25], which measures the inflation in the variances of the parameter estimates due to multicollinearity potentially caused by correlated predictors. Although there is no consensus as what cutoff based on values of VIF should be used to detect multicollinearity, VIF greater than 5 [25] is suggested for detecting multicollinearity.

To assess the accuracy of the prediction formula, we applied it to a separate cohort of 1974 patients. We defined differences less than 5 mg between the actual dose and estimated dose as "fitted to the formula (fitted group)" and otherwise defined as "unfitted to the formula (unfitted group)".

Age, height, weight, blood pressure, and drug use except vasopressor at induction and intubation were treated as continuous variables. Remaining covariates, namely ASA-PS scale (scores of 1 or 2 and 3 or 4), obesity (body mass index < 25 kg/m^2 and ≥ 25 kg/m^2), anesthesia start time (forenoon and afternoon), a clinical history of comorbidities (positive and negative), vasopressor (use [phenylephrine 0.05–0.1 mg or ephedrine 4-8 mg] or non-use) were treated as categorical variables. The 48 potential predictors as reported in the pre-existing literature, which may be associated with hemodynamic fluctuations in induction of general anesthesia, are shown in Table 1. All *P* values were 2-sided, and those less than 0.05 were considered statistically significant. All statistical analyses were performed using Stata version 14.1 software (StataCorp LP, College Station, Texas, USA).

Results

Of 2760 consecutive non-cardiac surgical patients 18 years or older who underwent general anesthesia induction using propofol, 192 did not have orotracheal intubation, 415 underwent repeated attempts at tracheal intubation and 56 were missing important covariate data. Exclusion of these patients resulted in a sample size of 2097 patients (Fig. 1). Enhanced hemodynamic fluctuations after induction of general anesthesia were observed in 482 patients (23.0%). Of these 482 patients, 287 (13.7%) developed hypotension, and 195 (9.3%) developed hypertension.

Tables 1 and 2 show differences in demographics and lifestyle-related and clinical features of the two fluctuation status groups. Age, history of ischemic heart disease, propofol dose, and fentanyl dose were significantly

Table 1 Demographic, lifestyle-related, physical and clinical characteristics of perioperative patients according to hemodynamic fluctuation status ($n = 2097$)

Variables	Hemodynamic fluctuation				P value
	≥30% ($n = 482$)	No.[a]	< 30% ($n = 1615$)	No.[a]	
Demographic and lifestyle-related					
Age (years), mean (range)	61.2 (18–96)	0	58.3 (18–93)	0	< 0.001
Female sex, n (%)	247 (51.2)	0	813 (50.3)	0	0.73
Height (cm), mean (95% CI)	160.5 (159.7–161.4)	0	161.0 (160.6–161.5)	3	0.29
Weight (kg), mean (95% CI)	59.3 (58.1–60.5)	0	60.1 (59.5–60.8)	0	0.23
BMI, n (%)		0		3	0.23
< 18	48 (29.6)		114 (70.4)		
≥ 18, < 25	316 (22.4)		1093 (77.6)		
≥25, < 35	110 (22.5)		379 (77.5)		
≥ 35	8 (23.5)		26 (76.5)		
Smoking history, n (%)	226 (46.9)	0	721 (44.8)	5	0.42
Physical status					
ASA-PS scale, n (%)		0		0	0.52
1 or 2	417 (86.5)		1415 (87.6)		
3 or 4	65 (13.5)		200 (12.4)		
Low exercise tolerability, n (%)	32 (6.7)	1	91 (5.7)	5	0.41
Clinical and laboratory data					
Arterial BP (mmHg) in the ward, mean (95% CI)					
Systolic BP	125 (123–126)	15	125 (124–126)	49	0.92
Diastolic BP	74 (73–75)	16	74 (74–75)	51	0.82
History of steroid use, n (%)	28 (5.8)	1	96 (6.0)	5	0.91
History of opioid use, n (%)	3 (0.6)	1	13 (0.8)	5	1.00[b]
Antithrombotic drug use, n (%)	66 (13.7)	1	184 (11.4)	5	0.17
Anemia, n (%)	172 (35.8)	1	573 (35.5)	2	0.93
Electrolyte imbalance, n (%)	4 (0.8)	3	12 (0.8)	6	0.77[b]
Hypoalbuminemia, n (%)	70 (14.6)	3	191 (11.9)	6	0.11
Elevated CRP, n (%)	133 (27.9)	5	413 (25.8)	14	0.36

Data are presented as *n* (%) for categorical variables, mean (95%CI) or mean (range) for continuous variables
BMI Body mass index, *ASA-PS* American Society of Anesthesiologists physical status, *BP* Blood pressure, *CI* Confidence interval, *CRP* C-reactive protein
[a]Number of missing patients
[b]Fisher's exact test

different between the two fluctuation status groups, whereas diabetes mellitus, peripheral vascular disease, and stroke appeared to be marginally significant. However, difference in two clinically important variables, namely ASA-PS score and sex, did not reach statistical significance.

Variables with a P value of less than 0.20 in univariate analyses or two clinically important variables were entered into the multivariate logistic regression model. The results of multivariate logistic regression analysis are shown in Table 3. Three potentially relevant ($P < 0.20$) variables with hemodynamic fluctuations, namely, ischemic heart disease (adjusted OR = 1.51, 95% CI = 0.93–2.46, $P = 0.10$), propofol dose (adjusted OR = 0.81, 95% CI = 0.65–1.01, $P = 0.06$), and fentanyl dose (adjusted OR = 0.84, 95% CI = 0.69–1.02, $P = 0.08$), were extracted.

SEM predicting enhanced hemodynamic fluctuations in preoperative patients is shown in Fig. 2 and Table 4. The path coefficients (r) indicated the direction and magnitude of the associations. Age ($r = -0.0113$, 95% CI = – 0.0126–0.010, $P < 0.001$), ASA-PS score ($r = -0.0788$, 95% CI = – 0.1431–0.0145, $P = 0.02$), sex ($r = 0.057$, 95% CI = 0.0149–0.9906, $P = 0.01$), and fentanyl dose ($r = 0.1087$, 95% CI = 0.0707–0.1467, $P < 0.001$) were significant factors that influenced the dose of propofol directly. The OR estimated using logistic

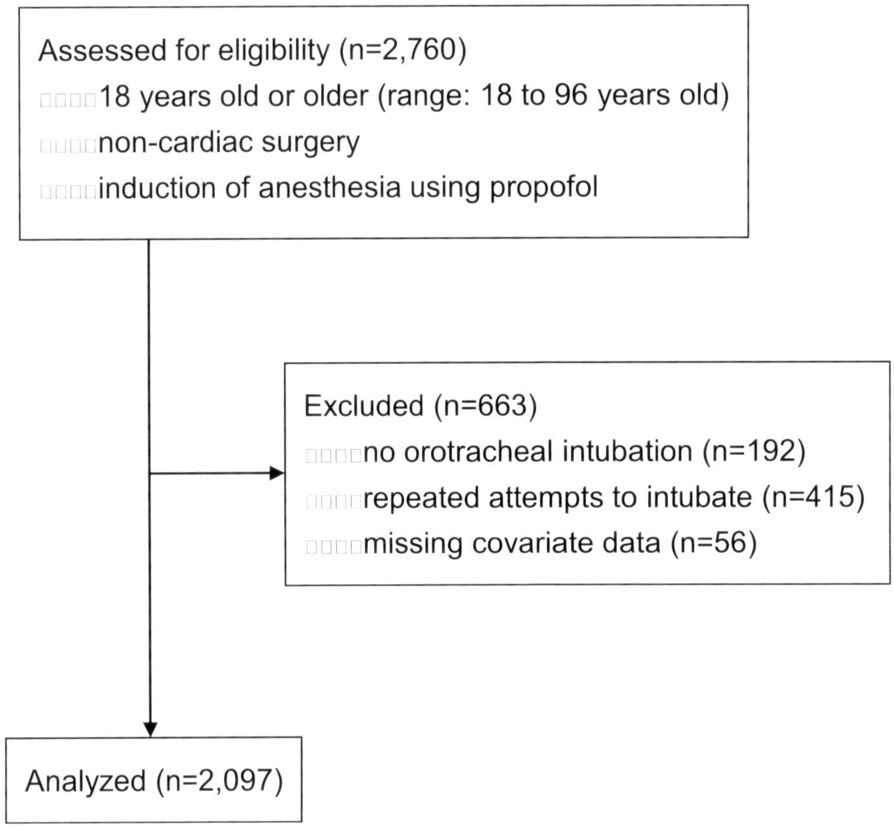

Fig. 1 Flow diagram of study subjects. All patients ($n = 2760$) underwent inpatient anesthesia and surgery. All patients were older than 18 years and underwent general anesthesia induction using propofol and tracheal intubation for non-cardiac surgery. Patients who had missing important covariates regarding intubation or hemodynamic data ($n = 56$), who did not receive oral intubation, or who underwent repeated attempts at intubation were excluded ($n = 607$). A total of 2097 participants were included in the analysis

regression in SEM of enhanced hemodynamic fluctuations was significantly increased per age increment (1.008, 95% CI = 1.001–1.015, $P = 0.03$). Conversely, ischemic heart disease (OR = 1.54, 95% CI = 0.99–2.38, $P = 0.06$), fentanyl dose (OR = 0.83, 95% CI = 0.69–1.01, $P = 0.06$), and propofol dose (OR = 0.81, 95% CI = 0.65–1.00, $P = 0.05$) were non-significant. Based on the data in Table 4, the prediction formula of propofol dose in induction is as follows:

$$\begin{aligned}\text{Propofol dose } (mg) = & [2.374 - 0.0113 \times \text{age (year)} \\ & - 0.0788(\text{if ASA}{-}PS \text{ 3 } or \text{ 4}) \\ & + 0.057 \text{ (if female)} + 0.1087 \\ & \times \text{fentanyl dose } (\mu g/kg)] \\ & \times \text{body weight (kg)}\end{aligned}$$

As a result of the application of this formula to a validation cohort, the prevalence of hemodynamic fluctuations in the unfitted group (26.7%, $n = 1654$) was significantly higher than that in the fitted group (19.7%, $n = 320$) ($P = 0.009$). Since all VIF values were lower than 2, we confirmed the absence of multicollinearity (data not shown).

Discussion

In our study, the prevalence of hemodynamic fluctuations after induction of general anesthesia was observed to be 23.0%. Age (OR = 1.008, 95% CI = 1.001–1.015, $P = 0.03$) was significantly associated with enhanced hemodynamic fluctuations. Whereas, ischemic heart disease (OR = 1.54, 95% CI = 0.99–2.38, $P = 0.06$), fentanyl dose (OR = 0.83, 95% CI = 0.69–1.01, $P = 0.06$), and propofol dose (OR = 0.81, 95% CI = 0.65–1.00, $P = 0.05$) were marginally associated. Conversely, age ($r = -0.0113$, 95% CI = −0.0126–0.010, $P < 0.001$), ASA-PS score ($r = -0.0788$, 95% CI = −0.1431–0.0145, $P = 0.02$), sex ($r = 0.057$, 95% CI = 0.0149–0.9906, $P = 0.01$), and fentanyl dose ($r = 0.1087$, 95% CI = 0.0707–0.1467, $P < 0.001$) were significant factors that influenced the dose of propofol directly.

A recent study found that the prevalence of hypotension (SBP < 80 for > 5 min) and hypertension

Table 2 Clinical history and anesthetic practice of perioperative patients according to hemodynamic fluctuation status (n = 2097)

Variables	Hemodynamic fluctuation				*P* value
	≥30% (*n* = 482)	No. [a]	< 30% (*n* = 1615)	No. [a]	
Clinical history, *n* (%)					
Diabetes mellitus	97 (20.1)	0	263 (16.3)	3	0.05
Hyperlipidemia	108 (22.4)	0	309 (19.2)	3	0.12
Hypertension	208 (43.2)	0	673 (41.2)	3	0.58
Ischemic heart disease	33 (6.9)	4	65 (4.0)	7	0.01
Congestive heart failure	5 (1.0)	0	18 (1.1)	3	0.88
Arrhythmia	19 (3.9)	0	70 (4.3)	3	0.70
Valvular heart disease	17 (3.5)	0	76 (4.7)	3	0.27
Cardiomyopathy	1 (0.2)	0	11 (0.7)	3	0.32[b]
Pulmonary hypertension	3 (0.6)	0	7 (0.4)	3	0.71[b]
Peripheral vascular disease	13 (2.7)	0	25 (1.6)	3	0.10
Aortic aneurysm	6 (1.2)	0	9 (0.6)	3	0.12
Stroke	35 (7.3)	0	84 (5.2)	3	0.09
Asthma	32 (6.6)	0	118 (7.3)	3	0.61
Sleep apnea syndrome	22 (4.6)	3	71 (4.4)	12	0.88
Chronic kidney disease	120 (25.1)	3	368 (22.9)	6	0.32
Liver dysfunction	9 (1.9)	5	28 (1.8)	16	0.84
Hyperthyroidism	4 (0.8)	1	12 (0.7)	3	0.85
Hypothyroidism	18 (3.7)	0	47 (2.9)	0	0.36
Rheumatoid arthritis	7 (1.5)	1	16 (1.0)	5	0.39
Gastrointestinal disorder	28 (5.8)	0	92 (5.7)	3	0.93
Operation and anesthesia, *n* (%)					
Emergency surgery	31 (6.4)	0	96 (5.9)	0	0.69
Combined epidural anesthesia	206 (42.7)	0	646 (40.0)	0	0.28
Anesthesia start time, *n* (%)		0		0	0.17
A.M.	294 (61.0)		1041 (64.5)		
P.M.	188 (39.0)		574 (35.5)		
Intubation method, *n* (%)		3		14	0.68
Direct	406 (84.8)		1369 (85.5)		
Video laryngoscope	73 (15.2)		232 (14.5)		
Operator of intubation, *n* (%)		0		0	0.61
Specialist	137 (23.7)		440 (76.3)		
Residents	345 (22.7)		1175 (77.3)		
Drug dosage at induction and intubation, mean (95%CI) or median (range)					
Propofol (mg/kg)	1.8 (1.7–1.8)	0	1.9 (1.9–1.9)	0	< 0.001
Fentanyl (μg/kg)	1.2 (1.2–1.3)	0	1.3 (1.3–1.3)	0	0.02
Remifentanil ($\mu g\ kg^{-1}\ min^{-1}$)	0.2 (0–0.5)	0	0.2 (0–0.5)	0	0.29
Sevoflurane (%)	0 (0–3.3)	0	0 (0–6.2)	0	0.70[c]
Desflurane (%)	0 (0–5.0)	0	0 (0–8.0)	1	0.74[c]
Midazolam (%)	0 (0–5.0)	0	0 (0–4.0)	1	0.17[c]
Vasopressor, *n* (%)	19 (3.9)	0	51 (3.2)	0	0.40

Data are presented as *n* (%) for categorical variables, mean (95%CI) or median (range) for continuous variables
A.M. Ante meridian, *P.M.* Post meridian, *CI* Confidence interval
[a]Number of missing patients
[b]Fisher's exact test
[c]Mann-Whitney U test

Table 3 Association between enhanced hemodynamic fluctuation (≥30%) and selected clinical factors

Variables	OR (95% CI)			
	Crude	*P* value	Adjusted[a]	*P* value
Age (year)	1.01 (1.01–1.02)	< 0.001	–	
Female sex	1.04 (0.85–1.27)	0.73	–	
ASA-PS scale, 3 or 4 vs. 1 or 2	1.10 (0.82–1.49)	0.53	0.87 (0.62–1.24)	0.45
Anesthesia start time, P.M. vs. A.M.	1.16 (0.94–1.43)	0.17	1.14 (0.92–1.41)	0.22
Ischemic heart disease	1.76 (1.14–2.71)	0.01	1.51 (0.93–2.46)	0.10
Peripheral vascular disease	1.76 (0.89–3.47)	0.11	1.39 (0.67–2.88)	0.38
Aortic aneurysm	2.25 (0.80–6.34)	0.14	1.55 (0.51–4.70)	0.44
Stroke	1.42 (0.95–2.14)	0.10	1.23 (0.77–1.95)	0.38
Diabetes mellitus	1.29 (0.99–1.67)	0.06	1.12 (0.85–1.48)	0.41
Hyperlipidemia	1.22 (0.95–1.56)	0.12	1.03 (0.79–1.35)	0.82
Hypoalbminemia	1.27 (0.95–1.71)	0.12	1.17 (0.85–1.61)	0.34
Antithrombotic drug use	1.23 (0.91–1.67)	0.18	0.91 (0.63–1.32)	0.62
Propofol (mg/kg)	0.71 (0.59–0.87)	< 0.001	0.81 (0.65–1.01)	0.06
Fentanyl (μg/kg)	0.80 (0.66–0.96)	0.02	0.84 (0.69–1.02)	0.08
Midazolam (mg)	0.75 (0.47–1.20)	0.18	0.79 (0.49–1.27)	0.33

[a]Mutually adjusted for all variables in Table 3
ASA-PS American Society of Anesthesiologists physical status, *OR* Odds ratio, *CI* Confidence interval

(SBP > 160 for > 5 min) were 26 and 20%, respectively [26]. Similarly, 25% of patients had arterial blood pressure fluctuations greater than 30% during anesthesia induction using propofol [27]. Therefore, the prevalence in our study of hemodynamic fluctuations after induction of general anesthesia was similar to the prevalence reported in other studies.

The recommended dose of propofol in induction is 2–2.5 mg/kg. Since geriatric patients and patients with ASA-PS scores of 3 or higher are more sensitive to the anesthetic and adverse effects, a dose reduction is recommended. In fact, predictors of hypotension after induction were ASA-PS score of 3 or 4 and age older than 50 years [1]. Also, age 65 years or older

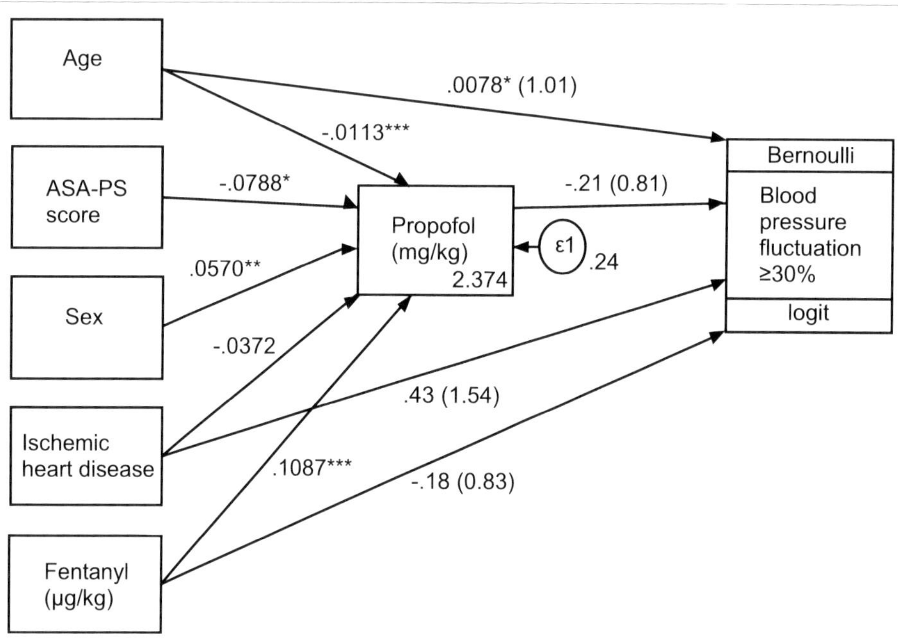

Fig. 2 Factors predicting enhanced blood pressure fluctuation with path coefficients and odds ratios (in parentheses) ($n = 2097$). ASA-PS American Society of Anesthesiologists physical status. Numbers by the arrow lines represent the estimated coefficients with significance level: $^{*}P < 0.05$; $^{**}P < 0.01$; $^{***}P < 0.001$. ε1: dependent variable

Table 4 Structural equation model of enhanced hemodynamic fluctuation (≥30%)

Variables	Model coefficient (95% CI)	*P* value
Propofol dose	Regression coefficient (r)	
Age (year, continuous)	−0.0113 (− 0.0126–0.0100)	< 0.001
ASA-PS scale	−0.0788 (− 0.1431–0.0145)	0.02
Sex	0.0570 (0.0149–0.9906)	0.01
Ischemic heart disease	−0.0372 (− 0.1388–0.0645)	0.47
Fentanyl (μg/kg)	0.1087 (0.0707–0.1467)	< 0.001
Constant	2.374 (2.275–2.473)	
Enhanced hemodynamic fluctuation (≥30%)	OR (95% CI)	P value
Age (year, continuous)	1.008 (1.001–1.015)	0.03
Ischemic heart disease	1.536 (0.990–2.382)	0.06
Fentanyl (μg/kg)	0.831 (0.687–1.005)	0.06
Propofol (mg/kg)	0.807 (0.652–1.000)	0.05

ASA-PS American Society of Anesthesiologists physical status, *CI* Confidence interval, *OR* Odds ratio

and higher dose of propofol were major two highly significant predictive factors for hypotension caused by propofol injection [2]. Additionally, the favorable induction dose of propofol in patients younger than 60 years was 2.25–2.5 mg/kg, whereas in patients older than 60 years was 1.5–1.75 mg/kg [21]. The induction dose of propofol should be adjusted for an individual patient's condition.

To determine the suitable dose of propofol to protect against hemodynamic fluctuations, we investigated the relation of propofol dose in induction to hemodynamic fluctuations. As shown in Table 4, age, sex, ASA-PS score, and fentanyl dose were associated with propofol dose to stabilize hemodynamic responses in induction.

Previous studies have provided consistent evidence for relationships between age and ASA-PS and enhanced hemodynamic fluctuation [1, 2, 21]. On the other hand, there was no difference that the effect of sex on the propofol dose in relation to loss of consciousness [28]. Similarly, a logistic regression model was used to predict blood pressure change caused by rapid injection of propofol during anesthesia induction [27]. It found that sex did not significantly contribute to blood pressure change. However, females were more likely to become hypotensive than males [2] and the half maximal effective concentration of propofol in males was significantly higher than females [29]. In our study, sex was not related to hemodynamic changes, but females required higher doses of propofol in induction than males.

Increasing the induction dose of fentanyl was a predictive factor for hypotension [1]. Similarly, concomitant use of opioids was a minor risk factor for hypotension caused by propofol [2]. Conversely, five μg/kg of fentanyl treatment caused a significant attenuation of the blood pressure response to laryngoscopy and intubation [30]. The magnitude of post-intubation hypertension was reported to be significantly less according to an increase in the fentanyl dose ($P < 0.05$ for 2 or 4 μg/kg vs. no fentanyl; $P < 0.05$ for 4 μg/kg vs. 2 μg/kg) [31].

Fentanyl was shown to cause and promote hypotension [1, 2]. On the other hand, the addition of fentanyl prior to propofol induction is used to decrease propofol dose and hypertensive response to tracheal intubation [30–32]. In our study, 1.3 μg/kg of fentanyl for the stable group (MAP change < 30%) and 1.2 μg/kg for the unstable group (MAP change ≥30%) were administered for anesthetic induction ($P < 0.001$). This result suggests that the preventive effect of fentanyl on hypertension is more dominant than the promoting effect of fentanyl on hypotension. Consequently, the propofol dose in induction increased with the increasing fentanyl dose (Table 4 and Fig. 2). Therefore, our formula indicating a positive association between propofol dose and fentanyl dose may be biologically plausible.

Our retrospective cohort study has several limitations. Generally, the researchers retrospectively identify the exposure and the outcome information. Selection bias would be possible if participation had been influenced by the physical status of patients. However, patients who had severe comorbidities could not be induced with general anesthesia using propofol. Moreover, data were entered manually during anesthesia (such as administration of medications and time of intubation). Since post-intubation blood pressure frequently reached its highest value at 0–1 min after intubation [30, 33], it may be a less reliable estimate of the exact time of induction and intubation. Because the timing of blood pressure measurement after intubation was unfixed, it may be also less reliable. Another limitation of our study is that outcome information could not be obtained using our current data system. Cooperation with other relevant diagnosis and treatment department is crucial in the future studies.

Advantages of our single-institution study are the large size of the study population, systematic consideration of potential confounders, and uniform collection of information about anesthetic practices. To estimate the generalizable prediction formula, almost all variables that affect hemodynamic fluctuations were considered; we also included a broad spectrum of patients in terms of surgical types and comorbidities. Several similar studies examining the relation of potential predictors to hemodynamic change have been reported [19, 27, 34–36]. However, since the variables to be entered in the prediction formula were either too few or too many, this was not clinically practical. Five variables, namely age, sex, ASA-PS score, fentanyl dose, and body weight, extracted from this study can be easily obtained from any patient and are essential factors for anesthesia. Therefore, our prediction formula is readily available at the time of anesthesia. A simple, generalized formula for choosing propofol dose should be required, especially for inexperienced anesthesiologists.

Conclusions

Age, ischemic heart disease, fentanyl dose and propofol dose were marginally or significantly associated with enhanced hemodynamic fluctuations in induction. The prediction formula derived to prevent hemodynamic fluctuations will help anesthesiologists tailor the dose of propofol in the induction of general anesthesia to each patient. Although the derived prediction formula is considered to be acceptable, future studies validating whether it can predict a patient's risk of enhanced hemodynamic fluctuations in clinical situations are necessary.

Abbreviations

ASA: American Society of Anesthesiologists; BMI: Body mass index; BP: Blood pressure; CI: Confidence interval; CRP: C-reactive protein; IRB: Institutional Review Board; MAP: Mean arterial blood pressure; OR: Odds ratio; PS: Physical status; SBP: Systolic blood pressure; SEM: Structural equation modeling; STROBE: Strengthening the Reporting of Observational Studies in Epidemiology; VIF: Variance inflation factor

Acknowledgements

Not applicable.

Authors' contributions

SK designs the study, acquire and analyze the data, and write the article. CK design and supervise the study, analyze the data, and write the article. ST supervise the study and data analysis. SH supervise the study and revise the article. All authors read and approved the final manuscript.

Competing interests

The authors declare that they have no competing interests.

Author details

[1]Department of Anesthesiology and Critical Care Medicine, Graduate School of Medical Sciences, Kyushu University, Maidashi 3-1-1, Higashi-ku, Fukuoka, Fukuoka, Japan. [2]Department of Preventive Medicine, Graduate School of Medical Sciences, Kyushu University, Maidashi 3-1-1, Higashi-ku, Fukuoka, Fukuoka, Japan. [3]Medical Information Center, Kyushu University Hospital, Maidashi 3-1-1, Higashi-ku, Fukuoka, Fukuoka, Japan.

References

1. Reich DL, Hossain S, Krol M, Baez B, Patel P, Bernstein A, et al. Predictors of hypotension after induction of general anesthesia. Anesth Analg. 2005;101:622–8 table of contents.
2. Hug CC Jr, McLeskey CH, Nahrwold ML, Roizen MF, Stanley TH, Thisted RA, et al. Hemodynamic effects of propofol: data from over 25,000 patients. Anesth Analg. 1993;77:S21–9.
3. Coates DP, Monk CR, Prys-Roberts C, Turtle M. Hemodynamic effects of infusions of the emulsion formulation of propofol during nitrous oxide anesthesia in humans. Anesth Analg. 1987;66:64–70.
4. Grounds RM, Twigley AJ, Carli F, Whitwam JG, Morgan M. The haemodynamic effects of intravenous induction. Comparison of the effects of thiopentone and propofol. Anaesthesia. 1985;40:735–40.
5. Aggarwal S, Goyal VK, Chaturvedi SK, Mathur V, Baj B, Kumar A. A comparative study between propofol and etomidate in patients under general anesthesia. Braz J Anesthesiol. 2016;66:237–41.
6. Group PS, Devereaux PJ, Yang H, Yusuf S, Guyatt G, Leslie K, et al. Effects of extended-release metoprolol succinate in patients undergoing non-cardiac surgery (POISE trial): a randomised controlled trial. Lancet. 2008;371:1839–47.
7. Bijker JB, Persoon S, Peelen LM, Moons KG, Kalkman CJ, Kappelle LJ, et al. Intraoperative hypotension and perioperative ischemic stroke after general surgery: a nested case-control study. Anesthesiology. 2012;116:658–64.
8. Walsh M, Devereaux PJ, Garg AX, Kurz A, Turan A, Rodseth RN, et al. Relationship between intraoperative mean arterial pressure and clinical outcomes after noncardiac surgery: toward an empirical definition of hypotension. Anesthesiology. 2013;119:507–15.
9. Bijker JB, van Klei WA, Vergouwe Y, Eleveld DJ, van Wolfswinkel L, Moons KG, et al. Intraoperative hypotension and 1-year mortality after noncardiac surgery. Anesthesiology. 2009;111:1217–26.
10. Monk TG, Bronsert MR, Henderson WG, Mangione MP, Sum-Ping ST, Bentt DR, et al. Association between intraoperative hypotension and hypertension and 30-day postoperative mortality in noncardiac surgery. Anesthesiology. 2015;123:307–19.
11. Forbes AM, Dally FG. Acute hypertension during induction of anaesthesia and endotracheal intubation in normotensive man. Br J Anaesth. 1970;42:618–24.
12. Prys-Roberts C, Greene LT, Meloche R, Foex P. Studies of anaesthesia in relation to hypertension. II. Haemodynamic consequences of induction and endotracheal intubation. Br J Anaesth. 1971;43:531–47.
13. Russell WJ, Morris RG, Frewin DB, Drew SE. Changes in plasma catecholamine concentrations during endotracheal intubation. Br J Anaesth. 1981;53:837–9.
14. Thomson IR. The haemodynamic response to intubation: a perspective. Can J Anaesth. 1989;36:367–9.
15. Rajbhandari PK. Lignocaine and Esmolol on stress response to laryngoscopy and intubation. JNMA J Nepal Med Assoc. 2014;52:775–9.
16. Edwards ND, Alford AM, Dobson PM, Peacock JE, Reilly CS. Myocardial ischaemia during tracheal intubation and extubation. Br J Anaesth. 1994;73:537–9.
17. Fox EJ, Sklar GS, Hill CH, Villanueva R, King BD. Complications related to the pressor response to endotracheal intubation. Anesthesiology. 1977;47:524–5.

18. Haku E, Hayashi M, Kato H. Anesthetic management of abdominal aortic surgery: a retrospective review of perioperative complications. J Cardiothorac Anesth. 1989;3:587–91.
19. Phillips AT, Deiner S, Mo Lin H, Andreopoulos E, Silverstein J, Levin MA. Propofol use in the elderly population: prevalence of overdose and association with 30-day mortality. Clin Ther. 2015;37:2676–85.
20. Steib A, Freys G, Beller JP, Curzola U, Otteni JC. Propofol in elderly high risk patients. A comparison of haemodynamic effects with thiopentone during induction of anaesthesia. Anaesthesia. 1988;43:Suppl:111–4.
21. Dundee JW, Robinson FP, McCollum JS, Patterson CC. Sensitivity to propofol in the elderly. Anaesthesia. 1986;41:482–5.
22. Bijker JB, van Klei WA, Kappen TH, van Wolfswinkel L, Moons KG, Kalkman CJ. Incidence of intraoperative hypotension as a function of the chosen definition: literature definitions applied to a retrospective cohort using automated data collection. Anesthesiology. 2007;107:213–20.
23. Goldman L, Caldera DL, Southwick FS, Nussbaum SR, Murray B, O'Malley TA, et al. Cardiac risk factors and complications in non-cardiac surgery. Medicine (Baltimore). 1978;57:357–70.
24. Kerlinger FN, Pedhazur EJ. Multiple regression in behavioral research. New York: Holt, Rinehart & Winston; 1973.
25. Kutner MH, Nachtsheim CJ, Neter J, Li W. Applied Linear Statistical Models 5th Edition. New York: McGraw-Hill/Irwin; 2004
26. Nair BG, Horibe M, Newman SF, Wu WY, Peterson GN, Schwid HA. Anesthesia information management system-based near real-time decision support to manage intraoperative hypotension and hypertension. Anesth Analg. 2014;118:206–14.
27. Rau RH, Li YC, Cheng JK, Chen CC, Ko YP, Huang CJ. Predicting blood pressure change caused by rapid injection of propofol during anesthesia induction with a logistic regression model. Acta Anaesthesiol Taiwanica. 2004;42:81–6.
28. Leslie K, Crankshaw DP. Lean tissue mass is a useful predictor of induction dose requirements for propofol. Anaesth Intensive Care. 1991;19:57–60.
29. Choi JJ, Kim JY, Lee D, Chang YJ, Cho NR, Kwak HJ. Male patients require higher optimal effect-site concentrations of propofol during i-gel insertion with dexmedetomidine 0.5 mug/kg. BMC Anesthesiol. 2016;16:20.
30. Dahlgren N, Messeter K. Treatment of stress response to laryngoscopy and intubation with fentanyl. Anaesthesia. 1981;36:1022–6.
31. Billard V, Moulla F, Bourgain JL, Megnigbeto A, Stanski DR. Hemodynamic response to induction and intubation. Propofol/fentanyl interaction. Anesthesiology. 1994;81:1384–93.
32. Li S, Yu F, Zhu H, Yang Y, Yang L, Lian J. The median effective concentration (EC50) of propofol with different doses of fentanyl during colonoscopy in elderly patients. BMC Anesthesiol. 2016;16:24.
33. Helfman SM, Gold MI, DeLisser EA, Herrington CA. Which drug prevents tachycardia and hypertension associated with tracheal intubation: lidocaine, fentanyl, or esmolol? Anesth Analg. 1991;72:482–6.
34. Kazama T, Ikeda K, Morita K, Kikura M, Ikeda T, Kurita T, et al. Investigation of effective anesthesia induction doses using a wide range of infusion rates with undiluted and diluted propofol. Anesthesiology. 2000;92:1017–28.
35. Adachi YU, Watanabe K, Higuchi H, Satoh T. The determinants of propofol induction of anesthesia dose. Anesth Analg. 2001;92:656–61.
36. Gurses E, Sungurtekin H, Tomatir E, Dogan H. Assessing propofol induction of anesthesia dose using bispectral index analysis. Anesth Analg. 2004;98:128–31 table of contents.

26

Nomogram for the prediction of postoperative hypoxemia in patients with acute aortic dissection

Huiqing Ge[1], Ye Jiang[1], Qijun Jin[1], Linjun Wan[1], Ximing Qian[2] and Zhongheng Zhang[3*]

Abstract

Background: Postoperative hypoxemia is quite common in patients with acute aortic dissection (AAD) and is associated with poor clinical outcomes. However, there is no method to predict this potentially life-threatening complication. The study aimed to develop a regression model in patients with AAD to predict postoperative hypoxemia, and to validate it in an independent dataset.

Methods: All patients diagnosed with AAD from December 2012 to December 2017 were retrospectively screened for potential eligibility. Preoperative and intraoperative variables were included for analysis. Logistic regression model was fit by using purposeful selection procedure. The original dataset was split into training and validating datasets by 4:1 ratio. Discrimination and calibration of the model was assessed in the validating dataset. A nomogram was drawn for clinical utility.

Results: A total of 211 patients, involving 168 in non-hypoxemia and 43 in hypoxemia group, were included during the study period (incidence: 20.4%). Duration of mechanical ventilation (MV) was significantly longer in the hypoxemia than non-hypoxemia group (41(10.5140) vs. 12(3.75,70.25) hours; $p = 0.002$). There was no difference in the hospital mortality rate between the two groups. The purposeful selection procedure identified 8 variables including hematocrit (odds ratio [OR]: 0.89, 95% confidence interval [CI]: 0.80 to 0.98, $p = 0.011$), PaO_2/FiO_2 ratio (OR: 0.99, 95% CI: 0.99 to 1.00, $p = 0.011$), white blood cell count (OR: 1.21, 95% CI: 1.06 to 1.40, $p = 0.008$), body mass index (OR: 1.32, 95% CI: 1.15 to 1.54; $p = 0.000$), Stanford type (OR: 0.22, 95% CI: 0.06 to 0.66; $p = 0.011$), pH (OR: 0.0002, 95% CI: $2*10^{-8}$ to 0.74; $p = 0.048$), cardiopulmonary bypass time (OR: 0.99, 95% CI: 0.98 to 1.00; $p = 0.031$) and age (OR: 1.03, 95% CI: 0.99 to 1.08; $p = 0.128$) to be included in the model. In an independent dataset, the area under curve (AUC) of the prediction model was 0.869 (95% CI: 0.802 to 0.936). The calibration was good by visual inspection.

Conclusions: The study developed a model for the prediction of postoperative hypoxemia in patients undergoing operation for AAD. The model showed good discrimination and calibration in an independent dataset that was not used for model training.

Keywords: Acute aortic dissection, Hypoxemia, Nomogram, Intensive care unit, Length of stay

* Correspondence: zh_zhang1984@zju.edu.cn
[3]Department of Emergency Medicine, Sir Run Run Shaw Hospital, Zhejiang University School of Medicine, No 3, East Qingchun Road, Hangzhou 310016, Zhejiang Province, China
Full list of author information is available at the end of the article

Background

Acute aortic dissection (AAD) represents a life-threatening condition that can be encountered in emergency and critical care setting [1]. Many factors can influence the clinical outcomes of these patients such as the comorbidities, complications, organ dysfunction and site of dissection. Surgical operation is usually needed to avert catastrophic complications of aortic dissection [2]. Postoperative hypoxemia has long been noted in substantial proportion of patients with AAD and has been found to be associated with poor clinical outcomes such as prolonged mechanical ventilation, increased length of stay (LOS) in the intensive care unit (ICU) and hospital [3–5]. Also, several studies have attempted to identify preoperative risk factor of hypoxemia [4, 5]. However, there is no report on training a model for early prediction of postoperative hypoxemia. Since early prediction of post-operative hypoxemia makes early intervention possible, it is of clinical utility to train and validate such a prediction model. The study aimed to develop a model for early prediction of postoperative hypoxemia. Discrimination and calibration of the model were validated in an independent dataset that was not used for model training. A nomogram was depicted for clinical use.

Methods

Study design and settings

The study was retrospective in design. All patients diagnosed as AAD from December 2012 to December 2017 were screened for potential eligibility. The patients were identified from the electronic healthcare record (EHR) of our hospital. Patients with initial suspected diagnosis of AAD as denoted by ICD9 code of 443.21 were identified. Exclusion criteria included one of the following items: 1) patients did not undergo surgery; 2) patients who were pregnant, or had neuromuscular disease, 3) confirmed complications such as heart failure, massive bleeding, pneumothorax, tracheal hemorrhage, atelectasis and pneumonia; and 3) patients had missing values on more than 50% variables. Data were extracted from EHR and deidentified before analysis. The study was approved by the ethics committee of Sir Run Run Shaw hospital (20180611–7). Informed consent was waived due to retrospective nature of the study.

Variables included for analysis

Demographic variables including age, gender, body weight, height, body mass index (BMI) were obtained for the hospital admission with surgical repair of the aorta artery. Past histories of smoking, hypertension and diabetes mellitus were also included. The admission type included emergency and non-emergency admissions.

Preoperative laboratory tests were obtained within 24 h before surgery, which included albumin, hematocrit (HCT), pH, lactate, PaCO2, PaO2/FiO2 ratio (P/F), serum creatinine (Scr), total bilirubin, white blood cell count (WBC), C-reactive protein (CRP), troponin, creatine kinase (CK), creatine kinase isoenzymes (CKMB), lactate dehydrogenase (LDH), aspartate aminotransferase (AST). If there were two or more measures of these variables before operation, the one nearest to the operation was employed.

Intraoperative variables included aortic clamping time, cardiopulmonary bypass (CPB) time, duration of the operation, fluid input and output during operation, and the minimum body temperature.

Clinical outcomes were LOS in ICU and hospital, duration of postoperative mechanical ventilation, and hospital mortality.

Postoperative hypoxemia was defined as P/F < 200 for the first 2 days after operation.

Statistical analysis

Continuous variables were expressed as mean and standard deviation for normally distributed data, and as median and interquartile range (IQR) for non-normal data. Categorical variables were expressed as number and percentage. Comparisons between hypoxemia and non-hypoxemia groups were performed using student t test or rank sum test as appropriate. Chi-square or Fisher's exact test was employed for categorical variables [6, 7].

Postoperative hypoxemia was employed as response variable assuming a binomial distribution, and covariates were included in the model if their p values were less than 0.05 in univariate analysis [8]. Other variables such as age, CPB time and pH were entered due to clinical expertise. Variables with $p > 0.2$ in the multivariable model were excluded. The initial dataset was randomly split into the training and validating dataset by 4:1 ratio (there were 36 cases of hypoxemia in the training set). The training set was used to develop the model, and the validating set was used to validate the model. Model discrimination was represented by the area under receiver operating characteristic curves (AUC), with an AUC greater than 0.8 indicating a good discrimination [9]. Model calibration was visually assessed by plotting fitted logistic calibration curve and a smooth nonparametric fit using lowess and grouped proportions vs. mean predicted probability in group [10]. Other statistics were also reported with the R package *Regression Modeling Strategies* (*rms*), such as Somers'D_{xy}, rank correlation between predicted probability and observed probability, Nagelkerke-Cox-Snell-Maddala-Magee R-squared index, the 0.9 quantile of same (E90), the Spiegelhalter Z-test for calibration accuracy, and its two-tailed *P*-value [11, 12].

A nomogram was drawn based on the fitted logistic regression model and each patient could be mapped onto the nomogram for the prediction of the occurrence of postoperative hypoxemia [13]. We drew the nomogram that converts each effect in the model to a 0 to 100 scale which is just proportional to the log odds. These points are added across predictors to derive the "Total Points," which are converted to linear predictor and then to predicted probabilities [12]. The distribution of covariates in the model, and of the total regression score, are superimposed on the nomogram scales. Also, the values of a sample patient were superimposed. Binomial distribution with logit link function was employed for the model fit.

All statistical analyses were performed using R (version 3.4.3). Two-tailed p value less than 0.05 was considered as statistical significance.

Results

Patient inclusion

A total of 287 patients with initial suspicion of AAD were initially identified from HER, and 49 were excluded because they did not undergo surgery during hospital stay, were ruled out for AAD, had neuromuscular disease. Furthermore, we excluded 27 patients with preoperative complications such as heart failure, massive bleeding, pneumothorax, atelectasis and pneumonia. As a result, a total of 211 patients were finally included for analysis (Fig. 1).

Baseline characteristics

There were 168 patients in the non-hypoxemia group and 43 in the hypoxemia group, with an incidence rate of 20.4%. Patients in the hypoxemia group appears to be elder than non-hypoxemia group, but the statistical significance was not reached (Table 1). Patients with hypoxemia showed significantly greater BMI than those in non-hypoxemia group (26.82 ± 3.84 vs. 24.94 ± 3.86 kg/m2, $p = 0.006$). All patients (100%) with hypoxemia were admitted from emergency setting, versus 86% for the non-hypoxemia group ($p = 0.005$).

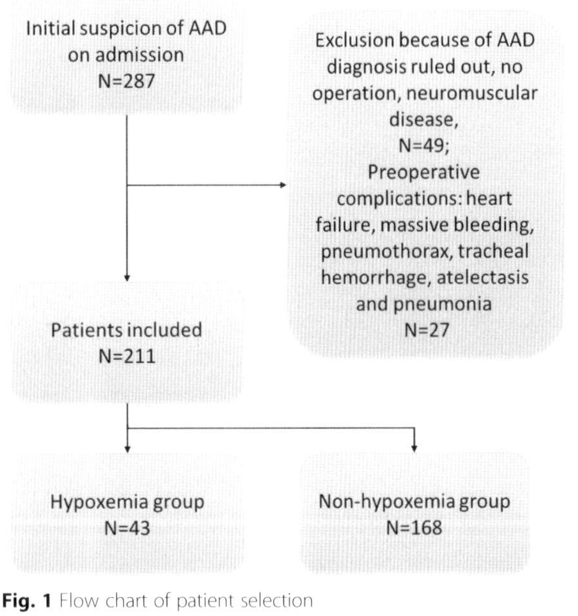

Fig. 1 Flow chart of patient selection

Preoperative laboratory test

For preoperative laboratory tests, hypoxemia patients showed significantly lower P/F ratio than non-hypoxemia patients (median, interquartile range [IQR]: 174(148.5237) vs. 249(183.75,367.25); $p < 0.001$). Other laboratory tests such as serum creatinine (103(77.5145) vs. 76.5(61,104) mmol/l; $p < 0.001$), total bilirubin (16.7(11.9,25) vs. 13.2(9.57,18.9) mmol/l; $p = 0.016$), WBC (12.9(9.3,15.5) vs. 8.9(6.8,11.65) ^10^9/l; $p < 0.001$), CRP (58.9(10.6118.3) vs. 23.4(4.57,60.38) mg/l; $p = 0.003$) and CK (109(62,228) vs. 72(48.75,136.25) U/l; $p = 0.023$) were significantly higher in the hypoxemia group than that in the non-hypoxemia group.

Intraoperative variables were not significantly different between hypoxemia and non-hypoxemia groups.

Clinical outcomes

The LOS in ICU (10(5.5,14) vs. 7(4,11) days; $p = 0.079$) and hospital (18(12.5,24) vs. 19(13,25) days; $p = 0.775$) were not significantly different between the two groups. Duration of MV was significantly longer in the hypoxemia than non-hypoxemia group (41(10.5140) vs. 12(3.75,70.25) hours; $p = 0.002$). There was no difference in the hospital mortality rate between the two groups (Table 1).

Model training

Logistic regression model was fit with the training set. The purposeful selection procedure included 8 variables as determined by clinical importance and statistical significance (Table 2). The preoperative HCT (odds ratio [OR]: 0.89, 95% confidence interval [CI]: 0.80 to 0.98, $p = 0.011$), P/F ratio (OR: 0.99, 95% CI: 0.99 to 1.00, $p = 0.011$), WBC (OR: 1.21, 95% CI: 1.06 to 1.40, $p = 0.008$), BMI (OR: 1.32, 95% CI: 1.15 to 1.54; $p < 0.001$), Stanford type (OR: 0.22, 95% CI: 0.06 to 0.66; $p = 0.011$), pH (OR: 0.0002, 95% CI: $2*10^{-8}$ to 0.74; $p = 0.048$), and CPB time (OR: 0.99, 95% CI: 0.98 to 1.00; $p = 0.031$) were significantly contributing to the prediction accuracy of the model. Age was not significantly associated with the outcome, but it remained in the model by clinical judgement.

Table 1 Comparison between hypoxemia and non-hypoxemia groups

	Total (*n* = 211)	Non-hypoxemia (*n* = 168)	Hypoxemia (*n* = 43)	p
Demographics				
Age, median (IQR) (years)	50 (43,63)	50 (42,64)	52 (46.5,59)	0.654
Male, n (%)	151 (0.72)	116 (0.69)	35 (0.81)	0.158
Height, median (IQR) (cm)	170 (163,174)	170 (162.75,174)	169 (165,174)	0.647
Weight, median (IQR) (kg)	70 (62,80)	70 (60,80)	80 (65,89.5)	0.005
BMI, mean ± SD (kg/m2)	25.32 ± 3.92	24.94 ± 3.86	26.82 ± 3.84	0.006
Smoking history, n (%)	59 (28)	47 (28)	12 (28)	0.998
Hypertension, n (%)	134 (64)	102 (61)	32 (74)	0.137
Diabetes, n (%)	13 (6)	11 (7)	2 (5)	0.998
Stanford A, n (%)	133 (63)	97 (0.58)	36 (84)	0.003
Emergency admission, n (%)	188 (89)	145 (86)	43 (1)	0.005
Laboratory tests before operation				
Albumin, mean ± SD (mg/l)	36.6 ± 4.65	36.75 ± 4.76	36 + 4.22	0.316
Hematocrit, mean ± SD (%)	36.09 ± 5.71	36.26 ± 5.4	35.41 ± 6.82	0.452
pH, median (IQR)	7.37 (7.34,7.4)	7.37 (7.34,7.4)	7.37 (7.32,7.38)	0.205
Lactate, median (IQR) (mmol/l)	2.1 (1.5,2.9)	2.05 (1.48,2.8)	2.30 (1.9,3.1)	0.082
PaCO2, median (IQR) (mmHg)	41 (37.55,45.55)	41 (37.88,45.23)	40.9 (36.5,47.7)	0.916
P/F ratio, median (IQR)	235 (176,355)	249 (183.75,367.25)	174 (148.5237)	< 0.001
Scr, median (IQR) (mmol/l)	81 (64,113)	76.5 (61,104)	103 (77.5145)	< 0.001
Total bilirubin, median (IQR) (mmol/l)	13.7 (10,22.25)	13.2 (9.57,18.9)	16.7 (11.9,25)	0.016
WBC, median (IQR) (^109/l)	9.5 (7.4,12.6)	8.9 (6.8,11.65)	12.9 (9.3,15.5)	< 0.001
CRP, median (IQR) (mg/l)	28.3 (5.75,68.75)	23.4 (4.57,60.38)	58.9 (10.6118.3)	0.003
Troponin, median (IQR) (ng/ml)	0.01 (0.01,0.01)	0.01 (0.01,0.01)	0.01 (0.01,0.12)	0.028
CK, median (IQR) (U/l)	78 (51,150.5)	72 (48.75,136.25)	109 (62,228)	0.023
CKMB, median (IQR) (U/l)	10 (8,16)	10 (8,16)	10 (6.5,14.5)	0.249
LDH, median (IQR) (U/l)	218 (171,283)	208.5 (165,274.25)	253 (196.5312.5)	0.013
AST, median (IQR) (U/l)	22 (16.5,34.5)	21 (15,31.25)	31 (18.5,44.5)	0.007
Intraoperative variables				
Aortic clamping time, mean ± SD (min)	127.91 + 40.82	128.84 ± 40.7	124.26 ± 41.59	0.519
CBP time, median (IQR) (min)	178 (140,211)	180 (146.75,210)	169 (132.5221)	0.749
Duration of operation, median (IQR) min	295 (120,390)	285 (90,390)	300 (242.5420)	0.072
Minimum temperature, median (IQR) (°C)	36.2 (35.6,36.55)	36.2 (35.4,36.6)	36.3 (36,36.5)	0.250
Input, median (IQR) (ml)	6250 (5150,7587.5)	6090 (5150,7332.5)	6380 (4775,8170)	0.651
Output, median (IQR) (ml)	4850 (3600,5800)	4900 (3575,6000)	4500 (3675,5600)	0.358
Clinical outcomes				
LOS in ICU, median (IQR) (days)	7 (4,12)	7 (4,11)	10 (5.5,14)	0.079
LOS in hospital, median (IQR) (days)	19 (13,24.5)	19 (13,25)	18 (12.5,24)	0.775
Duration of MV, median (IQR) (hours)	15 (5,82)	12 (3.75,70.25)	41 (10.5140)	0.002
Mortality, n (%)	7 (3)	6 (4)	1 (2)	0.997

Note: continuous variables were expressed as mean and standard deviation for normal data, and as median and interquartile range for non-normal data. Categorical variables were expressed as number and percentage. Comparisons between hypoxemia and non-hypoxemia groups were performed using student t test or rank sum test as appropriate. Chi-square or Fisher's exact test was employed for categorical variables

Abbreviations: *No.* number, *Prop.* proportion, *ICU* intensive care unit, *LOS* length of stay, *WBC* white blood cell count, *CRP* c-reactive protein, *Scr* serum creatinine, *BMI* body mass index, *CK* creatine kinase, *CKMB* creatine kinase isoenzymes, *LDH* lactate dehydrogenase, *AST* aspartate aminotransferase, *MV* mechanical ventilation, *CPB* cardiopulmonary bypass, *IQR* interquartile range, *SD* standard deviation

Table 2 Logistic regression model for the prediction of postoperative hypoxemia

Variables	Odds ratio	Lower limit of 95% CI	Upper limit of 95% CI	*P* value
BMI	1.32	1.15	1.54	< 0.001
PF	0.99	0.99	1.00	0.011
Stanford (A as reference)	0.22	0.06	0.66	0.011
WBC	1.21	1.06	1.40	0.008
Age	1.03	0.99	1.08	0.128
HCT	0.89	0.80	0.98	0.016
CBP time	0.99	0.98	1.00	0.031
pH	0.0002	$2*10^{-8}$	0.74	0.048

Note: The logistic regression model was selected by using stepwise forward selection procedure, AIC was used to decide the inclusion of a variable. The odds ratio was reported for each one unit increase for each variable

Abbreviations: *CI* confidence interval, *WBC* white blood cell count, *PF* PaO2/FiO2, *BMI* body mass index, *CBP* cardiopulmonary bypass, *HCT* hematocrit

Model validation in a separate dataset

In the validation dataset, the fitted model showed a good discrimination in distinguishing hypoxemia from non-hypoxemia patients (area under curve [AUC] = 0.869, 95% CI: 0.802 to 0.936). Model calibration was shown in Fig. 2. The non-parametric curve fits well to the ideal line, indicating the observed probability was in line with the predicted probability. However, the model may not predict well for patients with lower risk of postoperative hypoxemia. Also, the Fig. 3 shows that the predicted probability of hypoxemia is in agreement with the observed proportion.

Nomogram for predicting postoperative hypoxemia

Nomogram for the prediction of postoperative hypoxemia is shown in Fig. 4. The distribution of each variable was shown above each line. A representative patient was shown to illustrate how to use the nomogram. Given values of the 8 predictors, the patient can be mapped to the nomogram. Note there is a red dot in each line, representing the value of each of the 8 predictors for the patient. Regression coefficient of each predictor was scaled to points within the range of 0 to 100, and the relative importance (weight) of each predictor can be reflected by its

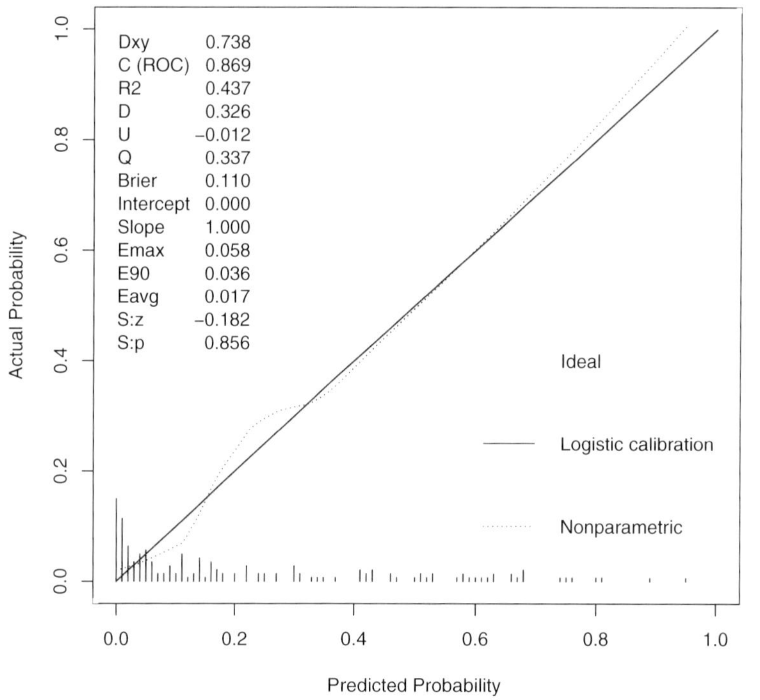

Fig. 2 Model calibration and discrimination. The predicted probability by the logistic regression model conforms well to the observed probability well. In the plot, the idea line is consistent with the Logistic calibration line. The discrimination was measured by AUC of 0.869 (95% CI: 0.802 to 0.936)

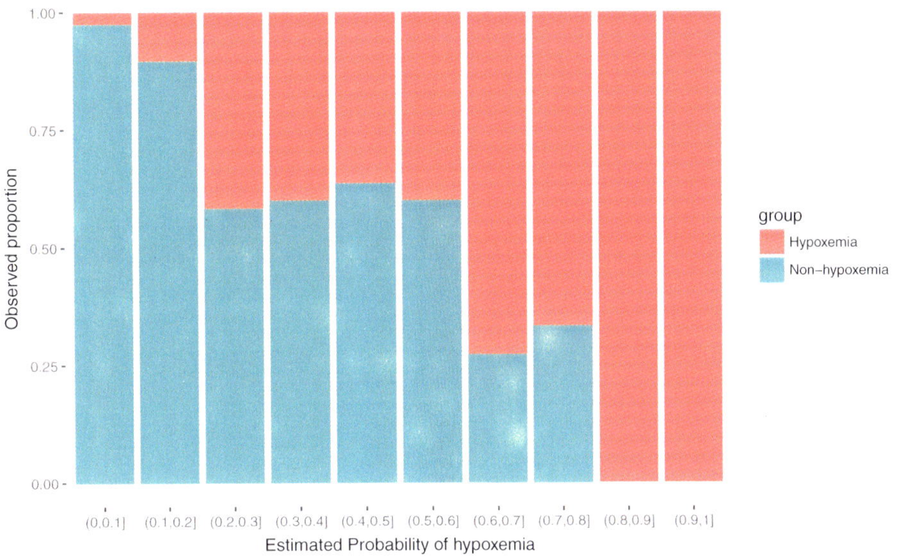

Fig. 3 Bar chart showing the agreement between predicted probability of hypoxemia and observed proportion

points. Points was translated into probability by logit transformation.

Discussion

The study included patients with AAD who had undergone operation for the repair of the dissection. Risk factors for postoperative hypoxemia were identified via purposeful selection procedure. These factors included age, lactate, preoperative P/F ratio, WBC, BMI and CRP. Internal validation was performed for the model, which showed good discrimination and calibration. A nomogram was established for clinical utility.

The incidence of hypoxemia was lower than those reported in the literature (20% vs. 30%) [4, 14]. Different definitions of postoperative hypoxemia may explain its different incidences. For example, Wang's study defined hypoxemia as P/F ratio less than 200 at 24 h after operation and they reported an incidence of 49.5% [5]. Several studies have been conducted to explore risk factors for postoperative hypoxemia. Consistent with our study, the study by Liu and colleagues also showed the preoperative P/F ratio and WBC were independently associated with postoperative hypoxemia [4]. It is not surprising that preoperative P/F ratio is independently associated with postoperative hypoxemia. Furthermore, WBC is a biomarker reflecting systemic inflammatory response, and higher responses may contribute to the respiratory dysfunction. There is empirical evidence that inflammatory response is associated with hypoxemia in patients with aortic dissection [15]. Furthermore, we also found CRP was associated with hypoxemia. CRP is a well-known biomarker of inflammatory response, which is more specific and sensitive than WBC [16, 17]. However, the effect of CRP disappeared after adjusting for covariates. Liu's study also included time from symptom onset and deep hypothermic circulatory arrest time in their regression model. None of the intraoperative variables were associated with hypoxemia in univariate analysis, but the CPB time was associated with hypoxemia in multivariable regression model. BMI was identified as an independent predictor of postoperative hypoxemia in the study, consistent with the study by Sheng and colleagues [14]. Actually, the association of obesity and hypoxemia is not limited to aortic surgery [18]. In a large cohort of noncardiac surgery, Kendale SM and colleagues found that the odds of experiencing hypoxemia increased significantly with increasing categories of BMI [19]. Similar results were documented in other studies [20, 21]. BMI is an important determinant of respiratory function and studies show morbidly obese patients have a typical restrictive pattern with a reduction of forced vital capacity (FVC), forced residual capacity (FRC) and total lung capacity (TLC) with a decreased expiratory reserve volume (ERV) [22–24]. Sex has been found to be related to postoperative hypoxemia in AAD (women were more likely to have hypoxemia than man), which was not replicated in our study. Most probably, the associated was confounded by other factors and the authors failed to adjust for these potential confounding factors [25].

An interesting finding in our study was that serum lactate was associated with postoperative hypoxemia in patients with AAD. Hyperlactatemia is an indicator of tissue ischemia [26]. In cardiac surgery patients, there is evidence that hyperlactatemia is associated with a

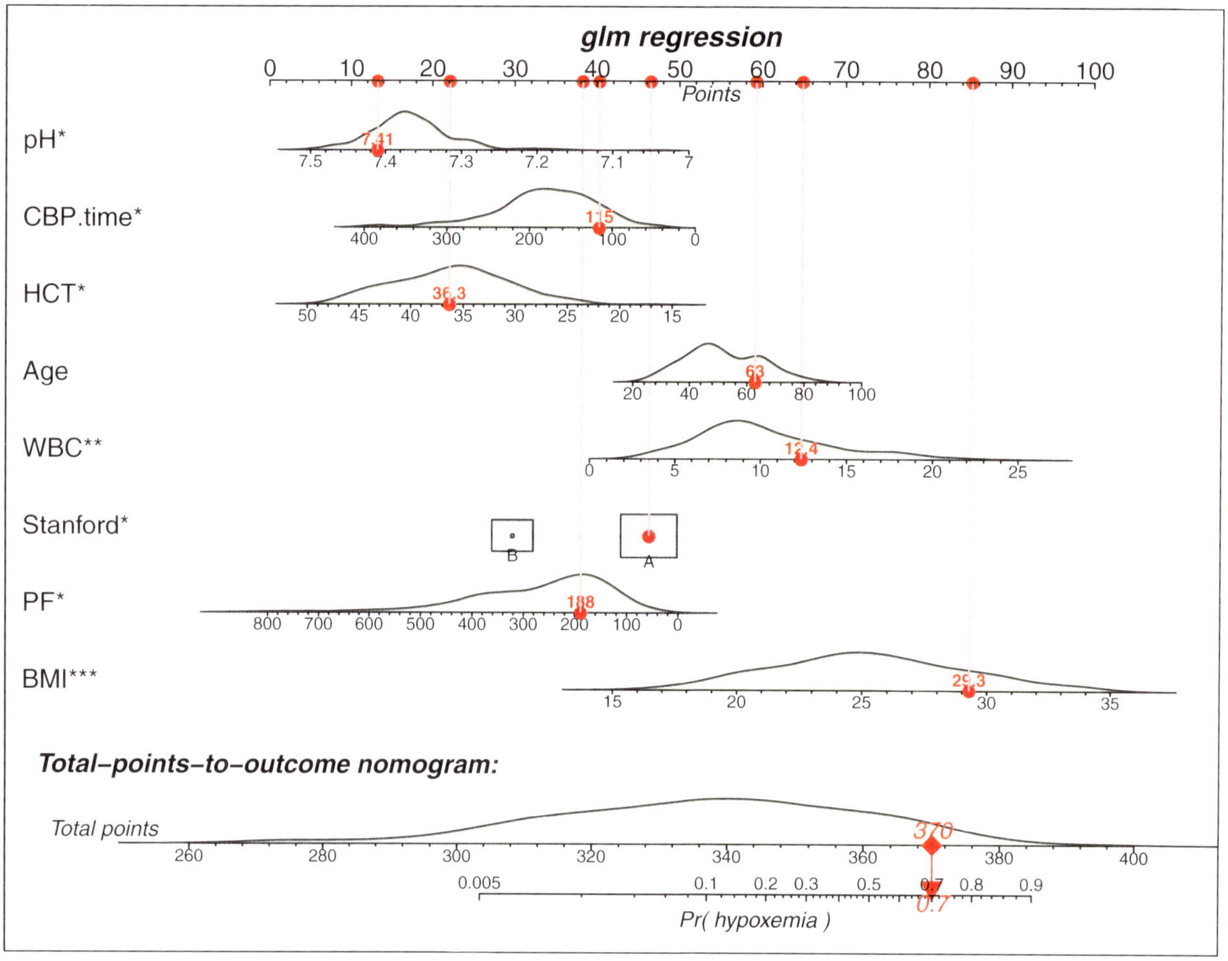

Fig. 4 Nomogram for the prediction of postoperative hypoxemia. The logistic regression model were described as a series of straight lines with a common linear scale in the nomogram, with the scale factors of the individual lines given by the coefficients (beta) of the covariates in the model.The distribution of each variable is superimposed on each scale. A representative patient was shown to illustrate how to use the nomogram. Given values of the eight predictors, the patient can be mapped onto the nomogram. Note there is a red dot at each scale, representing the value of each of the 8 predictors for the patient. The total point of the patient was 370, corresponding to a probability of 0.7 for developing postoperative hypoxemia

compromised respiratory function and prolonged mechanical ventilation. Also, hyperlactatemia can explain organ dysfunction in our study [27–29]. However, the effect of lactate disappeared in multivariable model, indicating that the effect could be explained by preoperative P/F ratio, as lactate was a biomarker of hypoxemia. Similarly, preoperative P/F ratio can explain the elevations of biomarkers of acute organ injury such as Scr, bilirubin and ALT. That was why the significant associations in univariate analysis disappeared in the multivariable regression model.

The potential utility of our prediction model is that interventions such as anti-inflammatory agents can be given to patients with high risk of postoperative hypoxemia. Furthermore, the model can be employed to design clinical trials to identify high risk patients who will benefit the most from treatment [30].

There were some limitations in the present study that must be acknowledged. First, the study was retrospective single center study. Although the prediction model was validated in a separate dataset that was not used for model training, its external validity was still unknown. In different cardiac centers, the healthcare process can be quite different and the predictive accuracy of a newly developed model needs to be tested [31, 32]. This is also our future work to perform a multicenter study to examine the external validity of the model. Second, postoperative hypoxemia reported in the study was defined by P/F ratio less than 200 for consecutive 2 days. While this definition was simple to perform, it suffers from case-mix. Some patients may have intensive respiratory support, and their P/F ratio is not comparable to those with spontaneous breathing. Thus, the definition of postoperative hypoxemia needs to be further explored.

However, in order to make our results comparable to that in the literature [4], we opt to use this simple definition. Third, the retrospective design of the study suffers from its inherent limitation of selection bias. Some patients were excluded because they did not perform operation in our hospital. They might go to other hospital for further evaluation. Thus, the included patients may not well represent the whole target population of AAD, but they represent those who are willing to undergo operation in our hospital. Finally, the sample size of the study was small that only 43 patients had the event of interest. As a rule of thumb, 10–20 events per variable should be used [33]. However, the primary purpose of this rule is to prevent overfitting [34]. We addressed the problem of overfitting by validating the model in a dataset that was not used for model training (e.g. an overfitting model performs poorly in the validation dataset). The results showed that the developed model can predict accurately in the validation dataset with an AUC of 0.869. Further studies by employing multicenter data are mandatory to endure generalizability of the model.

Conclusion

In conclusion, the study developed a model for the prediction of postoperative hypoxemia in patients undergoing operation for AAD. Eight variables of age, BMI, WBC, HCT, CPB time, pH, Stanford type and P/F ratio were included in the model. The model showed good discrimination and calibration in an independent dataset that was not used for model training.

Abbreviations

AST: Aspartate aminotransferase; BMI: Body mass index; CK: Creatine kinase; CKMB: Creatine kinase isoenzymes; CPB: Cardiopulmonary bypass; CRP: C-reactive protein; ICU: Intensive care unit; LDH: Lactate dehydrogenase; LOS: Length of stay; MV: Mechanical ventilation; Scr: Serum creatinine; WBC: White blood cell count

Acknowledgements

Not Applicable

Funding

Z.Z. received funding from The public welfare research project of Zhejiang province (LGF18H150005) and Scientific research project of Zhejiang Education Commission (Y201737841);

The funding body had no role in the design of the study and collection, analysis, and interpretation of data and in writing the manuscript.

Authors' contributions

HG and ZZ conceived of the study; YJ and QJ carried out data entry. LW participated in the data check and interpretation. XQ performed surgical operation and interpreted the results. ZZ performed statistical analysis and drafted the manuscript. All authors read and approved the final manuscript.

Competing interests

The authors declare that they have no competing interests.

Author details

[1]Department of Respiratory Care, Sir Run Run Shaw Hospital, Zhejiang University School of Medicine, Hangzhou, China. [2]Department of Cardiovascular Surgery, Sir Run Run Shaw Hospital, Zhejiang University School of Medicine, Hangzhou, China. [3]Department of Emergency Medicine, Sir Run Run Shaw Hospital, Zhejiang University School of Medicine, No 3, East Qingchun Road, Hangzhou 310016, Zhejiang Province, China.

References

1. McClure RS, Brogly SB, Lajkosz K, Payne D, Hall SF, Johnson AP. Epidemiology and management of thoracic aortic dissections and thoracic aortic aneurysms in Ontario, Canada: a population-based study. J Thorac Cardiovasc Surg. 2018; 155:2254–64.
2. Nienaber CA, Clough RE. Management of acute aortic dissection. Lancet. 2015;385:800–11.
3. Nakajima T, Kawazoe K, Izumoto H, Kataoka T, Niinuma H, Shirahashi N. Risk factors for hypoxemia after surgery for acute type a aortic dissection. Surg Today Springer-Verlag. 2006;36:680–5.
4. Liu N, Zhang W, Ma W, Shang W, Zheng J, Sun L. Risk factors for hypoxemia following surgical repair of acute type a aortic dissection. Interact Cardiovasc Thorac Surg. 2017;24:251–6.
5. Wang Y, Xue S, Zhu H. Risk factors for postoperative hypoxemia in patients undergoing Stanford a aortic dissection surgery. J Cardiothorac Surg BioMed Central. 2013;8:118.
6. Zhang Z, Gayle AA, Wang J, Zhang H, Cardinal-Fernández P. Comparing baseline characteristics between groups: an introduction to the CBCgrps package. Ann Transl Med. 2017;5:484.
7. Zhang Z. Univariate description and bivariate statistical inference: the first step delving into data. Ann Transl Med. 2016;4:91.
8. Zhang Z. Model building strategy for logistic regression: purposeful selection. Ann Transl Med. 2016;4:111.
9. Zhang Z. Residuals and regression diagnostics: focusing on logistic regression. Ann Transl Med. 2016;4:195.
10. Zhang Z, Zhang H, Khanal MK. Development of scoring system for risk stratification in clinical medicine: a step-by-step tutorial. Ann Transl Med. 2017;5:436.
11. Harrell FE. rms: Regression Modeling Strategies. 5 ed. 2018. https://cran.r-project.org/web/packages/rms/index.html.
12. Harrell FE. Regression Modeling Strategies. New York: Springer New York; 2001
13. Zhang Z, Kattan MWK. Drawing nomograms with R: applications to categorical outcome and survival data. Ann Transl Med. 2017;5:190–5.
14. Sheng W, Yang H-Q, Chi Y-F, Niu Z-Z, Lin M-S, Long S. Independent risk factors for hypoxemia after surgery for acute aortic dissection. Saudi Med J. 2015;36:940–6.
15. Duan X-Z, Xu Z-Y, Lu F-L, Han L, Tang Y-F, Tang H, et al. Inflammation is related to preoperative hypoxemia in patients with acute Stanford type a aortic dissection. J Thorac Dis. 2018;10:1628–34.
16. Castelli GP, Pognani C, Cita M, Stuani A, Sgarbi L, Paladini R. Procalcitonin, C-reactive protein, white blood cells and SOFA score in ICU: diagnosis and monitoring of sepsis. Minerva Anestesiol. 2006;72:69–80.
17. Zhang Z, Pan L, Deng H, Ni H, Xu X. Prediction of delirium in critically ill patients with elevated C-reactive protein. J Crit Care. 2014;29:88–92.
18. Kaw RK. Spectrum of postoperative complications in pulmonary hypertension and obesity hypoventilation syndrome. Curr Opin Anaesthesiol. 2017;30:140–5.
19. Kendale SM, Blitz JD. Increasing body mass index and the incidence of intraoperative hypoxemia. J Clin Anesth. 2016;33:97–104.
20. Aizawa K, Sakano Y, Ohki S, Saito T, Konishi H, Misawa Y. Obesity is a risk factor of young onset of acute aortic dissection and postoperative hypoxemia. Kyobu Geka. 2013;66:437–44.

21. Ranucci M, Ballotta A, La Rovere MT, Castelvecchio S, Surgical and Clinical outcome research (SCORE) group. Postoperative hypoxia and length of intensive care unit stay after cardiac surgery: the underweight paradox? PLoS One. 2014;9:e93992.
22. Zhou LN, Wang Q, Gu CJ, Li N, Zhou JP, Sun XW, et al. Sex differences in the effects of obesity on lung volume. Am J Med Sci. 2017;353:224–9.
23. Carey IM, Cook DG, Strachan DP. The effects of adiposity and weight change on forced expiratory volume decline in a longitudinal study of adults. Int J Obes Relat Metab Disord. 1999;23:979–85.
24. Salome CM, King GG, Berend N. Physiology of obesity and effects on lung function. J Appl Physiol. 2010;108:206–11.
25. Maitusong B, Sun H-P, Xielifu D, Mahemuti M, Ma X, Liu F, et al. Sex-related differences between patients with symptomatic acute aortic dissection. Medicine (Baltimore). 2016;95:e3100.
26. O'Connor E, Fraser JF. The interpretation of perioperative lactate abnormalities in patients undergoing cardiac surgery. Anaesth Intensive Care. 2012;40:598–603.
27. Zhang Z, Xu X. Lactate clearance is a useful biomarker for the prediction of all-cause mortality in critically ill patients: a systematic review and meta-analysis*. Crit Care Med. 2014;42:2118–25.
28. Zhang Z, Ni H. Normalized lactate load is associated with development of acute kidney injury in patients who underwent cardiopulmonary bypass surgery. PLoS One. 2015;10:e0120466.
29. Lee SM, Kim SE, Kim EB, Jeong HJ, Son YK, An WS. Lactate Clearance and Vasopressor seem to be predictors for mortality in severe Sepsis patients with lactic acidosis supplementing sodium bicarbonate: a retrospective analysis. PLoS One. 2015;10:e0145181.
30. Jin M, Cheng Y, Yang Y, Pan X, Lu J, Cheng W. Protection of xenon against postoperative oxygen impairment in adults undergoing Stanford type-a acute aortic dissection surgery: study protocol for a prospective, randomized controlled clinical trial. Medicine (Baltimore). 2017;96:e7857.
31. Riley RD, Ensor J, Snell KIE, Debray TPA, Altman DG, Moons KGM, et al. External validation of clinical prediction models using big datasets from e-health records or IPD meta-analysis: opportunities and challenges. BMJ. 2016;353:i3140.
32. Bos LD, Schouten LR, Cremer OL, DSY O, Schultz MJ, MARS consortium. External validation of the APPS, a new and simple outcome prediction score in patients with the acute respiratory distress syndrome. Ann Intensive Care. 2016;6:89.
33. Ogundimu EO, Altman DG, Collins GS. Adequate sample size for developing prediction models is not simply related to events per variable. J Clin Epidemiol. 2016;76:175–82.
34. Pavlou M, Ambler G, Seaman SR, Guttmann O, Elliott P, King M, et al. How to develop a more accurate risk prediction model when there are few events. BMJ. 2015;351:h3868.

A high risk of sleep apnea is associated with less postoperative cognitive dysfunction after intravenous anesthesia

Soeren Wagner[1,2*], Joerg Quente[1], Sven Staedtler[1], Katharina Koch[1,4], Tanja Richter-Schmidinger[3], Johannes Kornhuber[3], Harald Ihmsen[1] and Juergen Schuettler[1]

Abstract

Background: The obstructive sleep apnea syndrome (OSAS) is characterized by temporary cerebral hypoxia which can cause cognitive dysfunction. On the other hand, hypoxia induced neurocognitive deficits are detectable after general anesthesia.

The objective of this study was to evaluate the impact of a high risk of OSAS on the postoperative cognitive dysfunction after intravenous anesthesia.

Methods: In this single center trial between June 2012 and June 2013 43 patients aged 55 to 80 years with an estimated hospital stay of at least 3 days undergoing surgery were enrolled. Patients were screened for a high risk of OSAS using the STOP-BANG test. The cognitive function was assessed using a neuropsychological test battery, including the DemTect test for cognitive impairment and the RMBT test for memory, the day before surgery and within 36 h after extubation.

Results: Twenty-two of the 43 analyzed patients were identified as patients with a high risk of OSAS. Preoperatively, OSAS patients showed a significant worse performance only for the DemTect ($p = 0.0043$). However, when comparing pre- and postoperative test results, the OSAS patients did not show a significant loss in any test but significantly improved in RMBT test, whereas the control group showed a significant worse performance in three of eight tests. In five tests, we found a significant difference between the two groups with respect to the change from pre- to postoperative cognitive function.

Conclusion: Patients with a high risk of OSAS showed a less impairment of memory function and work memory performance after intravenous anesthesia. This might be explained by a beneficial effect of intrinsic hypoxic preconditioning in these patients.

Keywords: Cognitive dysfunction, Sleep apnea, Intravenous anesthesia, Preconditioning

* Correspondence: so.wagner@klinikum-stuttgart.de
[1]Department of Anesthesiology, University Hospital Erlangen, Friedrich-Alexander-University Erlangen-Nuremberg, Erlangen, Germany
[2]Department of Anesthesiology, Katharinenhospital Klinikum Stuttgart, Kriegsbergstrasse 60, D-70174 Stuttgart, Germany
Full list of author information is available at the end of the article

Background

The Obstructive Sleep Apnea Syndrome (OSAS) is the most common type of sleep apnea disorder. It is caused by an obstruction of the upper airway and causes dramatic arterial oxygen desaturation during sleep. The disease is characterized by repetitive episodes of hypopnea or apnea with intermittent arousals and considerable disruption of normal sleep architecture [1]. Epidemiological findings suggest that merely 2% of middle-aged (30–60 years of age) women and 4% of middle-aged (30–60 years of age) men are affected, however almost 75% of OSAS patients still remain undiagnosed [2]. OSAS patients are seriously affected by daytime sleepiness, fatigue and neuropsychological impairment compromising several areas of cognitive function including attention, vigilance, memory and executive function. Harmful hypoxemic intervals are also frequently observed in the immediate phase after general anesthesia procedures. The incidence of hypoxic episodes in the post anesthesia unit has been reported to be between 7.6% [3] and 13.5% [4]. These repeated episodes of desaturation often occur unrecognized and prolonged [5]. On the other hand, there is clinical evidence that exposure to intermittent hypoxia has beneficial effects such as increasing ischemia resistance and preserving cardiovascular and brain function, also described as ischemic preconditioning [6].

Ischemic preconditioning potentially affects postoperative function via numerous pathways, including the regulation of neurotrophin expression, strengthening the neurovascular network decreasing inflammation and apoptosis [7]. However, most studies were based on rodents and the translation to humans remains to be evaluated. On the other hand, the expression of brain derived neurotrophic factor (BDNF) is correlated positively with cognitive function in older adults [8]. Furthermore, intermittent hypoxia stimulates the expression of BDNF in the adult hippocampus [9] and enhances the process of learning [10]. Hence, intermittent hypoxia might result in an improvement in cognitive function. One may therefore hypothesize that the hypoxemic intervals associated with OSAS may have a beneficial effect on the postoperative cognitive function in terms of an ischemic preconditioning. We investigated this question in a pilot study in patients with a high risk of OSAS and in control patients undergoing non-cardiac surgery with total intravenous anesthesia.

Methods

In this prospective single-center study, two groups (OSAS group and a control group) were compared. The study was performed at the University Hospital of Erlangen, Germany between June 2012 and June 2013 in accordance with the guidelines for Good Clinical Practice and the Declaration of Helsinki. The study was approved by the local Ethics committee (Ethikkommission der Medizinischen Fakultät der Friedrich-Alexander-Universität Erlangen-Nürnberg, Erlangen, Germany) on 19.04.2012 (reference number: 87_12 B).

Patients

After written informed consent, 51 adult patients of both genders with an estimated hospital stay of at least 3 days undergoing surgery were enrolled in this study. Inclusion criteria were an age between 55 and 80 years and an American Society of Anesthesiologists physical status classification of I to III. Patients with a history of brain or head injury, cerebral ischemia, diseases of central nervous system, psychological disorder, alcohol or illegal drug abuse, neuroenhancing or neurocompromising medication, manifest diagnosis of pre-existing cognitive impairment or severe cardiovascular disorder were excluded from the study. Patients were assessed by a detailed screening examination and clinical interview. None of the included patients had been treated for OSAS. Cognitive function was assessed using a neuropsychological test battery on the day before surgery as a baseline measurement. The postoperative testing was performed after surgery on the first or second postoperative day.

Assessment of the risk for OSAS

The severity and classification of OSAS is most commonly characterized by measuring the apnea/hypopnea index (AHI) resulting from respiratory disturbances while the sleeping patient is monitored in a sleep laboratory. Oxygen desaturation far below the physiological range is the key clinical parameter to assume an apnea episode during sleep. In the present study, however, we used the STOP-BANG test to identify patients with a high risk for OSAS. The STOP-BANG test is a brief, well-known and international accepted questionnaire for sleep disorders [1]. This validated test detects patients with an increased risk for OSAS [11, 12]. The STOP BANG questionnaire asks for the incidence of snoring, fatigue and observed stop of breathing, and considers also data on blood pressure, body mass index, age, neck size and gender. Patients meeting the study criteria were asked to participate in the study. The assessors were blinded to the screened and enrolled patients. Patients were screened during premedication visit of the anesthesiology staff. Eligible patients were enrolled after written informed consent to the study. After consent, the patients were screened via the STOP Bang Test. If the resulting composite score (range 0 to 8) was 3 or higher, the patient was assigned to the OSAS group, otherwise the patient was assigned to the control group. The study was performed by two assessors to ensure a testing phase within the study schedule. There were no significant differences between both assessors regarding the results validity detected.

Clinical protocol

Preoperatively, we registered all medications, which had been prescribed and assured that no neuroenhancing or neurocompromising medication had been started recently or was given routinely. Benzodiazepines for premedication were strictly avoided in all patients, and instead 75 or 150 µg clonidine was given orally if needed. Total intravenous anesthesia with propofol and remifentanil was performed in all patients. Prior to intubation, patients received 0.1 mg fentanyl. Propofol and remifentanil were administrated as target controlled infusion (TCI). Rocuronium was given as neuromuscular blocking drug. Intraoperatively hemodynamic stability was adjusted in order to avoid hypotension and hypertension phases or fluctuations of blood pressure while surgery.

Hemoglobin oxygen saturation was monitored in all patients by pulse oximetry. Prior to in- and extubation, all patients received 100% oxygen for several minutes and were transferred quickly to the recovery room. If necessary, additional oxygen was supplied in the recovery room and patients were weaned of oxygen support prior discharge.

During the postoperative phase, control patients were monitored in the recovery room for at least two hours. Patients in the OSAS group were monitored overnight according to our hospital's clinical security guidelines. Pain was evaluated by the 11-point numerical rating scale (NRS, 0 = no pain, 10 = maximum pain). If the patient's pain score was greater than 4, an infusion with 7.5 or 15 mg piritramide was administrated over 20 min according to total body weight.

Assessment of cognitive function

Cognitive function was assessed using a neuropsychological test battery comprising six different cognitive test as a baseline measurement on the day before surgery. The postoperative testing was performed after surgery on the first or second postoperative day. All perioperative tests were carried out in a quiet and separate room during daytime and it was attempted to perform pre- and postoperative tests at matching times of the day. All tests required approximately 60 min per testing phase and patient. To avoid learning effects, tests were presented in two different versions if necessary. The following tests were performed:

DemTect

The DemTect is a highly sensitive psychometric screening test to identify patients with mild cognitive impairment and patients with dementia in the early stages of the disease [13]. The test consists of five tasks, which survey the functions "verbal memory", "verbal fluency", "cognitive flexibility" and "attention". The transformed total score with a range from 0 to 18 points is independent of age and education. DemTect helps in deciding whether cognitive performance is adequate for age (13–18 pts.) or whether mild cognitive impairment (9–12 pts.) respectively dementia (0–8 pts.) is likely.

Rivermead Behavioural memory test (RBMT)

The Rivermead Behavioural Memory test is a highly sensitive test of global memory impairment examining immediate and delayed recall [14]. It is designed to predict daily memory difficulties in people with an acquired and non-progressive brain injury in order to monitor their capability in the course of time. Regarding four parallel forms, learning effects can be avoided during the testing phases. We selected the subtest "story" for our study in which a nearly 55 word story is read out to the subject who has to recall the content immediately and after a 25 min interval. This subtest is known as a suitable evaluation of verbal memory function, logical memory and episodic memory. Maximum score is 84 points and a higher test value means a better performance.

Zahlen-Verbindungs-test (ZVT)

The ZVT measures general intelligence performance and analyzes non-verbal cognitive performance speed independent of education but influenced by genetics [15]. The corresponding ability is quantified as "liquid intelligence" or "perceptual or processing speed". The test represents a diagnostic tool that is used clinically in organic brain disease. Tested subjects have to connect 90 ascending numbers, arranged randomly on four different sheets of paper with a pen. The time needed is recorded, averaged and age-adjusted for interpretation. Thus, a higher test value means a worse performance.

Trail-making-test (TMT)

The Trail Making Test A/B attempts to test neurocognitive performance combined with psychomotor ability by using a setting in which the patient has to connect up scaling numbers in the correct order [16]. In the B version the test requires an additional task by switching between alternating numbers and letters. The time needed is recorded, and consequently longer total times reveal greater impairment. In our study we used TMT B, which provides information about visual search speed, scanning, speed of processing and mental flexibility, which are good parameters for executive function.

Digit span test

The Digit Span Test used in our study is a subtest of the Wechsler Memory Scale [17]. It consists of random number sequences presented orally to the patient. The single digits have to be repeated in the same order. If repeated correctly, a single digit will be added to the sequence. The examination is repeated twice forwards and twice backwards. Each examination uses six numerical series. Test scoring is based on the total digits recalled correctly. Each correct answer leads to one point. Maximum score is 24 and higher scores indicate better cognitive performance. The Digit Span Test investigates the patient's short term memory capacity (digit span forward) and verbal working memory (digit span backward).

Short cognitive performance test for assessing deficits of memory and attention (SKT)

The SKT assesses memory and attention deficits within a clinical setting [18]. It consists of nine subtests, which retrieve immediate and delayed verbal memory and attention, measured as the speed of information processing. Test samples are available in five parallel forms to avoid learning effects. Raw scores from each subtest are converted into norm values and a total score, which are age adjusted. Due to its subtest structure, memory and attention can be assessed separately. The scores range from 0 to 9 points for memory, and from 0 to 18 points for attention, respectively. Hence, the total score ranges from 0 to 27 points. Notable is that higher scores indicate more severe cognitive impairment, which is given gradually for each test result and related to the status of impairment.

Color-word-interference-test (FWIT)

The FWIT [19] is assembled from the three following parts: reading written color-words, naming the ink-color of a printed line and naming the ink-color of a written color-word instead of reading the word itself, which names a different color. In each part, processing time and the number of errors are recorded. Thus, a higher test value means a worse performance. The test measures nomination, alertness, and selectivity or rather interference. Recorded data allow the interpretation of executive function. The advantage of this test is that it is not subject to learning-effects upon repetition.

Statistical analysis

Outliers were identified using the Grubbs test. In this test, the value Xmax which shows the largest deviation from the population mean is identified as outlier and removed from the data set if the test statistic Z = abs (mean-Xmax)/SD is larger than a critical value which depends on the sample size. In our case with 21 and 22 patients in the two groups, the critical values for $p <$ 0.05 were 2.73 and 2.76, respectively. The procedure is iterated until no outliers are further detected. Categorical data were tested for differences between the two groups using the chi-square test. Continuous data were tested for deviations from the normal distribution using the Shapiro-Wilk test. The primary outcome parameter was the change of the cognitive function assessed by the difference between postoperative and preoperative test scores within a subject. The change from baseline values to post-anesthesia values within a group was tested for statistical significance using the paired t-test or the Wilcoxon test, respectively. The change of the cognitive function was further tested for significant differences between the two groups using the unpaired t-test or the Mann-Whitney test, respectively. In order to account for a different distribution of males and females within the two groups, we also analyzed the change of the cognitive function by ANOVA with the factors "gender" and "group". The level of significance was defined as $p < 0.01$.

The sample size was estimated based on published results for the DemTect [13]. A standard deviation of approximately 3 points was reported for the score. We assumed a difference of at least 4 points between the two groups as clinically relevant. Therefore, we needed at least 19 subjects per group to detect such a difference with an α-error of 0.01 and a power of 0.9. As we expected a 25% dropout rate for the postoperative testing we aimed a study size of at least 25 patients per group.

Categorical data are reported as numbers, continuous data are reported as median and range if not stated else. Statistical analysis was performed using Statistica software (Statistica Version 6, Tulsa/USA).

Results

Demographics and clinical data

We recruited a total of 51 patients, out of which seven patients did not complete the second test phase. Reasons for study dropouts were pain, discomfort and inconveniences leading to time shifts in the second phase test protocol. From the remaining patients, one patient was identified as outlier. Demographic and related clinical data of finally 43 patients used for analysis are given in Table 1. The twenty-two patients assigned to the OSAS group had a median score of 5 (3–7) points in the STOP BANG test and therefore a high risk for OSAS, compared with the patients in the control group with a median score of 2 (1–2) points. OSAS patients and control patients did not differ in age, but the percentage of males was significantly higher in the OSAS group. However, this distribution reflects the epidemiology of sleep apnea, which is far more frequent in males. Correspondingly, the patients in the OSAS group had a significantly higher weight and height. As expected, we also found a significant difference in BMI, since obesity is an important risk factor for sleep apnea and both parameters are used in the STOP BANG questionnaire.

The main type of surgery was otorhinolaryngologic surgery. There were no significant differences regarding dosage and anesthesia procedure between the OSAS and the control group. There were also no differences in oximetry parameters in both groups, although it's notable

Table 1 Patients'data

	Control ($n = 21$)	OSAS ($n = 22$)	P value
Demographics			
Age (yrs.)	64 (57–72)	66 (60–76)	0.50
Gender (female/male)	13/8	4/18	0.004
Body weight (kg)	74 (61–100)	90 (74–112)	0.0002
Height (cm)	168 (155–183)	177 (159–188)	0.006
Body mass index (kg m^{-2})	27 (22–35)	29 (23–38)	0.037
ASA classification (I/II/III)	2/16/3	0/16/6	0.23
STOP-BANG score	2 (1–2)	5 (3–7)	
Comorbidities			
History of smoking	6	10	0.48
Diabetes mellitus	1	4	0.16
Surgery			
Otorhinolaryngologic surgery	13	12	
Other type of Surgery	8	10	
Operation data			
Duration of operation (min)	70 (25–186)	76 (17–195)	0.61
Duration of anaesthesia (min)	113 (39–330)	140 (42–236)	0.38
SpO_2 before procedure (%)	97 (92–100)	96 (92–100)	0.059
SpO_2 at extubation (%)	99 (91–100)	100 (81–100)	0.97
SpO_2 at arrival intermediate care (%)	96 (88–100)	93 (88–98)	0.080
SpO_2 lowest level (%)	91 (70–98)	92 (72–99)	0.72
Propofol dose (mg kg^{-1} h^{-1})	6.18 (5.45–11.7)	5.84 (0.84–7.03)	0.11
Remifentanil dose (μg kg^{-1} min^{-1})	0.16 (0.11–0.33)	0.17 (0.09–0.23)	0.64

Data are reported as number or as median (range). SpO_2 is the oxygen saturation measured by pulse oximetry. P value is the significance level of the difference between the two groups

that we found a slightly more pronounced desaturation in the OSAS subjects after transfer to the recovery room, when the mean oxygen saturation was 96% in the control group and 93% in the OSAS group, respectively.

Neuropsychological testing

Cognitive function was assessed using a combination of neuropsychological tests on the day before surgery as a baseline measurement. The same test battery was repeated on the first or second postoperative day. Thirty five patients out of 43 patients were tested on the first postoperative day and only eight (three control and five OSAS patients) on the second postoperative day. The pre- and postoperative test results are summarized in Table 2. Preoperatively, significant differences between the two groups were found only for the DemTect, where the patients in the OSAS group showed a significant worse performance compared to the control group ($p = 0.0043$). When comparing pre- and postoperative values within the control group, there was a significant decrease in three of the tests (DemTect, RMBT, and SKT). In contrast, the patients in the OSAS group did not show a significant loss in any of the tests but even a significantly improved performance in the RMBT test. The differences between the two groups were more obvious when not the absolute values but the difference of the post- and the preoperative values were compared (Table 3). In five of the eight tests (DemTect, RMBT, Digit span forward and backward, and SKT), we found a significant difference between the two groups with respect to the change from pre- to postoperative cognitive function. This statistical significance was confirmed by the ANOVA which revealed high significance for the factor "group" but no significance for the factor "gender" and the interaction between the two factors.

Discussion

It was the aim of this study to evaluate the impact of a high risk of OSAS on the postoperative cognitive dysfunction after intravenous anesthesia. Patients susceptible for a high risk of OSAS were identified using the STOP BANG questionnaire, which is recommended for screening patients with moderate to severe risk for OSAS [20–22]. Recently, Kim and co-workers published

Table 2 Results of the pre- and postoperative neurocognitive testing

Test	Control group			OSAS group		
	Pre	Post	P value	Pre	post	P value
DemTect (points)	18 (13–18)	14 (8–18)	< 0.0005	16 (12–18)	15 (12–18)	0.81
RBMT (points)	39 (14–58)	25 (6–47)	0.0024	35 (16–51)	37 (15–58)	0.0041
ZVT (mm:ss)	02:00 (01:13–03:32)	01:47 (00:55–2:51)	0.019	01:47 (01:06–2:59)	01:43 (01:03–2:49)	0.0055
TMT (mm:ss)	01:59 (00:47–03:49)	02:14 (00:53–3:20)	0.11	01:43 (00:42–04:30)	01:32 (00:34–3:34)	0.22
Digit Span Forwards (points)	9 (6–12)	7 (4–12)	0.010	8 (5–11)	9 (4–12)	0.033
Digit Span Backwards (points)	7 (3–10)	5 (3–10)	0.011	6 (4–11)	8 (3–11)	0.050
SKT (points)	1 (0–7)	5 (1–9)	< 0.0005	3 (0–8)	3 (1–7)	0.24
FWIT (mm:ss)	00:56 (00:40–01:19)	00:58 (00:43–1:16)	0.31	00:57 (00:45–01:15)	00:55 (00:48–1:24)	0.09

Data are reported as median (range). The *p* value is the significance level of the difference between pre- and postoperative values within a group

a very high sensitivity of 97% for the STOP BANG questionnaire [23]. However, its specificity was low (19%). More important for our purpose was the finding that the positive predictive value was quite high with 86%. Thus, this test seems to be able to detect patients with an at least moderate risk for OSAS. Moreover, several other recently published validation studies revealed fairly good positive predictive values to identify patients with sleep breathing disorder [24–26]. Furthermore, in a systematic review prepared as a part of the Society of Anaesthesia and Sleep Medicine (SASM) publication for the Preoperative Assessment of Patients with Sleep Disordered-Breathing, Opperer and co-workers analyzed how the diagnosis OSA was elucidated. Based on the SASM consensus group criteria for OSAS, 17 publications referred to the diagnosis via polysomnographic results and 15 published articles on screening questionnaires [27]. Chung and co-workers reported that a STOP-Bang score of 5–8 identified patients with a high probability of moderate or severe OSAS in a surgical population [22]. Therefore, we assumed that the patients in our OSAS group were highly suspected of having intermittent hypoxemic episodes.

To account for possible interindividual variation with respect to education levels, we focused on the change in test results prior to and after surgery between OSAS and control patients. In most tests performed, we found significant differences in the change of memory function between OSAS patients and control group patients. OSAS patients in general showed a significantly less decrease or even an increase of the performance compared to the control group.

In this study six separate cognitive test were used to detect different aspects of cognitive impairment as described above. While some tests address a single cognitive function, like the Digit Span test in terms of memory or the RMBT in terms of several aspects of memory, other tests address multiple aspects of cognitive function. Gagnon and colleagues summarized that OSAS patients elicited in all cognitive functions an impaired ability compared to controls [28]. Focusing on the attention aspect, the DemTect and SKT in our study elicited a decrease in attention performance. Moreover, executive function was tested with both tests, DemTect and SKT. Executive function is a complex system of skills including behavioral inhibition, mental flexibility, and working memory. We found impairments in executive function in the preoperative testing phase in OSAS patients compared to controls as described by others [28]. Focusing on executive function, which was tested

Table 3 Change of cognitive functions, expressed as the difference between post- and preoperative values

Test	Control	OSAS	P_{MWU}	P_{ANOVA}
DemTect (points)	−4 (−8–0)	0 (− 4–6)	< 0.0001	< 0.0001, 0.56
RBMT (points)	−15 (− 25–25)	5 (−9–16)	< 0.0001	< 0.0001, 0.91
ZVT (min)	− 0.17 (− 1.55–0.29)	−0.16 (− 0.63–0.29)	1.00	0.26, 0.32
TMT (min)	0.19 (−1.44–0.79)	- 0.11 (− 1.67–1.16)	0.049	0.37, 0.35
Digit Span Forwards (points)	−1 (− 6–2)	1 (− 2–3)	0.0013	0.0010, 0.74
Digit Span Backwards (points)	−1 (− 4–3)	2 (−3–5)	0.0025	0.0019, 0.91
SKT (points)	3 (−3–6)	1 (− 6–5)	0.0022	0.026, 0.31
FWIT (min)	0.03 (−0.18–0.26)	−0.02 (− 0.23–0.33)	0.055	0.28, 0.59

Data are reported as median (range). P_{MWU} is the significance level of the difference between the two groups obtained by the Mann-Whitney test. P_{ANOVA} are the significance levels of the factors "group" and "gender" obtained by analysis of variance separately by the FWIT, the OSAS group presented diminished results in our study preoperatively. Working memory was tested separately by the Digit Span test, which likewise showed impaired results in the OSAS group preoperatively. Psychomotor speed was analyzed via TMT und ZVT which revealed decreased results in OSAS patients. Memory function was evaluated using the RMBT, in which the OSAS subjects elicited decreased results in comparison to controls. These results of the present study are in accordance with previously reported findings [28].

Postoperatively, the DemTect revealed a decrease in verbal memory performance in control patients but not in OSAS patients. Using the RBMT, verbal function was also found to be impaired significantly in control patients, whereas it even improved significantly in the OSAS group. Working memory and memory capacity as assessed by the Digit Span Test were also characterized by an impairment in controls but an improvement in OSAS patients. A similar aspect of memory function is the quality of attention capability, as rated by the SKT test. Again, the test performance of the OSAS group improved after surgery, whereas the performance of the control patients clearly deteriorated. On the other hand, the Color Word Interference Test, which investigates the ability of nomination, alertness and selectivity or interference respectively executive function, did not reveal significant differences between both groups. Moreover, the ZVT did not detect any differences between both groups representing liquid intelligence or processing speed. Finally, using the TMT, which aimed at detecting processing speed as well as rating executive function, we found only minor differences between both groups' test performance.

It is well believed that OSAS patients have impaired cognitive function [29]. There is, however, controversy regarding the grade of impairment. As there is a wide variety in neurocognitive test systems it is difficult to compare the results [30]. The patients in our OSAS group showed indeed a worse preoperative performance in the Demtect test. However, these patients stayed at this level whereas the patients in the control group showed a significantly reduced test performance postoperatively than reported in the literature [31]. Regarding memory function ability, we used the Rivermead Behavioural Memory Test to focus on logical and episodic memory function. In the literature, memory function has been assessed differently and different aspects of memory function are emphasized. While some reviews found impairments in short-term memory function [32], others reported deficits in verbal and visual delayed long-term memory in OSAS patients [33]. On the other side, no effect was found analyzing the severity of OSAS and its influence on memory function [34]. We found that individuals with a high risk of OSAS performed significantly better in a combination of logical and episodic test settings than control subjects. We concentrated on verbal memory using the subtest "story" in its immediate and delayed version. While we found an increase in verbal memory performance between both test intervals, others described a decrease regarding verbal episodic memory tasks [35].

The observation that the OSAS patients in our study generally showed a less postoperative decrease or even an increase of the cognitive function might be explained by the phenomenon of hypoxic preconditioning. It is well known that OSAS patients show nocturnal oxygen desaturation [2]. Affected patients present significant consequences including excessive daytime sleepiness. Experimental studies in healthy adults with sleep deprivation lead to the assumption that sleepiness negatively influences neurocognitive performance [36, 37]. Others reported that sleep deprivation tolerance in young adults might compensate alteration of cognitive capabilities [38]. Further investigations demonstrated the existence of an ample cognitive reserve and cerebral recruitment enabling individuals to maintain cognitive performance and to resist sleep deprivation induced impairment [39, 40]. Functional imaging studies confirmed this protective mechanism in OSAS patients [41]. This observation might explain the finding that patients affected by mild or moderate OSAS can present a normal cognitive function [42]. On the other hand, the severity of hypoxemia altered processing and motor speed performance [42]. It is well known that severe unrecognized and unanticipated desaturation phases may occur following general anesthesia [5]. In both study groups we detected oxygen desaturation after the surgical intervention (Table 1). While our postoperative observations mostly revealed a single hypoxic stimulus following anesthesia randomly, OSAS patients are exposed to multiple hypoxic stimuli per night. Given the assumption that OSAS patients might have adapted to those numerous desaturation events, a single, fortuitous ischemic strike might not negatively affect the neurocognitive performance in these patients. Beneficial effects of prior episodes of ischemia on brain function were found in patients with transient ischemic attack [43]. Hoth and co-workers reported that subjects with a more pronounced hypoxemia performed better in learning and memory tasks compared to those with less severe levels of hypoxemia [44]. These findings led to the assumption that ischemic preconditioning might have protective effects on brain function. Consequently, remote preconditioning approaches have been proposed [45, 46]. However, a recently published study failed to prove beneficial effects of remote ischemic preconditioning on postoperative neurocognitive dysfunction in patients who underwent cardiac surgery [47]. On the other hand, lately published data suggest that remote ischemic preconditioning prevent a short-term postoperative cognitive function decline after cardiac surgery [48]. Moreover, He and co-workers published recently that remote ischemic preconditioning improved cognitive function in elderly patients [49]. Already in 2013, Schega and colleagues assumed that additional intermittent hypoxic training and physical exercise enhance cognitive function and quality of life in elderly [50]. Recently in a review published by Li and co-workers, it was summarized that ischemic preconditioning techniques could prevent organ damage and play a neuroprotective role [51]. Therefore, we assume that endogenous hypoxic training might be a favorable cerebral preconditioning factor in OSAS patients and leads to clinical relevance in future.

However, there are some study limitations that should be paid attention to. We merely screened the risk for an OSAS which leads to apnea phases while sleep. Patients have not been diagnosed for OSAS using a sleep laboratory tests or polysomnographic studies. However, the STOP BANG test is an international well established screening tool to quantify the risk for having the OSAS. Although patients were comparable regarding surgical procedures, surgery duration time and severity, they were different in weight and body mass index due to the risk factors for OSAS. The patients of the two groups were of similar age, but the gender distributions were different with a significant higher proportion of males in the OSAS group. However, a two-way ANOVA with gender and group as factors revealed that the observed differences in the change of the cognitive function could be attributed to the factor group whereas the gender did not show a significant effect. Moreover, the study focused on non-cardiac surgery patients only. As O'Brien and colleges summarized that intraoperative hypotension is an intrinsic risk factor of postoperative cognitive dysfunction [52], intraoperatively hemodynamic stability was considered conscientiously in this study. We did not observe hypotension, defined as systolic blood pressure values below 80 mmHg [3]. However, brief hypotension phases between the measurement intervals might remain undetected and even small periods of hypotension are clearly associated with worse cognitive function in the postoperative phase. Furthermore it is notable that the heterogeneous results reported in literature could be explained by the various severity of OSAS and the wide range in subjects' intellectual function and education. Lastly, this study included only total intravenous anesthesia to avoid an additional confounding factor. However, volatile anesthesia should also be tested and analyzed as cognitive impairment is possible in both general anesthesia regimens.

Conclusions

In conclusion, this is the first prospective study that elicited indications for beneficial effects of possible intrinsic hypoxic preconditioning in patients suspected of being at high risk for OSAS on the early postoperative cognitive function. Focusing on memory function and work memory performance after anesthesia for non-cardiac surgery, we discovered significant differences between patients suspect to sleep apnea and control patients. In a clinical setting, the DemTect or SKT can be recommended to assess cognitive impairment in a fast and valid manner. Cognitive reserve and learning ability might play a role in compensating deficits in executive function. Further investigations are needed to address the impact of the anesthesia regimen.

Abbreviations

AHI: Apnoea/Hypopnea Index; ASA: American Society of Anesthesiologists physical status classification; BDNF: Brain Derived Neurotrophic Factor; FWIT: Color-Word-Interference-Test; NRS: Numerical Rating Scale; OSAS: Obstructive Sleep Apnea Syndrome; RBMT: Rivermead Behavioural Memory Test; SASM: Society of Anaesthesia and Sleep Medicine; SKT: Short Cognitive Performance Test; STOP-BANG: Snoring, Tired, Observed, Pressure, Body mass index, Age, Neck size, Gender; TCI: Target Controlled Infusion; TMT: Trail-Making-Test; ZVT: Zahlen-Verbindungs-Test

Authors' contributions

SW helped to design and to conduct the study, to analyze the data and write the manuscript. JQ conducted the study and helped to analyze the data. KK conducted the study and helped to analyze the data and write the manuscript. SS, JK, JS helped to conduct the study. TRS helped to design the study. HI helped to analyze the data and write the manuscript. All authors read and approved the final manuscript.

Competing interests

The authors declare that they have no competing interests.

Author details

[1]Department of Anesthesiology, University Hospital Erlangen, Friedrich-Alexander-University Erlangen-Nuremberg, Erlangen, Germany. [2]Department of Anesthesiology, Katharinenhospital Klinikum Stuttgart, Kriegsbergstrasse 60, D-70174 Stuttgart, Germany. [3]Department of Psychiatry and Psychotherapy, University Hospital Erlangen, Friedrich-Alexander-University, Erlangen, Germany. [4]Department of Anaesthesiology, Klinikum Oldenburg AöR, University Hospital Oldenburg, Oldenburg, Germany.

References

1. American Academy of Sleep Medicine Task Force. Sleep-related breathing disorders in adults: recommendations for syndrome definition and measurement techniques in clinical research. Sleep 1999; 22:667-89.
2. Young T, Palta M, Dempsey J, Skatrud J, Weber S, Badr S. The occurrence of sleep-disordered breathing among middle-aged adults. N Engl J Med. 1993;328(17):1230–5.
3. Belcher AW, Leung S, Cohen B, Yang D, Mascha EJ, Turan A, et al. Incidence of complications in the post-anesthesia care unit and associated healthcare utilization in patients undergoing non-cardiac surgery requiring neuromuscular blockade 2005-2013: a single center study. J Clin Anesth. 2017;43:33–8.
4. Aust H, Kranke P, Eberhart LH, Afshari A, Weber F, Brieskorn M, et al. Impact of medical training and clinical experience on the assessment of oxygenation and hypoxaemia after general anaesthesia: an observational study. J Clin Monit Comput. 2015;29(3):415–26.
5. Froese AB. From the journal archives: be alert to the risk of unexpected prolonged postoperative hypoxemia! Can J Anaesth. 2014;61(4):379–82.
6. Manukhina EB, Downey HF, Mallet RT. Role of nitric oxide in cardiovascular adaptation to intermittent hypoxia. Exp Biol Med. 2006;231(4):343–65.

7. Wang Y, Reis C, Applegate R 2nd, Stier G, Martin R, Zhang JH. Ischemic conditioning-induced endogenous brain protection: applications pre-, per- or post-stroke. Exp Neurol. 2015;272:26–40.
8. Gunstad J, Benitez A, Smith J, Glickman E, Spitznagel MB, Alexander T, et al. Serum brain-derived neurotrophic factor is associated with cognitive function in healthy older adults. J Geriatr Psychiatry Neurol. 2008;21(3):166–70.
9. Zhu XH, Yan HC, Zhang J, Qu HD, Qiu XS, Chen L, et al. Intermittent hypoxia promotes hippocampal neurogenesis and produces antidepressant-like effects in adult rats. J Neurosci. 2010;30(38):12653–63.
10. Xie H, Leung KL, Chen L, Chan YS, Ng PC, Fok TF, et al. Brain-derived neurotrophic factor rescues and prevents chronic intermittent hypoxia-induced impairment of hippocampal long-term synaptic plasticity. Neurobiol Dis. 2010;40(1):155–62.
11. Chung F, Yegneswaran B, Liao P, Chung SA, Vairavanathan S, Islam S, et al. STOP questionnaire: a tool to screen patients for obstructive sleep apnea. Anesthesiology. 2008;108(5):812–21.
12. Vasu TS, Doghramji K, Cavallazzi R, Grewal R, Hirani A, Leiby B, et al. Obstructive sleep apnea syndrome and postoperative complications: clinical use of the STOP-BANG questionnaire. Arch Otolaryngol Head Neck Surg. 2010;136(10):1020–4.
13. Kalbe E, Kessler J, Calabrese P, Smith R, Passmore AP, Brand M, et al. DemTect: a new, sensitive cognitive screening test to support the diagnosis of mild cognitive impairment and early dementia. Int J Geriatr Psychiatry. 2004;19(2):136–43.
14. Bollo-Gasol S, Pinol-Ripoll G, Cejudo-Bolivar JC, Llorente-Vizcaino A, Peraita-Adrados H. Ecological assessment of mild cognitive impairment and Alzheimer disease using the Rivermead Behavioural memory test. Neurologia. 2014;29(6):339–45.
15. Metternich B, Schmidtke K, Hull M. How are memory complaints in functional memory disorder related to measures of affect, metamemory and cognition? J Psychosom Res. 2009;66(5):435–44.
16. Reitan RM. The relation of the trail making test to organic brain damage. J Consult Psychol. 1955;19(5):393–4.
17. Cheng Y, Wang YJ, Yan JC, Zhou R, Zhou HD. Effects of carotid artery stenting on cognitive function in patients with mild cognitive impairment and carotid stenosis. Exp Ther Med. 2013;5(4):1019–24.
18. Stemmler M, Petermann F, Daseking M, Siebert J, Schott H, Lehfeld H, et al. The assessment and course of development of cognitive abilities in the elderly. Gesundheitswesen. 2013;75(11):761–7.
19. Dittrich WH, Johansen T. Cognitive deficits of executive functions and decision-making in obsessive-compulsive disorder. Scand J Psychol. 2013;54(5):393–400.
20. Vana KD, Silva GE, Goldberg R. Predictive abilities of the STOP-bang and Epworth sleepiness scale in identifying sleep clinic patients at high risk for obstructive sleep apnea. Res Nurs Health. 2013;36(1):84–94.
21. Auckley D, Bolden N. Preoperative screening and perioperative care of the patient with sleep-disordered breathing. Curr Opin Pulm Med. 2012;18(6):588–95.
22. Chung F, Subramanyam R, Liao P, Sasaki E, Shapiro C, Sun Y. High STOP-bang score indicates a high probability of obstructive sleep apnoea. Br J Anaesth. 2012;108(5):768–75.
23. Kim B, Lee EM, Chung YS, Kim WS, Lee SA. The utility of three screening questionnaires for obstructive sleep apnea in a sleep clinic setting. Yonsei Med J. 2015;56(3):684–90.
24. Chung F, Yang Y, Brown R, Liao P. Alternative scoring models of STOP-bang questionnaire improve specificity to detect undiagnosed obstructive sleep apnea. J Clin Sleep Med. 2014;10(9):951–8.
25. Nagappa M, Liao P, Wong J, Auckley D, Ramachandran SK, Memtsoudis S, et al. Validation of the STOP-bang questionnaire as a screening tool for obstructive sleep apnea among different populations: a systematic review and meta-analysis. PLoS One. 2015;10(12):e0143697.
26. Chiu HY, Chen PY, Chuang LP, Chen NH, Tu YK, Hsieh YJ, et al. Diagnostic accuracy of the Berlin questionnaire, STOP-BANG, STOP, and Epworth sleepiness scale in detecting obstructive sleep apnea: a bivariate meta-analysis. Sleep Med Rev. 2017;36:57–70.
27. Opperer M, Cozowicz C, Bugada D, Mokhlesi B, Kaw R, Auckley D, et al. Does obstructive sleep apnea influence perioperative outcome? A qualitative systematic review for the Society of Anesthesia and Sleep Medicine Task Force on preoperative preparation of patients with sleep-disordered breathing. Anesth Analg. 2016;122(5):1321–34.
28. Gagnon K, Baril AA, Gagnon JF, Fortin M, Decary A, Lafond C, et al. Cognitive impairment in obstructive sleep apnea. Pathol Biol. 2014;62(5):233–40.
29. Boland LL, Shahar E, Iber C, Knopman DS, Kuo TF, Nieto FJ, et al. Measures of cognitive function in persons with varying degrees of sleep-disordered breathing: the sleep heart health study. J Sleep Res 2002;11(3):265–272.
30. Decary A, Rouleau I, Montplaisir J. Cognitive deficits associated with sleep apnea syndrome: a proposed neuropsychological test battery. Sleep. 2000;23(3):369–81.
31. Fulda S, Schulz H. Cognitive dysfunction in sleep disorders. Sleep Med Rev 2001;5(6):423–45.
32. Saunamaki T, Jehkonen M. A review of executive functions in obstructive sleep apnea syndrome. Acta Neurol Scand. 2007;115(1):1–11.
33. Wallace A, Bucks RS. Memory and obstructive sleep apnea: a meta-analysis. Sleep. 2013;36(2):203–20.
34. Aloia MS, Arnedt JT, Davis JD, Riggs RL, Byrd D. Neuropsychological sequelae of obstructive sleep apnea-hypopnea syndrome: a critical review. J Int Neuropsychol Soc. 2004;10(5):772–85.
35. Twigg GL, Papaioannou I, Jackson M, Ghiassi R, Shaikh Z, Jaye J, et al. Obstructive sleep apnea syndrome is associated with deficits in verbal but not visual memory. Am J Respir Crit Care Med. 2010;182(1):98–103.
36. Dinges DF, Pack F, Williams K, Gillen KA, Powell JW, Ott GE, et al. Cumulative sleepiness, mood disturbance, and psychomotor vigilance performance decrements during a week of sleep restricted to 4-5 hours per night. Sleep. 1997;20(4):267–77.
37. McCoy JG, Strecker RE. The cognitive cost of sleep lost. Neurobiol Learn Mem. 2011;96(4):564–82.
38. Mu Q, Nahas Z, Johnson KA, Yamanaka K, Mishory A, Koola J, et al. Decreased cortical response to verbal working memory following sleep deprivation. Sleep. 2005;28(1):55–67.
39. Drummond SP, Meloy MJ, Yanagi MA, Orff HJ, Brown GG. Compensatory recruitment after sleep deprivation and the relationship with performance. Psychiatry Res. 2005;140(3):211–23.
40. Alchanatis M, Zias N, Deligiorgis N, Amfilochiou A, Dionellis G, Orphanidou D. Sleep apnea-related cognitive deficits and intelligence: an implication of cognitive reserve theory. J Sleep Res. 2005;14(1):69–75.
41. Yaouhi K, Bertran F, Clochon P, Mezenge F, Denise P, Foret J, et al. A combined neuropsychological and brain imaging study of obstructive sleep apnea. J Sleep Res. 2009;18(1):36–48.
42. Quan SF, Wright R, Baldwin CM, Kaemingk KL, Goodwin JL, Kuo TF, et al. Obstructive sleep apnea-hypopnea and neurocognitive functioning in the sleep heart health study. Sleep Med. 2006;7(6):498–507.
43. Weih M, Kallenberg K, Bergk A, Dirnagl U, Harms L, Wernecke KD, et al. Attenuated stroke severity after prodromal TIA: a role for ischemic tolerance in the brain. Stroke. 1999;30(9):1851–4.
44. Hoth KF, Zimmerman ME, Meschede KA, Arnedt JT, Aloia MS. Obstructive sleep apnea: impact of hypoxemia on memory. Sleep Breath. 2013;17(2):811–7.
45. Dave KR, Saul I, Prado R, Busto R, Perez-Pinzon MA. Remote organ ischemic preconditioning protect brain from ischemic damage following asphyxial cardiac arrest. Neurosci Lett. 2006;404(1–2):170–5.
46. Ren C, Gao X, Steinberg GK, Zhao H. Limb remote-preconditioning protects against focal ischemia in rats and contradicts the dogma of therapeutic time windows for preconditioning. Neuroscience. 2008;151(4):1099–103.
47. Meybohm P, Renner J, Broch O, Caliebe D, Albrecht M, Cremer J, et al. Postoperative neurocognitive dysfunction in patients undergoing cardiac surgery after remote ischemic preconditioning: a double-blind randomized controlled pilot study. PLoS One. 2013;8(5):e64743.
48. Hudetz JA, Patterson KM, Iqbal Z, Gandhi SD, Pagel PS. Remote ischemic preconditioning prevents deterioration of short-term postoperative cognitive function after cardiac surgery using cardiopulmonary bypass: results of a pilot investigation. J Cardiothorac Vasc Anesth. 2015;29(2):382–8.
49. He Z, Xu N, Qi S. Remote ischemic preconditioning improves the cognitive function of elderly patients following colon surgery: a randomized clinical trial. Medicine. 2017;96(17):e6719.
50. Schega L, Peter B, Torpel A, Mutschler H, Isermann B, Hamacher D. Effects of intermittent hypoxia on cognitive performance and quality of life in elderly adults: a pilot study. Gerontology. 2013;59(4):316–23.
51. Li S, Hafeez A, Noorulla F, Geng X, Shao G, Ren C, et al. Preconditioning in neuroprotection: from hypoxia to ischemia. Prog Neurobiol. 2017;157:79–91.
52. O' Brien H, Mohan H, Hare CO, Reynolds JV, Kenny RA. Mind over matter? The hidden epidemic of cognitive dysfunction in the older surgical patient. Ann Surg. 2017;265(4):677–91.

Permissions

All chapters in this book were first published in BA, by BioMed Central; hereby published with permission under the Creative Commons Attribution License or equivalent. Every chapter published in this book has been scrutinized by our experts. Their significance has been extensively debated. The topics covered herein carry significant findings which will fuel the growth of the discipline. They may even be implemented as practical applications or may be referred to as a beginning point for another development.

The contributors of this book come from diverse backgrounds, making this book a truly international effort. This book will bring forth new frontiers with its revolutionizing research information and detailed analysis of the nascent developments around the world.

We would like to thank all the contributing authors for lending their expertise to make the book truly unique. They have played a crucial role in the development of this book. Without their invaluable contributions this book wouldn't have been possible. They have made vital efforts to compile up to date information on the varied aspects of this subject to make this book a valuable addition to the collection of many professionals and students.

This book was conceptualized with the vision of imparting up-to-date information and advanced data in this field. To ensure the same, a matchless editorial board was set up. Every individual on the board went through rigorous rounds of assessment to prove their worth. After which they invested a large part of their time researching and compiling the most relevant data for our readers.

The editorial board has been involved in producing this book since its inception. They have spent rigorous hours researching and exploring the diverse topics which have resulted in the successful publishing of this book. They have passed on their knowledge of decades through this book. To expedite this challenging task, the publisher supported the team at every step. A small team of assistant editors was also appointed to further simplify the editing procedure and attain best results for the readers.

Apart from the editorial board, the designing team has also invested a significant amount of their time in understanding the subject and creating the most relevant covers. They scrutinized every image to scout for the most suitable representation of the subject and create an appropriate cover for the book.

The publishing team has been an ardent support to the editorial, designing and production team. Their endless efforts to recruit the best for this project, has resulted in the accomplishment of this book. They are a veteran in the field of academics and their pool of knowledge is as vast as their experience in printing. Their expertise and guidance has proved useful at every step. Their uncompromising quality standards have made this book an exceptional effort. Their encouragement from time to time has been an inspiration for everyone.

The publisher and the editorial board hope that this book will prove to be a valuable piece of knowledge for researchers, students, practitioners and scholars across the globe.

List of Contributors

Peng Zhang, Jun-Hao Lei, Xin-Jun Su and Xing-Huan Wang
Department of Urology, Zhongnan Hospital, Wuhan University, 169 Donghu load, Wuchang district, Wuhan 430071, Hubei, People's Republic of China

Hyun-Jung Shin, Jung-Won Hwang, Sang-Hwan Do and Hyo-Seok Na
Department of Anesthesiology and Pain Medicine, Seoul National University Bundang Hospital, 82, Gumi 173, Bundang, Seongnam, Gyeonggi 13620, South Korea

Eun-Young Kim
Department of Anesthesiology and Pain Medicine, Daerim St. Mary's Hospital, Seoul, South Korea

Maliwan Oofuvong, Thitikan Kunapaisal, Orarat Karnjanawanichkul, Nussara Dilokrattanaphijit and Jaranya Leeratiwong
Department of Anesthesiology, Faculty of Medicine, Prince of Songkla University, 15 Kanjanavanich Road, Songkhla 90112, Thailand

Hong Yu, Lu Zhang and Hai Yu
Department of Anesthesiology, West China Hospital of Sichuan University, Chengdu 610041, People's Republic of China

Ye Ma
Department of Anesthesiology, China-Japan Friendship Hospital, Beijing 100029, People's Republic of China

Marc Kriege, Nina Pirlich, Thomas Ott, Eva Wittenmeier and Frank Dette
Department of Anesthesiology, University Medical Center of the Johannes Gutenberg-University, Langenbeckstraße 1, 55131 Mainz, Germany

Seon-Hee Oh
School of Medicine, Chosun University, 309 Pilmundaero, Dong-gu, Gwangju 501-759, South Korea

Myung Ha Yoon
Department of Anesthesiology and Pain Medicine, Medical School, Chonnam National University, 42 Jebongro, Donggu, Gwangju 501-757, South Korea

Kyung Joon Lim, Byung Sik Yu and Ki Tae Jung
Department of Anesthesiology and Pain Medicine, School of Medicine, Chosun University, Chosun University Hospital, 365 Pilmun-daero, Dong-gu, Gwangju 61453, South Korea

In Gook Jee
Department of Anesthesiology and Pain Medicine, Chosun University Hospital, 365 Pilmun-daero, Dong-gu, Gwangju 61453, South Korea

Byung Seop Shin, Young Hee Shin, Nam-Su Gil, Ye Na Oh and Ji Seon Jeong
Department of Anesthesiology and Pain Medicine, Samsung Medical Center, Sungkyunkwan University school of Medicine, 81 Irwon-ro, Gangnam, Seoul 06352, South Korea

RyungA Kang
Department of Anesthesiology and Pain Medicine, Samsung Medical Center, Sungkyunkwan University school of Medicine, 81 Irwon-ro, Gangnam, Seoul 06352, South Korea
Department of Anesthesiology and Pain Medicine, Kangwon National University School of Medicine, Chuncheon, South Korea

Hans Bahlmann and Lena Nilsson
Department of Medical and Health Sciences, Linköping University, University Hospital, 58185 Linköping, Sweden
Department of Anesthesiology and Intensive Care, Linköping University, University Hospital, 58185 Linköping, Sweden

Robert G. Hahn
Department of Medical and Health Sciences, Linköping University and Research Unit, Södertälje Hospital, 152 86 Södertälje, Sweden

Jean Wong, Enoch Lam, Najia Hasan and Frances Chung
Department of Anesthesiology and Pain Medicine, Toronto Western Hospital, University Health Network, University of Toronto, Toronto, ON, Canada

George Ho
Department of Anesthesiology and Pain Medicine, Toronto Western Hospital, University Health Network, University of Toronto, Toronto, ON, Canada
Faculty of Medicine, University of Toronto, Toronto, ON, Canada

Crispiana Cozowicz
Department of Anesthesiology, Hospital for Special Surgery, Weill Cornell Medical College, New York, NY, USA
Perioperative Medicine and Intensive Care Medicine, Paracelsus Medical University, Salzburg, Austria

Mandeep Singh
Department of Anesthesiology and Pain Medicine, Toronto Western Hospital, University Health Network, University of Toronto, Toronto, ON, Canada
Toronto Sleep and Pulmonary Centre, Toronto, ON, Canada

Stavros G. Memtsoudis
Department of Anesthesiology, Hospital for Special Surgery, Weill Cornell Medical College, New York, NY, USA

Eva E. Mörwald
Department of Anesthesiology, Hospital for Special Surgery, Weill Cornell Medical College, New York, NY, USA
Perioperative Medicine and Intensive Care Medicine, Paracelsus Medical University, Salzburg, Austria

Zhenqing Liu, Menglu Jiang, Tongsheng Xu and Hao Hua
Department of Anesthesiology, The Ninth People's Hospital of Wuxi, No.999 Liangxi Road, Wuxi 214062, China

Michał Borys, Klaudia Zyzak, Katarzyna Gałaszkiewicz, Agata Kłaput, Kai Wróblewski, Justyna Miękina and Mirosław Czuczwar
The Second Department of Anaesthesiology and Intensive Therapy, Medical University of Lublin, ul. Staszica 16, 20-081 Lublin, Poland

Agata Hanych
The Department of Anaesthesia and Intensive Therapy, The Podkarpackie Center of Lung Disease, Rzeszów, Poland

Michał Domagała
The Department of Anaesthesia and Intensive Therapy, Saint Lukash Hospital, Końskie, Poland

Piotr Gałkin
The Department of Anaesthesia and Intensive Therapy, Jedrzej Sniadecki Hospital, Białystok, Poland

Dariusz Onichimowski
The Department of Anaesthesia and Intensive Therapy, University of Warmia and Mazury, Olsztyn, Poland

Maliwan Oofuvong, Siriwimol Ratprasert and Thavat Chanchayanon
Department of Anesthesiology, Faculty of Medicine, Prince of Songkla University, 15 Kanjanavanich Road, Songkhla 90112, Thailand

Weilin Zhu, Yuansi Huang, Yuqiong Ye and Yafeng Wang
Department of Anesthesia, People's Hospital of Guangxi Zhuang Autonomous Region, Nanning 530021, China

Lena M. Mayes, Ana Fernandez-Bustamante and Karsten Bartels
Department of Anesthesiology, University of Colorado School of Medicine, 12401 E. 17th Avenue Leprino Office Building, 7th Floor, MS B-113, Aurora, CO 80045, USA

Cynthia A. Wong
Department of Anesthesia, University of Iowa Carver College of Medicine, Iowa City, IA, USA

Shanta Zimmer
Department of Medicine, University of Colorado School of Medicine, Aurora, CO, USA

Weijuan Zhu, Riyong Zhou, Lulu Chen, Yuanqing Chen, Lvdan Huang and Xuzhong Xu
Department of Anesthesiology, The First Affiliated Hospital of Wenzhou Medical College, 2 Fuxue Road, Wenzhou City, Zhejiang Province 325000, China

Yun Xia
Department of Anesthesiology, The Ohio State University Medical Center, Columbus, OH, USA

Thomas J. Papadimos
Department of Anesthesiology, The University of Toledo College of Medicine and Life Sciences, Toledo, OH, Spain

Zhijian Fu
Department of Pain Management, Shandong Provincial Hospital affiliated to Shandong University, 324 Jingwu Road, Jinan 250021, China

Chengyu Wang, Yi Lu and Mengmeng Huang
Department of Anesthesiology, Critical Care and Pain Medicine, The 2nd Affiliated Hospital & Yuying Children's Hospital of WenZhou Medical University, Wenzhou, China

Fang Chen
Department of Pain Management, Shandong Provincial Hospital affiliated to Shandong University, 324 Jingwu Road, Jinan 250021, China
Department of Anesthesiology, Critical Care and Pain Medicine, The 2nd Affiliated Hospital & Yuying Children's Hospital of WenZhou Medical University, Wenzhou, China

Wei Yu, Zijian Wang, Dapeng Gao, Wei Zhang, Wen Jin, Xuesong Ma and Sihua Qi
Department of Anaesthesiology, Fourth Affiliated Hospital of Harbin Medical University, 37 Yiyuan Road, Harbin 150001, Heilongjiang Province, China

Lucia Mirabella, Antonella Cotoia, Davide D'Antini, Franca Valentino, Livio Tullo and Gilda Cinnella
Department of Anesthesia and Intensive care, University of Foggia, Viale Pinto, 1-71100 Foggia, Italy

Salvatore Grasso
Department of Anesthesia and Intensive care, University of Bari, Bari, Italy

Savino Spadaro
Department of Anesthesia and Intensive care, University of Ferrara, Ferrara, Italy

Francesco Sollitto and Domenico Loizzi
Department of Thoracic Surgery, University of Foggia, Foggia, Italy

Michela Rauseo
Department of Anesthesia and Intensive care, University of Foggia, Viale Pinto, 1-71100 Foggia, Italy
Interdepartmental Division of Critical Care Medicine, University of Toronto, Toronto, ON, Canada

Pablo Cruces
Pediatric Intensive Care Unit, Hospital El Carmen de Maipú, Santiago, Chile
Centro de Investigación de Medicina Veterinaria, Escuela de Medicina Veterinaria, Facultad de Ecología y Recursos Naturales, Universidad Andres Bello, Santiago, Chile

Sebastián González-Dambrauskas and Javier Martínez
3Pediatric Intensive Care Unit, Centro Hospitalario Pereira Rossell, Montevideo, Uruguay.

Federico Cristiani and Ronnie Henderson
Department of Anesthesiology, Centro Hospitalario Pereira Rossell, Montevideo, Uruguay

Franco Díaz
Unidad de Cuidados Intensivos Pediátricos, Clínica Alemana de Santiago, Avda. Vitacura, 5951 Santiago, Chile
Facultad de Medicina Clínica Alemana Universidad del Desarrollo, Santiago, Chile
Area de Cuidados Críticos, Hospital Padre Hurtado, Santiago, Chile

Benjamin Erranz
Unidad de Cuidados Intensivos Pediátricos, Clínica Alemana de Santiago, Avda. Vitacura, 5951 Santiago, Chile

Thomas Wiesmann, Lilli Hoff, Lara Prien, Alexander Torossian, Leopold Eberhart, Hinnerk Wulf and Carsten Feldmann
Department of Anesthesiology and Intensive Care Medicine, Philipps University Marburg, University Hospital Marburg (UKGM - Campus Marburg), Baldinger Strasse, 35033 Marburg, Germany

Chuanbing Wen
Department of Pain Management, Sichuan Academy of Medical Sciences and Sichuan Provincial People's Hospital, Chengdu, Sichuan Province 610072, People's Republic of China

Ling Ye and Hui Liu
Department of Pain management, West China Hospital, Sichuan University, Chengdu, Sichuan Province 610041, People's Republic of China

Lei Chen, Liangrong Wang, Qiong Zhang, Feifei Chen, Liling Li and Lina Lin
Department of Anesthesiology, The First Affiliated Hospital of Wenzhou Medical University, Wenzhou, Zhejiang Province, China

Qian Zhuo
Wenzhou People's Hospital, Wenzhou, Zhejiang Province, China

Lanqi Guo, Jianfeng Xie, Yingzi Huang, Chun Pan, Yi Yang, Haibo Qiu and Ling Liu
Department of Critical Care Medicine, Zhongda Hospital, School of Medicine, Southeast University, Nanjing, Jiangsu, China

Henok Mulugeta and Mezinew Sintayehu
Department of Nursing, College of Health Science, Debre Markos University Debre Markos, Ethiopia

Mulatu Ayana
Department of Public Health, College of Health Science, Debre Markos University, Debre Markos, Ethiopia

Getenet Dessie
Department of Nursing, School of Health Science, College of Medicine and Health Science, Bahir Dar University, Bahir Dar, Ethiopia

Tesfu Zewdu
Department of Nursing, College of Health Science, Assosa University, Assosa, Ethiopia

Sho Kawasaki
Department of Anesthesiology and Critical Care Medicine, Graduate School of Medical Sciences, Kyushu University, Maidashi 3-1-1, Higashi-ku, Fukuoka, Fukuoka, Japan
Department of Preventive Medicine, Graduate School of Medical Sciences, Kyushu University, Maidashi 3-1-1, Higashi-ku, Fukuoka, Fukuoka, Japan

Sumio Hoka
Department of Anesthesiology and Critical Care Medicine, Graduate School of Medical Sciences, Kyushu University, Maidashi 3-1-1, Higashi-ku, Fukuoka, Fukuoka, Japan

Chikako Kiyohara
Department of Preventive Medicine, Graduate School of Medical Sciences, Kyushu University, Maidashi 3-1-1, Higashi-ku, Fukuoka, Fukuoka, Japan

Shoji Tokunaga
Medical Information Center, Kyushu University Hospital, Maidashi 3-1-1, Higashi-ku, Fukuoka, Fukuoka, Japan

Huiqing Ge, Ye Jiang, Qijun Jin and Linjun Wan
Department of Respiratory Care, Sir Run Run Shaw Hospital, Zhejiang University School of Medicine, Hangzhou, China

Ximing Qian
Department of Cardiovascular Surgery, Sir Run Run Shaw Hospital, Zhejiang University School of Medicine, Hangzhou, China

Zhongheng Zhang
Department of Emergency Medicine, Sir Run Run Shaw Hospital, Zhejiang University School of Medicine, No 3, East Qingchun Road, Hangzhou 310016, Zhejiang Province, China

Joerg Quente, Sven Staedtler, Harald Ihmsen and Juergen Schuettler
Department of Anesthesiology, University Hospital Erlangen, Friedrich-Alexander-University Erlangen-Nuremberg, Erlangen, Germany

Soeren Wagner
Department of Anesthesiology, University Hospital Erlangen, Friedrich-Alexander-University Erlangen-Nuremberg, Erlangen, Germany
Department of Anesthesiology, Katharinenhospital Klinikum Stuttgart, Kriegsbergstrasse 60, D-70174 Stuttgart, Germany

Tanja Richter-Schmidinger and Johannes Kornhuber
Department of Psychiatry and Psychotherapy, University Hospital Erlangen, Friedrich-Alexander-University, Erlangen, Germany

Katharina Koch
Department of Anesthesiology, University Hospital Erlangen, Friedrich-Alexander-University Erlangen-Nuremberg, Erlangen, Germany
Department of Anaesthesiology, Klinikum Oldenburg AöR, University Hospital Oldenburg, Oldenburg, Germany

Index